Monoclonal Antibodies

METHODS IN MOLECULAR BIOLOGY™

John M. Walker, SERIES EDITOR

METHODS IN MOLECULAR BIOLOGY™

Monoclonal Antibodies

Methods and Protocols

Edited by

Maher Albitar

Department of Hematopathology,
Quest Diagnostics Nichols Institute, San Juan Capistrano, CA

HUMANA PRESS ✳ TOTOWA, NEW JERSEY

© 2007 Humana Press Inc.
999 Riverview Drive, Suite 208
Totowa, New Jersey 07512

www.humanapress.com

All papers, comments, opinions, conclusions, or recommendations are those of the author(s), and do not necessarily reflect the views of the publisher.

This publication is printed on acid-free paper. ∞
ANSI Z39.48-1984 (American Standards Institute)

Permanence of Paper for Printed Library Materials.

Production Editor: Tara L. Bugg

Cover design by Nancy K. Fallatt
Cover illustration: *(Background)* From Chapter 8, Fig. 8. *(Foreground)* From Chapter 2, Fig. 2.

For additional copies, pricing for bulk purchases, and/or information about other Humana titles, contact Humana at the above address or at any of the following numbers: Tel.: 973-256-1699; Fax: 973-256-8341; E-mail: orders@humanapr.com; or visit our website at www.humanapress.com.

Printed in the United States of America. 10 9 8 7 6 5 4 3 2 1

E-ISBN 978-1-59745-323-3

ISSN 1064-3745

Library of Congress Cataloging in Publication Data

Monoclonal antibodies : methods and protocols / edited by Maher Albitar.
    p. ; cm. -- (Methods in molecular biology, ISSN 1064-3745 ; 378)
  Includes bibliographical references and index.
  ISBN 1-58829-567-2 (alk. paper)
  1. Monoclonal antibodies--Laboratory manuals. 2. Immunodiagnosis--Laboratory manuals. I. Albitar, Maher. II. Series: Methods in molecular biology (Clifton, N.J.) ; v. 378.
  [DNLM: 1. Antibodies, Monoclonal--Laboratory Manuals. QW 525 M7515 2007]
  RB46.5.M66 2007
  616.07'98--dc22
                              2006017633

Preface

The concept of monoclonal antibodies was first suggested more than 100 yr ago by Paul Ehrlich, who envisioned them as a "magic bullet" for the treatment of various diseases. Early on, immunization of animals was used mainly to generate tumor-specific polyclonal antibodies. Generation of monoclonal antibodies for use in laboratory research and medical tests commenced in the mid-1970s. Not until the mid 1990s did technological advances allow the generation of monoclonal antibodies that were clinically useful as therapeutic agents. Monoclonal antibodies now constitute an integral component of laboratory diagnostics and are used in most laboratories that offer clinical testing.

The goal of *Monoclonal Antibodies: Methods and Protocols* is to provide a collection of methods that employ monoclonal antibodies in the clinical setting. The book starts with a chapter describing the gold standard method for generating mouse monoclonal antibodies through hybridoma technology. Chapter 2 takes us to the future and describes methods for engineering recombinant and humanized antibodies. The authors describe the use of phage display and bacterial systems to generate monoclonal antibodies without the need for animal immunization. They also present methods for using these antibodies not only as therapeutic agents, but in laboratory experiments and clinical testing as well. Along the same lines, Chapter 3 describes a method for engineering soluble Fc fusion proteins. The Fc portion of monoclonal antibodies can be used to generate and purify large quantities of proteins that have the potential to be used for immunization as well as in clinical testing and patient monitoring.

The next chapters focus on laboratory methods that employ monoclonal antibodies. Chapter 4 describes the use of monoclonal antibodies in the context of flow cytometry for the diagnosis and classification of hematological diseases. The authors provide detailed methods for staining and detecting specific antigens using flow cytometry, and discuss the use of algorithms to diagnose and classify hematological diseases. Chapter 5 provides methods for flow cytometric quantification of antigens present on the surface of cells. Quantifying the expression levels of these cell-surface antigens allows for a better understanding of the biology underlying antibody-based treatments, and has the potential to improve monitoring of such therapy. Chapter 6 discusses methods for quantifying CD13 and CD10 expression on granulocytes using the same quantitative flow cytometry approach, and shows how these levels can be used to monitor immune system function.

The use of flow cytometry has recently expanded from cell surface analysis to intracellular protein analysis. Measuring intracellular protein is particularly important for therapies that target the activity of specific oncoproteins (i.e., targeted therapy). These intracellular proteins must be monitored and quantified before and during therapy. Chapter 7 describes methods for the permeabilization and quantitative monitoring of intracellular proteins and their activity (phosphorylation).

Changing direction from flow cytometry to immunohistochemistry, Chapter 8 depicts methods that have transformed morphological evaluation and anatomical pathology from guesswork to objective science. The authors describe how monoclonal antibodies can be used in immunohistochemistry to diagnose hematological diseases. This approach is also applicable to other tumors and reactive diseases that can manifest with histological changes.

Although monoclonal antibodies have been used extensively in standard enzyme-linked immunosorbent assays (ELISAs), the recent adaptation of polystyrene beads in place of microtiter plates as the solid surface for capture of antibody binding has allowed the introduction of new classes of testing with flow cytometry or Luminex® platforms. This bead-based technology has several advantages over routine ELISAs, most importantly the ability to multiplex and analyze several analytes simultaneously. Chapter 9 illustrates methods for the use of beads to measure cytokines, chemokines, and other soluble proteins. Similarly, Chapter 10, which explores the detection of FLT-3 and its phosphorylation, represents a method for immunoprecipating cellular proteins on beads and using flow cytometry to measure these proteins and their phosphorylation. Chapter 11, which focuses on measuring levels of almetuzumab, a humanized rat antibody used for treatment of lymphoid cells that express CD52, describes a bead-based method for quantifying the humanized antibody, CD52, and the almetuzumab/CD52 immune complexes that can be seen free in circulation. The most recent innovation using bead-based immunoassays with flow cytometry in detecting chromosomal translocations is presented in Chapter 12 with the quantitation of the BCR-ABL fusion protein, which results from a translocation between chromosomes 9 and 22. The authors also describe a method for quantifying BCR-ABL phosphorylation, which may have clinical implications when patients with chronic myeloid leukemia are treated with ABL-specific kinase inhibitors.

This volume also contains chapters selected to provide additional examples of methodologies that employ monoclonal antibodies. Chapter 13 concentrates on detecting multidrug-resistance (MDR) in tumor cells presenting an approach for not only detecting the MDR protein, but also for demonstrating the active efflux that allows cytotoxic drugs to be pumped out of cells. Chapter 14 presents a method for detecting human antibodies directed against therapeutic mouse antibodies; detection of these antibodies has significant clinical implications for the course of therapy. Although humanization of therapeutic antibodies has reduced the incidence of developing anti-mouse antibodies, the issue remains a serious concern. Finally, Chapter 15 illustrates methods that depend on highly automated instruments for detection of IgE in patients suffering from an allergy.

In summary, *Monoclonal Antibodies: Methods and Protocols* provides descriptions of methods that cover a wide spectrum of applications in the field of monoclonal antibodies. This field will continue to expand and provide new and innovative techniques, not only in the laboratory, but also as a basis that complements targeted therapy.

Maher Albitar

Contents

Contributors

MAHER ALBITAR • *Department of Hematopathology, Quest Diagnostics Nichols Institute, San Juan Capistrano, CA*

JOHN APGAR • *Cell Signaling Research, BD Biosciences, San Diego, CA*

ROBYN S. ARIAS • *Department of Pathology, Keck School of Medicine, University of Southern California, Los Angeles, CA*

HUAI EN HUANG CHAN • *Department of Hematopathology, Quest Diagnostics Nichols Institute, San Juan Capistrano, CA*

RICHARD CHANG • *Department of Hematopathology, Quest Diagnostics Nichols Institute, San Juan Capistrano, CA*

ROY CHEN • *Applications Development, BD Biosciences, San Jose, CA*

MARIEL DONZEAU • *Department of Research, MorphoSys AG, Martinsried, Germany*

ALAN L. EPSTEIN • *Department of Pathology, Keck School of Medicine, University of Southern California, Los Angeles, CA*

MEG L. FLANAGAN • *Department of Pathology, Keck School of Medicine, University of Southern California, Los Angeles, CA*

M. MICHAEL GLOVSKY • *Department of Immunology, Quest Diagnostics Nichols Institute, San Juan Capistrano, CA*

PEISHENG HU • *Department of Pathology, Keck School of Medicine, University of Southern California, Los Angeles, CA*

IMAN B. JILANI • *Department of Hematopathology, Quest Diagnostics Nichols Institute, San Juan Capistrano, CA*

LESLIE A. KHAWLI • *Department of Pathology, Keck School of Medicine, University of Southern California, Los Angeles, CA*

ACHIM KNAPPIK • *Global Head of Research, MorphoSys AG, Martinsried, Germany*

EUGENE MECHETNER • *Department of Research and Development, Oncotech Inc., Tustin, CA and Department of Radiological Sciences, College of Medicine, University of California–Irvine, Irvine, CA*

DENNIS P. O'MALLEY • *Department of Pathology, Indiana School of Medicine, Indianapolis, IN and Laboratory Director, Immunohistochemistry Laboratory, Indianapolis, IN*

ATTILIO ORAZI • *Department of Pathology and Laboratory Medicine, Indiana University School of Medicine, Indianapolis, IN*

DAGMAR REIMANN • *Institute of Medical Immunology, Martin Luther University Halle–Wittenberg, Halle, Germany*

JOCHEN REINSBERG • *Department of Gynecological Endocrinology and Reproductive Medicine, University of Bonn, Bonn, Germany*

ARNIM SABLOTZKI • *Department of Anesthesiology, Martin Luther University Halle–Wittenberg, Halle, Germany*

PATRICK SCHROETER • *Institute of Medical Immunology, Martin Luther University Halle–Wittenberg, Halle, Germany*

HOMERO SEPULVEDA • *Department of Applications Development, BD Biosciences, San Diego, CA*

MOHAMMAD-REZA SHEIKHOLESLAMI • *Department of Hematopathology, Quest Diagnostics Nichols Institute, San Juan Capistrano, CA*

RUDOLF VARRO • *Department of Applications Development, BD Biosciences, San Jose, CA*

1

Development and Characterization of Mouse Hybridomas

Eugene Mechetner

Summary

Cell fusion protocols that were developed by Kohler and Milstein in the mid-1970s and aimed at producing and characterization of mouse monoclonal antibodies (MAbs) remain the gold standard of hybridoma development. Despite tremendous progress in using MAbs in multiple research, diagnostic, and therapeutic areas, major experimental flaws in designing and carrying out hybridoma experimentation often result in the production of hybridomas exhibiting poor growth parameters and secreting low-specificity and low-affinity antibodies. This methodology chapter is built around the conventional hybridoma protocol, with a special emphasis on tissue culture and biochemical techniques aimed at producing truly monospecific and highly active mouse MAbs.

Key Words: Hybridoma; monoclonal antibodies; MAbs; mouse; tissue culture.

1. Introduction

Tremendous progress in the development, characterization, and manufacturing of monoclonal antibodies (MAbs) has been made since 1976, the year when George J. F. Kohler and Cesar Milstein published their seminal paper (1) on the production of MAbs by producing hybrids between mouse splenocytes with their myeloma fusion partner. Kohler's and Milstein's outstanding contribution, for which they were awarded together with Niels K. Jerne the 1984 Nobel Prize in Physiology or Medicine, and—beyond all—their deliberate (and, alas, incomprehensible by today's standards) decision not to patent the hybridoma technology resulted in the rapid and widespread adoption of MAbs by both academia and industry.

As shown in **Table 1**, over the last 30 yr two new types of MAbs, recombinant and synthetic, have been developed and validated. Recombinant MAbs can be

From: *Methods in Molecular Biology, vol. 378: Monoclonal Antibodies: Methods and Protocols*
Edited by: M. Albitar © Humana Press Inc., Totowa, NJ

Table 1
Progress in Antibody Development Since 1976

	1976	2006
Antibody types	Polyclonal Monoclonal (animal)	Polyclonal Monoclonal (animal) Monoclonal (recombinant) Monoclonal (synthetic)
Diversity platform	Amino acids	Amino acids Nonamino acid-based (e.g., aptamers)
Monoclonal antibodies: host species	Mouse	Mouse Rat Hamster Rabbit Human Chicken Algae
Expression systems	Mouse cells	Mouse and other mammalian cells Bacteria Yeast Plants (algae, higher plants)
Applications	Research Diagnostics	Research Diagnostics Imaging Therapeutics Nanotechnology
Therapeutic indications	None	Cancer Transplant rejection Inflammatory diseases Cardiovascular diseases Antiviral

produced in transgenic mice that carry human antibody gene loci inserted in their germ line *(2)*, through bacteriophage display-based technologies yielding high quantities of high-affinity antibodies *(3,4)*, and ribosome mRNA displays allowing for construction of high-member, high-affinity human immune repertoire antibody libraries *(5)*. Synthetic antibodies (diabodies, triabodies, tetrabodies) are generated using chemical or molecular biological cross-linking to produce di-, tri-, and tetrameric multivalent conjugates exhibiting enhanced specificity and functional activity *(6)*. Successful attempts have been made to replace amino acids by other biological molecules to create chemical diversity and produce nucleic acid-based molecules mimicking the most fundamental property—specific binding to target antigens—of natural MAbs *(7)*. In the "classical" MAb family, the range of host species expanded from mouse–mouse hybridomas to mono- and heterohybridomas originating in mice, rats, hamsters, rabbits, humans, chickens, and plants. All these developments, accompanied by major breakthroughs in manufacturing processes (including highly efficient and animal-free expression bacterial systems) and regulatory environment made initially by Idec (Rituximab) and Genentech (Trastuzumab), led to drastic expansion of MAb-based diagnostics and therapeutics in several areas of modern medicine *(8,9)*.

However, it has to be emphasized that mouse MAbs remain the primary "work horse" in the vast majority of research and diagnostics applications. According to broad antibody industry surveys, more than 95% of research MAbs are represented by mouse MAbs *(10)*. The very process of generating mouse MAbs practically did not change since the early 1980s *(11)*, and Kohler and Milstein's P3X63Ag8.653 myeloma fusion partner is still the gold standard in hybridoma development. The real challenge for a researcher entering the hybridoma field is not in reproducing routine cell fusion and protein purification protocols, but in avoiding common experimental mistakes resulting in the production of low- or nonspecific hybridomas with poor growth characteristics and low-affinity antibodies. For example, many research antibody Reagent companies continue manufacturing MAbs using mouse ascitic fluids. This approach, although seemingly attractive and inexpensive in the short term, results in the production (and subsequent use by these companies' customers in academia and industry) of MAbs irreversibly contaminated by (1) irrelevant and (2) immunologically active immunoglobulins originating from the host serum. Another example is provided by Reagent companies using affinity chromatography protocols that include very low pH elution buffers, thereby leading to high yields of mostly inactive MAbs. Not only do these flaws in experimental design defeat the idea of monospecific and uniformly functional MAbs, but they cannot be quantified and accounted for in all downstream MAb applications. Therefore, this methodology chapter is built around the conventional and widely accepted hybridoma protocol, with a special emphasis on tissue culture and biochemical techniques aimed at producing truly monospecific and highly active mouse MAbs.

2. Materials

1. Use 20- to 30-wk-old -30 BALB/c mice to generate routine mouse or mouse–rat hybridomas; Sprague-Dawley rats are used for rat–rat MAb antibody production.
2. P3X63Ag8.653 (ATTC, Manassas, VA, cat. no. CRL-1580) murine myeloma cell line; other mouse, as well as human and rat hybridoma fusion partners, are listed on the ATCC web page www.atcc.org/common/products/HybridDev.cfm.
3. Dulbecco's (DMEM)- or Iscove's-modified Eagle's medium, supplemented with 10–20% preselected fetal bovine serum (FBS), 4 mM L-glutamine, 1 mM sodium pyruvate, nonessential amino acids, 50 U penicillin, 50 µg streptomycin, and 50 µM

β-mercaproehtanole in the absence or presence of Hypoxanthine–Aminopterin–Thymidine (HAT) or hypoxanthine/thymidine (HT) for selection (all from Invitrogen, Carlsbad, CA). PFHM II (Invitrogen) or UltraDOMA-PF™ (Cambrex, East Rutherford, NJ) protein-free media can be used to grow hybridoma cells to produce supernatants with high MAb concentrations. Hybri-Care cell culture medium (ATCC) is used to grow fastidious hybridoma clones.

4. 500X concentrates of HAT and HT (ATCC, cat. nos. 69-X and 71-X) and premade stocks of 8-azaguanine (Sigma, St. Louis, MO, cat. no. A5284) are used to select hybridoma clones and myeloma partner cells, respectively. Polyethylene glycol solution (PEG) 50% (w/v), mol wt 1450 (Sigma, cat. no. P7181) made up in a protein-free medium is used for hybridoma fusion protocols requiring 40–50% PEG. Use 0.4% Trypan Blue solution (Sigma; cat. no. T8154) for counting viable cells and hybridoma-grade DMSO (dimethyl sulfoxide; Sigma, cat. no. P2650) for cryopreservation.

5. Complete Freund's adjuvant (Sigma, cat. no. F5881), Incomplete Freund's adjuvant (Sigma, cat. no. F5506), or Ribi Adjuvant System (Ribi ImmunoChem Research, Inc., Hamilton, MT) (MPL+TDM) are widely utilized in immunization protocols. Use Pristane (2,6,10,14-tetramethylpentadecane; Sigma; cat. no. P1403) to produce hybridoma ascites.

6. Use an antibody-capturing strip based kit (Sigma, cat. no. ISO1) for rapid and specific isotyping of MAbs. Quantitative determination of MAb concentration in hybridoma supernatants is performed using the Standard Vectastatin ABC kit (Vector Labs, Burlingame, CA, cat. no. PK-4000). Protein A, Protein G, and other affinity chromatography reagents used to purify MAbs from protein-free supernatants and ascitic fluids, as well as numerous thoughtful and detailed biochemical protocols, are available from www.piercenet.com (Pierce Biotechnology, Inc., Rockford, IL).

7. Low-tox rabbit complement (CL3051) is from Cedarlane Laboratories (Hornby, ON, Canada). AMICON Centriprep 100 (Millipore, Billerica, MA) concentration units are utilized to concentrate IgG MAbs from tissue culture supernatants.

8. Standard laboratory equipment and supplies: sterile 96-well plates, tissue culture flasks, Petri dishes, conical tubes (15 and 50 mL), multichannel pipets, microsurgery dissection instruments, glass spleen crusher/homogenizer, hemocytometers, water baths, sterile tissue culture hoods, cell centrifuges, inverted and direct light microscopes, other equipment and supplies required for screening procedures.

3. Methods

3.1. Immunization

1. An efficient immunization protocol resulting in the availability of high numbers of highly proliferating antigen-secreting B-cells is one of the most significant factors in generating successful hybridomas.

2. Complete Freund's adjuvant (0.2–0.5 mL) or Ribi Adjuvant System (0.1 mL), at 1:1 mixtures with antigenic material, are used as i.p. injections for initial

immunization to boost the immune response. Incomplete Freund's adjuvant (1:1) is used in subsequent immunizations via s.c., i.m., or i.p. administration.

3. Immunization protocols vary widely, depending on the investigator's experimental objectives, model, and personal style. Typically, 50–100 μg of protein or 10^6–10^7 cells mixed with the adjuvant of choice are used for initial immunization, followed by booster injections containing 10–50 μg of protein or 10^5–10^6 cells in 1:1 ration with incomplete adjuvant. To avoid neutralization of the injected antigen by circulating antibodies, the following immunization schedule is most commonly utilized:

    Day 0—primary immunization, i.p.
    Day 14—1st boost, s.c.
    Day 28—2nd boost, s.c.
    Day 36—serum collection and titration
    Day 42—3rd boost, s.c.
    Day 56—final boost, i.v.
    Day 59—serum collection, harvest of splenocytes, cell fusion

4. Blood for subsequent serum titration is collected (not to exceed 0.5 mL) from the retro-orbital sinus under IACUC-approved anesthesia guidelines. The timeline for the fusion is determined based on the most recent serum titration data obtained using the screening method of the investigator's choice.

3.2. Maintenance of the Myeloma Fusion Partner

1. P3X63Ag8.653 murine myeloma (or another fusion partner of choice) should be thawed in advance and propagated in flasks or roller bottles for at least 2 wk at $<10^6$/mL in DMEM with HT, 8-azaguanine and 10–20% FBS preselected for superior growth in preliminary experiments and other supplements, as described in the previous sections.

2. Grow myeloma cells in the presence of both selection drugs, cryopreserve every 10–14 d, and use these cells (kept in 8-azaguanine-free and HT-free medium for 7 d) for the fusion procedure.

3.3. Cell Fusion

1. Grow 8-azaguanine-resistant P3X63Ag8.653 myeloma cells at a maximum concentration of 0.5×10^6/mL for 3 d; refresh medium 24 h before fusion. Harvest and wash the cells immediately before fusion, wash them twice in large volumes of serum-free medium (e.g., 50-mL conical tubes with ice-cold DMEM), and keep on ice until fusing with splenocytes. It is imperative that myeloma cells remain highly viable and completely free of protein in the medium.

2. Place and keep tube with 1.5 mL of 50% PEG solution in serum-free DMEM. In water bath or incubator at 37°C until fusion.

3. Euthanize the animal, collect as much blood as possible, prepare nonhemolyzed serum, aliquot, and keep at –20°C for further analysis.

4. Under aseptic conditions, remove the spleen, cut off the pancreas, and transfer the spleen into a sterile Petri dish with 10 mL of cold DMEM. Using sterile

forceps wash the spleen in two additional Petri dishes containing 10 mL of cold DMEM.

5. Transfer the spleen into a sterile glass spleen crusher/homogenizer with 5–7 mL of cold DMEM, wait until it falls on the bottom, and move the pestle down to press hard on the spleen to squeeze out splenocytes. Repeat one or two times to remove all splenocytes in the suspension; the spleen will then acquire a whitish color. It is critical to avoid any circular motions of the pestle.

6. Using a wide-mouth 10-mL pipet, carefully remove the splenocytes suspension into a 15-mL conical tube and carefully pipet on the tube wall four to eight times to break down large cell clumps. Let the debris to settle down and collect debris-free splenocytes. At all times keep the suspension on ice and maintain high cell viability.

7. Wash twice at $200g$ for 10 min in a 50-mL conical tube with ice-cold DMEM.

8. Resuspend P3X63Ag8.653 myeloma and splenocytes cell pellets in 10 mL of DMEM and calculate cell concentrations using a hemocytometer. Although a large range of splenocytes-to-myeloma cells ratios (from 1:1 to 20:1) and total cell numbers (from 5×10^7 to 5×10^8 of splenocytes and myeloma cells per tube) has been reported, the most commonly utilized protocols recommend a 5:1 ratio and approx 10^8 cells per fusion.

9. Combine 5×10^7 splenocytes and 5×10^7 myeloma cells in a 50-mL conical tube, resuspend in prewarmed (to 37°C) protein-free DMEM, and spin down in a bucket rotor centrifuge at $200g$ for 10 min to obtain a loose cell pellet that is evenly spread on the bottom of the 50-mL tube.

10. Quickly aspirate the supernatant and dissociate the cell pellet by gently flicking (up to five times) on the bottom of the 50-mL tube. Using a 2-mL pipet, over a period of 2 min, add 1 mL of the warm PEG solution drop-wise to the cell pellet, while gently tapping on the bottom of the 50-mL tube to constantly mix the cell pellet with PEG. Make sure that the full 1 mL of the viscous PEG solution is added.

11. Immediate after adding PEG, use a 10-mL pipet to drop-wise add 20 mL of warm (37°C) serum-free DMEM to the cells, while gently swirling the 50-mL tube after every 5 mL of DMEM added to the tube. After the first 20 mL of warm DMEM, slowly add another 20 mL of warm DMEM.

12. Centrifuge at $200g$ for 10 min, aspirate the supernatant using a 10-mL pipet, add 10 mL of warm (37°C) complete HAT medium with serum and supplements (*see* **Subheading 2.**), gently pipet 10 times on the tube wall to form a uniform cell suspension, and transfer in a bottle containing 190 mL of warm (37°C) complete HAT medium.

13. Using a multichannel pipet with 0.2-mL tips, transfer the cells into 10 96-well flat-bottom plates, 0.2 mL per well. Gently stir the bottle after completing each 96-well plate to ensure even distribution of the cell suspension between the plates.

14. Incubate at 37°C in 5% CO_2 in a humidified incubator, changing 0.1–0.15 mL of complete HAT medium once every 2 or 3 d. Under the described conditions, approx 50% of the wells exhibit clonal growth of hybridoma cells.

3.4. Screening

1. Use sera from immunized animals, control sera from nonimmunized animals, and supernatants from empty wells to control and, if needed, adjust screening protocols. All experimental conditions have to be pretested and optimized in preliminary experiments.
2. Start screening 10–12 d after the fusion when wells containing hybridoma clones are 25–50% confluent. The entire screening procedure should yield final results no later than 48 h to avoid overgrowth and death of the tested clones.
3. Transfer 150 µL of the hybridoma supernatant from the top of positive wells into empty prelabeled sterile 96-well plates. Replace the wells with 150 µL of complete HAT medium.

3.5. Cloning by Limiting Dilutions, Cell Propagation, and Archiving

1. Every primary hybridoma clone requires at least three consecutive rounds of recloning.
2. Examine 96-well plates containing hybridoma clones on an inverted microscope (low magnification). Reclone all positive wells after primary fusion and only the largest single colonies (5–10 colonies per one primary hybridoma clone) in subsequent rounds of cloning.
3. Reserve two flat-bottom 96-well plates per each well to be recloned; add 100 µL of complete hybridoma medium 1 h prior to the recloning procedure. This will result in higher plating efficiency due to absorption of serum proteins on the plastic.
4. Using an automatic pipet with a 200-µL tip, pipet the desired well to generate a single-cell suspension, immediately aspirate 45 µL of this suspension and mix it with 5 µL of Trypan Blue. Calculate the concentration and total number of viable hybridoma cells in the well; calculate the volume and dilutions required for plating hybridoma cells at 1 or 0.25 cells per well in one of the two reserved plates.
5. Using an automatic pipet with a 200-µL tip, mix and then aspirate the needed volumes from the plate, dilute with complete medium if needed, and add the required volumes to a Petri dish containing 10 mL of complete hybridoma medium. Using a multichannel pipet, add 100 µL to each well of each of the two reserved 96-well plates.
6. Analyze each of the two plates containing 1 or 0.25 cells per well for single colonies using an inverted microscope every 2 to 3 d. On days 8–12, select the largest 15–20 colonies, test them utilizing the screening procedure of choice, select 5–10 of the best colonies, and repeat the recloning procedure. At each recloning step, cryopreserve all colonies that will be included in the next round of cloning.
7. Use complete HAT hybridoma medium for the first round of recloning. In the second round, start replacing HAT with complete HT medium after 3 d of culture by replacing 50% of the well volume every 2–3 d. In the third round of recloning, use HT medium to fill initial wells and start replacing HT medium with regular complete DMEM-based hybridoma medium according to the same schedule. Continue functional testing and cryopreserving each clone at each step.

8. Select at least five of the best clones for each primary hybridoma; transfer cells into 24-well plates and, upon achieving active and stable growth, into T25 and T75 flasks. Test and cryopreserve clones from each selection/adaptation cell culture step. After the growth of mass hybridoma populations is well established in T75 flasks, perform functional testing again, confirm the desired functional parameters, select one clone for future work, freeze down large numbers of these cells, and proceed to mass production in multiwell plates, tissue culture flasks, roller bottles, cell factories, etc.

9. Even highly selected hybridoma cell lines need to be periodically retested to confirm their specificity and recloned to protect the population from overgrowing by hybridoma revertants with "throw-out genes" that produce no MAb immunoglobulin.

10. Do not keep selected hybridoma clones growing for over 2 mo; ideally, each mass production procedure should be initiated using frozen cells from earlier passages.

11. Hybridoma cells are typically cryopreserved using standard tissue culture procedure in a freshly prepared mixture of 90% FBS and 10% tissue-culture-grade DMSO, with at least 10^6 viable cells per cryovial.

12. In most labs, thawing of hybridoma cultures involves initial transfer of cells into 15-mL conical tubes, drop-wise addition of complete hybridoma medium, gentle centrifugation at $200g$ for 8–10 min, aspiration of the supernatant, addition of 2 mL of fresh complete medium, gentle pipetting, and transfer of different volumes of the resulting cell suspension into six 24-well plates containing full hybridoma medium. Growth of the thawed cells should be monitored on an inverted microscope.

3.6. Determining Isotypes and Complement-Fixation Activity

1. Determining a class and subclass of a MAb, as well as the ability to bind and activate complement, are major MAb parameters that affect its performance in the desired application. As such, early and definitive testing of MAbs for these parameters is an essential part of the hybridoma selection process.

2. Multiple isotyping kits are available commercially, ranging from the more than 50 yr old Ouchterlony immunodiffusion agar-based assays to the highly sensitive ELISA tests, for identifying class and subclass composition in different species. In the vast majority of cases, all these kits provide reliable qualitative data, and, therefore, can be used in both primary and advanced screening. One example of such a simple, inexpensive, quick (less than 1 h), and adequately sensitive (1 µg/mL) kit is Sigma's Immunotype ISO1 Mouse Monoclonal Antibody Isotyping Kit based in incubating nitrocellulose membrane strips bound to inert support with 2 mL of the supernatant in question, followed by secondary detection using a self-descriptive avidin–biotin detection system. Although more than 90% of murine immunoglobulins contain κ light chains, the κ vs λ light structure should be also determined for each MAb.

3. Test the ability of the MAb in question to fix and activate complement using rabbit low-Tox-M complement from Cedarlane Laboratories (*see* **Subheading 2.**). First, make sure the concentration of the MAb in the tested material (typically,

hybridoma supernatant from 24-well plates) is equal or greater that 1 µg/mL. Quantitate MAb concentration in ELISA using the Standard Vectastatin ABC kit according to the manufacturer's recommendations. If needed, adjust the supernatant to pH 7.2–7.4. Incubate 10^6 washed viable target cells exposing the antigen in question on their membrane with 1 mL of the hybridoma supernatant at 4°C for 1 h or complete hybridoma medium (negative control). After two washes in prewarmed serum-free medium, incubate target cells with 1 mL of prediluted rabbit complement at the concentrations recommended by the manufacturer for the complement lot used in the experiment. After incubation, immediately determine the percentage of cell death in the hybridoma supernatant vs the negative control sample. This experiment must be repeated at least three times with different lots and concentrations of the complement.

3.7. Production of Ascitic Fluids in Mice

1. Prime BALB/c mice with 0.5 mL of Pristane injected i.p. prior to hybridoma cell injection.
2. 7 d after Pristane administration, inject i.p. 5×10^6 to 5×10^7 prewashed (twice in serum-free DMEM) hybridoma cells.
3. Check inoculated mice for abdominal distension every 3–5 d until the abdomen is filled completely with ascitic fluid (typically, 3–4 wk). Drain ascitic fluid from the abdomen using an 18-gage needle.
4. Clear ascitic fluids by centrifugation at 500g for 10 min; remove the yellowish layer of fat on the top of the ascitic fluid and clotted material from other areas of the tube.
5. Aspirate the supernatant, aliquot, and keep at –20°C until further analysis and MAb purification.
6. Collect the cell pellet and use it one or two times to induce ascites in the next group of Pristane-primed animals. Do not use ascitic cells more than twice.
7. In most labs, one mouse produces 5–10 mL of ascitic fluid containing 5–20 mg/mL of the MAb.

3.8. Production of MAbs in Protein-Free Medium

1. In this section, we describe our experience of selecting a hybridoma clone capable of secreting high MAb concentrations when growing in a serum-, protein-free medium. *See* Chapter 13 for a detailed description of the uses of this MAb for the detection of MDR1 P-glycoprotein expression and functional activity.
2. A subclone of the UIC2 hybridoma, termed UIC2/A (ATCC; cat. no. HB11287), was developed by gradually replacing the original growth medium (DMEM supplemented with 10% FBS and penicillin-streptomycin) with PFHM II protein-free hybridoma medium *(12)*. Complete DMEM-based medium was replaced by PFHM II supplemented by 10% FBS during the fourth round of recloning, according to the timeline described in **Subheading 3.5.**
3. Subsequently, the hybridoma was cultured in 25-mL flasks on complete PFHM II medium. The concentration of FBS was gradually reduced to 0% by replacing 25% of complete PFHM II medium with unmodified PFHM II. After 1 mo of

cultivation in the protein-free medium, all cells had lost their ability to grow while attached to the flask surface, and were growing in PFHM II as a suspension culture in clusters consisting of 8–20 cells.

4. At that point, hybridoma cells were cloned by serial dilution in unmodified PFHM II in 96-well plates (*see* **Subheading 3.5.**), and supernatants from the best wells were tested for antibody production by indirect immunofluorescence. A clone that gave the strongest immunofluorescence signal was selected, transferred to a 25-mL flask, and the cell line was further expanded.

5. This cell line, designated UIC2/A (ATCC; cat. no. HB11287), was then passaged as a suspension culture in PFHM II medium in 25-mL, to 75-mL, and, finally, to 175-mL flasks. When supplemented with 25 m*M* HEPES, UIC2/A could be then cultivated in roller bottles, which resulted in high antibody titers (0.2–0.4 mg/mL).

6. As repeatedly verified by indirect immunofluorescence, the UIC2/A hybridoma produced MAb with the specificity and isotype (IgG2a) identical to those produced by the parental UIC2.

7. The data shown in **Fig. 1** demonstrates that the UIC2 MAb present in UIC2/A supernatants was about 80% pure IgG without any purification (lanes 6–9). After a single-step purification on a protein-A affinity column, the purity of the UIC2/A MAb was close to 100% (lanes 3 and 4), similar to that of the protein A-purified MAb from ascitic fluids produced by parental UIC2 hybridoma (lanes 1 and 2). The concentration of the UIC2 antibody in UIC2/A supernatants varied between 200 and 350 µg/mL, based on the yield determined after affinity purification and sodium dodecyl sulfate-polyacrylamide gel electrophoresis.

8. The ability of the UIC2/A cell line to grow in suspension (including permanent rotation in roller bottles), the high titers of the UIC2 MAb produced, and the small amount of extraneous proteins make this cell line particularly useful for industrial-scale production of the UIC2 MAb. Additionally, in many applications (e.g., immunofluorescent and Immunohistochemistry (IHC) staining of cells and tissues, cell separation, immunoprecipitation, and so on) UIC2/A supernatant fluids may be used without purification or concentration.

9. When licensed to Chemicon International (Temecula, CA) and manufactured as a commercial research reagent, gram amounts of the UIC2/A antibody were readily produced using the INTEGRA (Chur, Switzerland) cell line perfusion system and the Cellex (Minneapolis, MN) ACUSYST-miniMAX bioreactor.

3.9. Purification of MAbs

1. Protein A- and Protein G-based commercially available purification kits are most commonly used to purify MAbs from ascitic fluids, supernatants, and other MAb preparations. These proteins are isolated from the cell wall of several micro-organisms and naturally binds to the Fc portion of immunoglobulins from several mammalian species, including murine MAbs, at pH 8.2 (Protein A) and pH 5.0 (Protein G).

2. All murine IgG subclasses, except IgG1, bind strongly to both Protein A and Protein G and can be purified using either of these two systems. Because of better

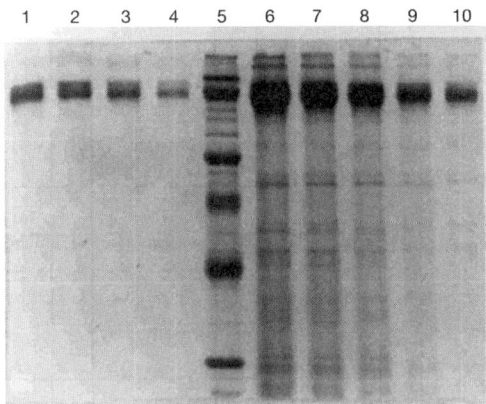

Fig. 1. Sodium dodecyl sulfate-polyacrylamide gel electrophoresis separation under nonreducing conditions of the proteins present in UIC2 and UIC2/A monoclonal antibody preparations. Lanes 1 through 4 show immunoglobulins purified on a Protein A affinity column (1.2 µg of protein in lanes 1–3, 0.4. µg in lane 4) after harvesting from the ascitic fluid of the UIC2 hybridoma (lane 1), tissue culture supernatant fluid of UIC2 cells grown in medium containing 10% fetal bovine serum (lane 2), and tissue culture supernatants of UIC2/A hybridoma cells grown in PFHM II protein-free media (lanes 3 and 4). Lane 5 in the figure contains Bio-Rad molecular mass markers (200, 116, 97, 66, and 45 kDa). Lanes 6 through 9 show unfractionated proteins from the tissue culture supernatant from UIC2/A cells concentrated by centrifugation using AMICON Centriprep 100 concentration units and electrophoresed at the following amounts: 50 µg in lane 6; 25 µg in lane 7; 12.5 µg in lane 8; 6.25 µg in lane 9. Lane 10 contains 4 µg of unpurified and unconcentrated protein from the UIC2/A suspension culture supernatant.

stability of mouse MAbs at slightly basic pH, Protein A-based purification systems are more advantageous than those based on Protein G. Mouse IgG1 and IgM MAbs can be isolated using Protein L-based purification kits.

4. Notes

1. It is absolutely essential that myeloma cells are resistant to 8-azaguanine and, therefore, are not capable of producing Hypoxanthine-guanine phosphoribosyl-transferase (HGPRT) and using hypoxanthine contained in after-fusion selective hybridoma medium. This can be achieved by growing cells in a media containing 8-azaguanine and HT. Resistance to 8-azaguanine results in the elimination of all HGPRT+ revertants, whereas HT preselection leads to optimal survival and growth of primary hybridoma clones in HAT after-fusion medium.

2. The unused splenocytes can be aliquoted, cryopreserved, and, upon careful thawing, utilized for future cell fusions. This could be a very valuable resource to improve the specificity, sensitivity, isotype, and other parameters of the desired

antibody, including changing the origin and even species specificity of the fusion partner.

3. In this chapter, we are not attempting to describe typical screening protocols — these differ very significantly between different hybridoma projects, based on the objectives and resources of each research group. The most important general rule here is to build primary and secondary screening protocols exactly in accordance with the intended application of the desired MAb and, if possible, perform screening procedures using experimental techniques closely linked to the intended application. In other words, if you are planning to develop a MAb for immunohistochemistry staining, it would be not a good idea to use ELISA for the selection of hybridoma clones. Although tempting for experimentators who are new to the hybridoma field, these seemingly straightforward and inexpensive strategies rarely work well in the long run, resulting in selecting numerous clones with unfavorable parameters in the desired application.

4. The objective of recloning is not only to ensure the clonality of resulting subclones and ensuing hybridoma mass population used to produce and manufacture large amounts of the desired MAb, but also to select for the most stable, quickly growing, and highly producing MAb subclones. This approach ultimately results in generating durable and reliable hybridoma cell banks that can be used for large-scale production on highly active MAb immunoglobulins.

5. As discussed in **Subheadings 1.** and **4.**, generating MAbs in tissue culture is a viable and increasingly popular alternative to growing ascites in BALB/c and *nude* mice. The former approach does not require animal use and allows the full realization of the potential of MAbs by avoiding nonspecific antibody contaminants.

6. Similarly to the immunization and screening protocols, every research group uses its own approach and methodology for purifying MAbs. Therefore, in this paper we are not attempting to present a detailed purification protocol that would be acceptable for all experimental models and objectives.

References

1. Kohler, G. and Milstein, C. (1976) Derivation of specific antibody-producing tissue culture and tumor lines by cell fusion. *Eur. J. Immunol.* **6,** 511–519.
2. He, Y., Honnen, W. J., Krachmarov, C. P., et al. (2002) Efficient isolation of novel human monoclonal antibodies with neutralizing activity against HIV-1 from transgenic mice expressing human Ig loci. *J. Immunol.* **169,** 595–605.
3. Hoogenboom, H. R. and Chames, P. (2000) Natural and designer binding sites made by phage display technology. *Immunol. Today* **21,** 371–378.
4. Liu, B., Huang, L., Sihlbom, C., Burlingame, A., and Marks, J. D. (2002) Towards proteome-wide production of monoclonal antibody by phage display. *J. Mol. Biol.* **315,** 1063–1073.
5. Hanes, J., Schaffitzel, C., Knappik, A., and Pluckthun, A. (2000) Picomolar affinity antibodies from a fully synthetic naive library selected and evolved by ribosome display. *Nat. Biotechnol.* **18,** 1287–1292.

6. Tomlinson, I. and Holliger, P. (2000) Methods for generating multivalent and bispecific antibody fragments. *Methods Enzymol.* **326,** 461–479.
7. Proske, D., Blank, M., Buhmann, R., and Resch, A. (2005) Aptamers—basic research, drug development, and clinical applications. *Appl. Microbiol. Biotechnol.* **69,** 367–374.
8. Hudson, P. J. and Souriau, C. Engineered antibodies. (2003) *Nat. Med.* **9,** 129–134.
9. Jain, K. K. (2005) Personalised medicine for cancer: from drug development into clinical practice. *Expert Opin. Pharmacother.* **6,** 1463–1476.
10. Bioinfomatics (2004) The market for antibodies: keys to success for commercial suppliers. Report #04-049.
11. de StGroth, S. F. and Scheidegger, D. (1980) Production of monoclonal antibodies: strategy and tactics. *J. Immunol. Methods* **35,** 1–21.
12. Mechetner, E. and Roninson, I. (1998) Monoclonal antibody to a human MDR1 multidrug resistance gene product, and uses. US Patent no. 5,773,280.

2

Recombinant Monoclonal Antibodies

Mariel Donzeau and Achim Knappik

Summary

Recombinant antibody technology is a rapidly evolving field that enables the study and improvement of antibody properties by means of genetic engineering. Moreover, the functional expression of antibody fragments in *Escherichia coli* has formed the basis for antibody library generation and selection, a powerful method to produce *human* antibodies for therapy. Because in vitro-generated antibodies offer various advantages over traditionally produced monoclonal antibodies, such molecules are now increasingly used for standard immunological assays. This chapter will give a short review on how recombinant antibodies are generally be produced and engineered, and how typical immunoassays are performed.

Key Words: Recombinant antibodies; antibody engineering; Fab; scFv; antibody libraries; phage display.

1. Introduction

Although the development of hybridoma technology (*see* Chapter 1) was a critical breakthrough in life science research, the technology has a number of limitations. It requires considerable time, expense, and expertise, as well as specialized cell culture facilities, and relies on the use of animals. Additionally, many molecules are not immunogenic in mammals or are toxic and cannot be used as antigens. Most seriously for therapeutic application of antibodies, standard methods of producing monoclonal antibodies (MAbs) yield rodent antibodies that are rejected by the human immune system. Various approaches to overcome this limitation have been attempted, such as combining the DNA that encodes the binding site of mouse MAbs with DNA that encodes human antibodies. This generates antibodies known as either chimeric antibodies or humanized antibodies, depending on how large a part of the mouse antibody is used. Another approach is to use mice that are genetically engineered to produce antibodies with human antibody sequences.

From: *Methods in Molecular Biology, vol. 378: Monoclonal Antibodies: Methods and Protocols*
Edited by: M. Albitar © Humana Press Inc., Totowa, NJ

Developments in the fields of bacterial expression of functional antibodies and methods to select genes from a library by using the phenotype of the encoded polypeptide between 1985 and 1988 have been a breakthrough in antibody technology.

This chapter summarizes some of the methodologies commonly used to select, identify, and engineer antibody fragments for particular properties and apply them in typical immunoassays.

1.1. Antibody Libraries and Phage Display

Nowadays, phage display in combination with antibody gene libraries is widely used to select *Escherichia coli* host cells that express desired antibody fragments. Such gene libraries are typically produced either from natural sources (e.g., from the spleen of an immunized animal or from plasma cells of human donors) or generated by genetic engineering. The latter has been used to create naïve libraries based on one or more antibody VH and VL gene segments that are diversified by cassette mutagenesis or similar approaches. Such libraries are typically unbiased and can be used for any given antigen (*1–4*). Modern naïve libraries are generally large (more than 10^{10} members), contain only few nonfunctional members, yield antibodies that are well expressed in *E. coli* (more than 1 mg/L of purified material), and are designed to allow further affinity maturation, if needed. Phage display is then most often used to select desired antibodies from such libraries (for reviews, *see* **refs. 5** and **6**). First, *E. coli* host cells are transformed with the library that has been inserted into phagemid vectors bearing the antibody gene fragments fused to the phage gene III that will later be part of the phage particle. Host cells carrying the phagemid are selected with an antibiotic-resistance marker. For phage display, the culture is infected with a helper phage that will deliver all necessary components for phage production. During infection, the cloned antibody sequences are transcribed, and the sequences are produced as a fusion protein, consisting of a bacterial "leader sequence," the antibody gene fragment(s), and the gIII phage coat protein. The leader sequence directs the proteins to the periplasmic space, where the fused antibody fragment is incorporated into viable phage particles via the coat protein. Phages are secreted through the bacterial outer membrane and display one to three copies of the encoded antibody fragment on their outer surfaces. Such phages can be easily isolated and stored for later use.

1.2. Antibody Selection and Production

Once the phage library has been generated, the panning process begins by incubating the phage population with an immobilized antigen. Such "phage panning" or "bio-panning" is similar to a solid-phase immunoassay. In this process, the antigen of interest is immobilized on microplate wells or magnetic beads, or is biotinylated and later captured in the process. Also, selection on cells, on membrane fractions or on tissue sections has been shown. After extensive washing to remove all unbound phage, the bound phage are eluted and amplified by replication in new host cells. The selection procedure is repeated typically one to three times, resulting in a population that consists mostly of phage that display the desired antibodies, i.e., antibodies with affinity to the used antigen. After these selection steps, the antibody genes are isolated and inserted into an expression vector. Schematic expression cassettes *(7,8)* for single-chain antibodies and for Fab fragments (*see* **Below**), which are based on the lac-promoter, are shown in **Fig. 1**. The Fab expression cassette is mostly arranged as a bicistronic unit, whereby the antibody light chain gene is located upstream. This arrangement ensures that there is more light chain present than heavy chain because heavy chains are prone to aggregation without a light chain partner, whereas light chains are soluble.

To produce soluble antibody fragments after selection, the antibody genes cloned into the phagemid are then expressed without the phage coat protein, which is usually achieved by either removing the DNA encoding the phage coat gene III protein from the vector or by subcloning the whole pool of enriched antibody genes into an expression vector. At this step, the transformed cells are isolated as single colonies, each producing a defined and therefore monoclonal antibody. A number of colonies are separately picked, grown in microtiter plates, and antibody expression is induced.

Because antibodies contain disulfide bonds that are necessary for maintaining their overall structure and binding activity, the folding of the molecule has to take place under oxidizing conditions. Gram-negative *E. coli* provides an oxidizing compartment between the cytoplasmic and outer membrane, the so-called periplasmic space. Hence, the attachment of bacterial leader sequences to the N-terminus of an antibody fragment directs the translated antibody chain(s) into the periplasmic space by the bacterial transport apparatus, where folding can take place under oxidizing conditions.

After induction of antibody expression, cells are subsequently lysed (either gently by an osmotic shock procedure or simply by adding lysozyme) and the antibody-containing lysates can be tested by enzyme-linked immunosorbent assay (ELISA) or other methods for the presence of antigen-specific antibody material. Screening by ELISA is one of the most used and well-established methods to screen antibody-expressing clones. Target molecules can be directly coated onto 96- or 384-well microtiter plates, or biotinylated target antigens can be captured onto streptavidin plates. Bacterial extracts are added to the microtiter plates and bound antibody fragments are detected with enzyme-conjugated polyclonal antiserum or with antibodies directed against the C-terminal tags provided by the vector (*see* **below**). Often, positive hits are

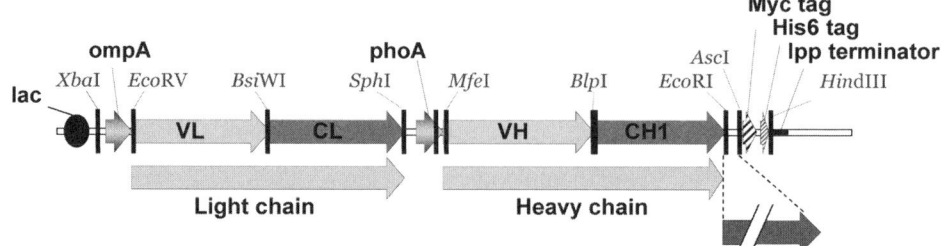

Fig. 1. Design of HuCAL® Fab antibody expression unit (*see* **ref. 2**). The bicistronic operon is under control of the lac promoter/operator, so expression can be induced with Isopropyl β-D-1-thiogalactopyranoside. Both L and H gene segments are preceded by signal sequences (derived from the *Escherichia coli ompA* and the *phoA* genes) that ensure transport to the periplasmic space. The elements that are located downstream of the heavy chain gene segment between the *Eco*RI and *Hind*III restriction sites determine what valency the final product will have and what tags or fusion partners will be attached to the Fab molecule. Note the modularity of the gene segments resulting from the location of unique restriction sites, whereby each segment can be easily exchanged by compatible modules.

sequenced to determine the number of unique antibodies from a selection. The process previously described can be automated to a large extent using standard pipetting robots, thereby enabling massive increase in throughput, one of the advantages over animal-based methodologies.

Target molecules presenting therapeutic interests can be receptors expressed on the surface of a particular eukaryotic cell line. Screening of recombinant antibody fragments on whole cells has been successfully applied, for example, to isolate binders targeting the fibroblast growth factor receptor 3, which belongs to a family of cell surface receptor tyrosine kinases, or the intercellular adhesion molecule 1 *(7,8)*. Specific antibody fragments binding to a receptor molecule in ELISA can be further tested for their binding capacity on the surface of the eukaryotic cells. Cells expressing the endogenous molecule or cells transiently transfected with an eukaryotic vector expressing the target molecule can be used. In both cases, incubation steps of bacterial extract containing antibody fragments and cells are carried out at 4°C.

At this step, the panning method has typically resulted in the isolation of a number of different antigen-specific MAb fragments starting from the original large library of antibody genes. The procedure overall takes about 4–6 wk, albeit massive reduction in timelines have also been reported. Now the antibodies can be individually expressed and purified in larger scale. Soluble antibody fragments produced by bacterial colonies isolated as previously explained are typically purified by one-step affinity chromatography using peptide tags that have been fused to the C-terminus of the antibody fragment. After purification, the material is mostly aliquoted and stored frozen, similar to traditional MAbs.

1.3. Selection Strategies

Because the selection process takes place in vitro, as opposed to animal immunization where the immune response is not under control of the experimentator, the panning conditions can be adjusted to drive the selection toward desired antibody properties. Typical examples for guided selections include the way of presenting the antigen to the phage library (native, denatured, captured, masked), the stringency of washing (which determines the affinity range of enriched antibodies), the method of phage elution (e.g., by competition with free antigen), the simulation of assay conditions during panning (e.g., by adding denaturants to select for highly stable antibodies, *see* **ref. 9** as an example), the selection of cross-reactive antibody by alteration of two or more antigens during the panning rounds, and last but not least the selection of epitope-specific antibodies by blocking or subtracting the library with a related antigen. The latter can be used, for instance, to select phospho-specific antibodies (*see* **Fig. 2**). Such methods have been shown to reliably enrich desired antibody properties, thereby dramatically reducing the subsequent screening effort.

1.4. Recombinant Antibody Engineering

The major types of recombinant antibody fragments that are usually expressed in *E. coli* are named Fv, dsFv, scFv, and Fab (**Fig. 3**). Fv (fragment variable) fragments consists of only the variable domains of the heavy and light chains (VH and VL) and are the smallest units that retain binding properties to a given antigen *(10)*. VH and VL expressed in *E. coli* assemble spontaneously into Fv fragments through noncovalent interactions. However, the VH–VL interaction is usually weak, and therefore these dimeric proteins are sometimes prone to dissociation and aggregation, depending on the antibody sequence. Recombinant DNA techniques have been used to either create an interdisulfide bond between VH and VL (leading to the dsFv antibody fragment) or to introduce a short peptide linker between VH and the VL to create a single polypeptide chain folding into the so-called scFv antibody fragment. While the dsFv needs site-directed mutagenesis within the framework and/or Complementarity Determining Region (CDR) region of a given antibody, the creation of scFv is a generally applicable method. It has been shown that shortening the linker between the two variable domains leads to so-called diabodies *(11)*, which pair with the complementary domains of another scFv chain and thereby promote the assembly of dimeric or bispecific molecules with two functional antigen-binding sites.

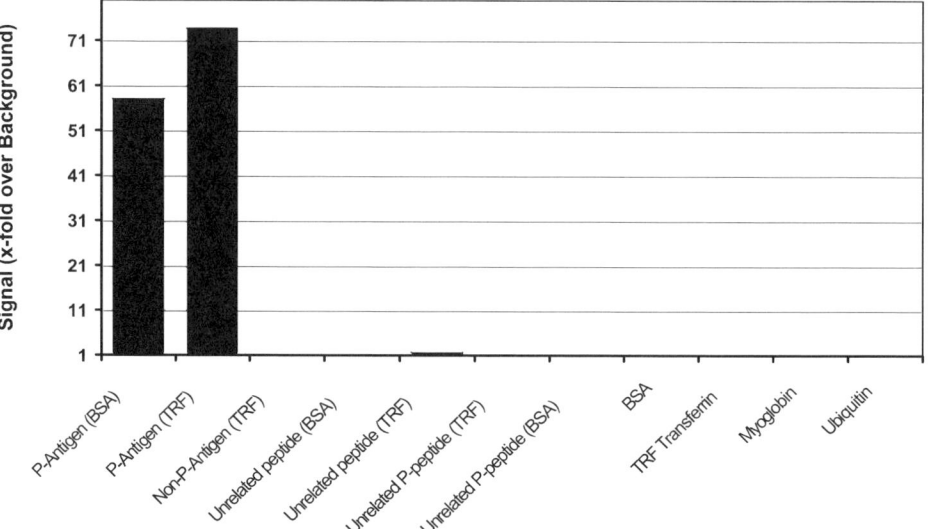

Fig. 2. Specificity ELISA of an antibody (bivalent Fab-dHLX fragment) selected from the HuCAL® library on a phosphorylated peptide with the sequence RKSAPpSTGG-C (P-antigen), coupled to the carrier proteins bovine serum albumin (BSA) and human transferring (TRF) and immobilized on a microtiter well. Prior to selection, the antibody library was incubated with the nonphosphorylated counterpart RKSAPSTGG-C (non-P-antigen), thereby blocking antibody specificities toward the nonphosphorylated form. During the panning, the peptide-carrier conjugate was alternated between TRF in rounds 1 and 3, and BSA in round 2, thereby removing carrier-specific antibodies. One of selected antibodies was purified and tested in ELISA (2 µg/mL) for binding to a range of immobilized peptides and proteins (5 µg/mL each). Detection was performed with horseradish peroxidase-conjugated mouse anti-His-tag antibody (1:500 diluted) and Quanta-Blue as substrate. As can be seen in the figure, the antibody recognizes the phosphorylated antigen and does neither bind to the nonphosphorylated counterpart nor to the carrier proteins. In addition, unrelated peptides (with or without a phosphorserine group) or unrelated proteins are also not bound.

Another commonly used recombinant antibody fragment is the Fab fragment, which is composed of the truncated heavy chain containing the variable and the first constant region, and the entire light chain composed of the variable and constant domain. These two polypeptides are either covalently linked by disulfide bridges at the C-terminus, or are produced in higher yields without those, which nevertheless lead to highly stable H/L heterodimers *(8)*. The Fab fragment is truly monovalent (which is not always the case with scFv fragments), it does not contain an artificial linker sequence which might interfere with the antigen binding site, and well-established anti-Fab detection antibodies can be used.

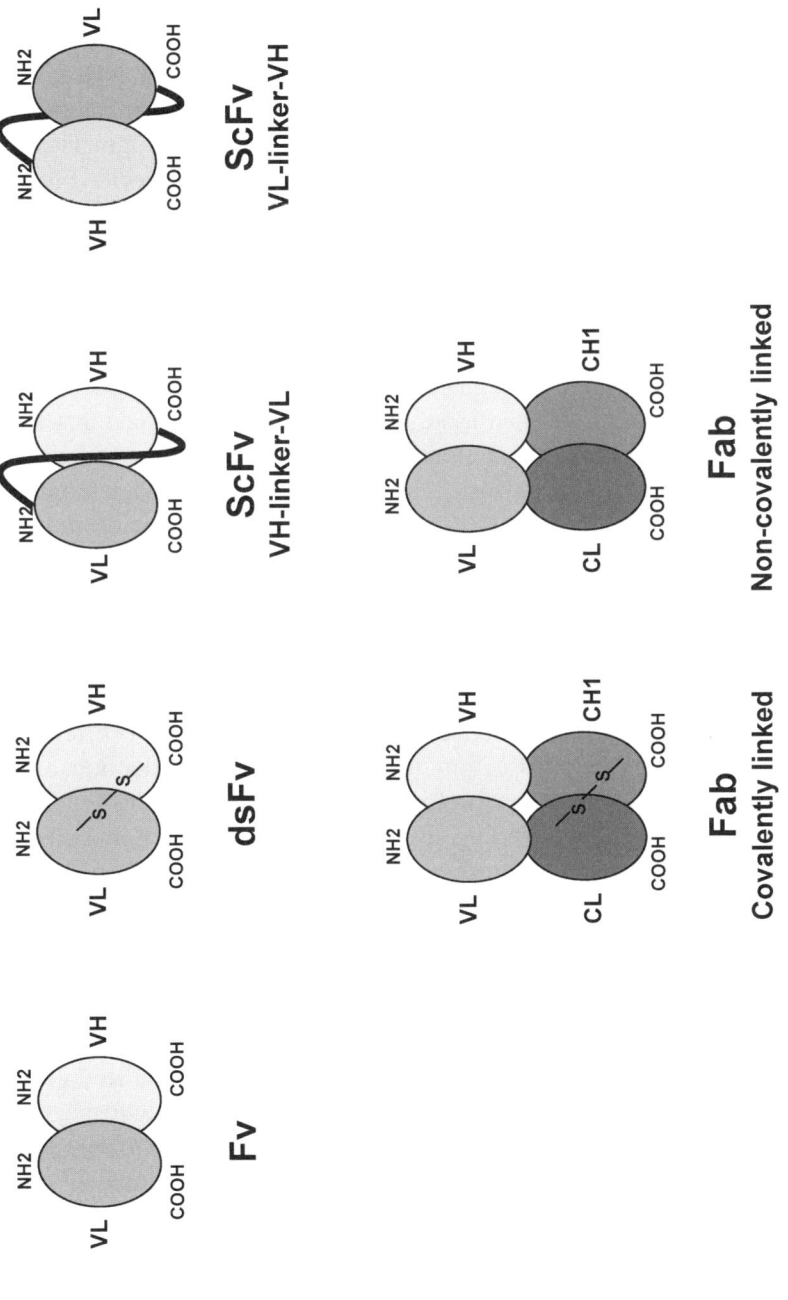

Fig. 3. Antibody fragments commonly expressed in *Escherichia coli*. The Fv, dsFv, and Fab formats are expressed as two distinct polypeptide chains and assemble after folding in the periplasm to functional antibody fragments. The Fab format can be either covalently linked by a C-terminal disulfide bond or associated by noncovalent forces. The scFv formats are expressed as one polypeptide chain, whereby the two variable domains are connected with a Gly_4Ser linker of variable length. Both orientations (VH-linker-VL or VL-linker-VH) have been described.

Recombinant antibodies offer many advantages that are only beginning to be explored. These advantages stem from two properties: the ability to assess the antibody DNA within an *E. coli* environment that allows the use of well-known genetic engineering methodologies, and the use of antibody fragments rather than intact IgG molecules because of the small size of Fab and scFv fragments, and because of the absence of the Fc domain. The latter eliminates nonspecific binding to cellular Fc receptors and avoids other nonspecific effects caused by the Fc part of intact IgG, which for instance induces cytokine release in functional assays with immunocompetent cells. In addition, nonspecific binding to the Fc region in immunocytochemical applications is eliminated, which often leads to lower background, better signal-to-noise ratio, and increased sensitivity. Moreover, fragments diffuse better through tissue and through cell membranes than intact IgG because of its small size, leading to faster and more efficient staining. The fact that scFv and Fab perform monovalent interactions is important when avidity effects should be avoided, e.g., when the intrinsic binding affinity needs to be determined. In fluorescent or enzyme conjugates, Fab or scFv fragments provide reduced hydrophobicity, reduced steric hindrance (improved stoichiometry because more markers can bind to the presented antigens), and less interference with serum factors and macromolecules (which mostly bind to the Fc region). Cocrystallization of target proteins with antibodies also requires smaller antibody fragments.

Generation of antibodies in vitro enables manipulation of their sequences, for instance by linking desired sequences to the antibody framework regions. Examples are peptide tags for purification, immobilization, and detection, enzymatic activities like alkaline phosphatase for direct detection, modules for multimerization to create multimeric-binding sites with increased functional affinity (avidity), modules that lead to heterodimerization, thereby creating bispecific antibodies, and, last but not least, toxins for the elimination of tumor cells in therapeutic applications. Typically, such fusions are cloned in-frame at the 3'-end of the antibody gene, leading to a maximum distance in the native fusion protein between the antigen-binding site and the additional functionality. A few such fusions will be highlighted here.

Peptide tags are mostly used for affinity purification purposes. Most tags that have been generally developed for recombinant protein purification will also work for antibodies. A typical example is the His-tag, a series of five to six histidines that bind to affinity media such as Nitrilotriacetic acid (NTA)-agarose or Talon resin, when metal ions (nickel or cobalt) are bound. His-tagged proteins bind with millimolar affinity to the column and are gently eluted with 150–300 mM imidazole. Another such tag is the StrepII-tag, which shows affinity to streptavidin- or streptactin-sepharose (streptactin is a genetically engineered streptavidin with higher affinity to the Strep-tag). Antibodies to both tags are available, so the tags can be used for detection purposes as well. Other detection tags like the V5-tag

(GKPIPNPLLGLDST), which is derived from a small epitope present on the P/V proteins of the paramyxovirus, SV5, or the myc-tag (EQKLISEEDL), which correspond to residues 408–439 of the human p62 c-myc protein are also frequently used because specific high-affinity MAbs are commercially available. The FLAG-tag (DYKDDDDK) is of special interest because a MAb (termed M1) exists that only binds to the tag when the N-terminus is free and not involved in a peptide bond. This has been used to monitor cleavage of signal sequences during *E. coli* antibody expression *(12)*.

Site-directed immobilization of recombinant antibodies should improve functional activity in array- or bead-based applications because it has been shown that random passive adsorption of whole antibodies on plastic surfaces results in major loss of protein function *(13)*. Indeed, in a comparative study it was shown that specifically oriented Fab fragments that had been immobilized via a C-terminal thiol group had an up to 10-fold higher capture capacity compared with surfaces which randomly oriented capture agents *(14)*. Recombinant antibodies with a C-terminal cysteine residue can easily be engineered.

Antibody fragments usually have the same antigen-binding specificity as the corresponding intact antibody because the complete antigen-binding site is present. However, multivalency is a very general nature of antibodies. IgG contain two binding sites per molecule, which increases the apparent affinity (avidity) compared with a Fab antibody fragment in cases where the antigen contains multiple epitopes or where multiple antigens are bound to a surface. The most noticeable example is IgM, which carries 10 recognition binding sites. For particular applications, bivalency might be advantageous or even required. Thus, bivalency and further multivalency have been also engineering for recombinant antibody fragments (**Fig. 4**). Dimeric mini-antibodies have been created using small "association domains," which are fused to the C-terminal portion of Fab or scFv antibody fragments *(15)*. For example, the leucine zipper from the yeast transcription factor GCN4 has been shown to be suitable as a dimerization device. Such "mini-antibodies" have been shown to display identical functional affinities as a whole parent antibody. Antibody fragments fused to the small tetramerization domain of p53 can form tetrameric molecules. In general, the expression yields are not reduced with such constructs.

Genetic fusions to enzymes like bacterial alkaline phosphatase (BAP) connect the binding and detection capability into one molecule. Such fusions lead to molecules the size of full-length antibodies to be expressed in *E. coli* with the same yields as smaller antibody fragments. Because the BAP is a homo-dimer, the resulting molecules are bivalent (*see* **Fig. 4**). Many other antibody fusions for various applications have been desribed in the literature, such as core streptavidin for avidity increase, β-lactamase for prodrug activation, or interleukin-8 fusion for neutrophil activation, to name a few. Cleary this field is still in its infancy.

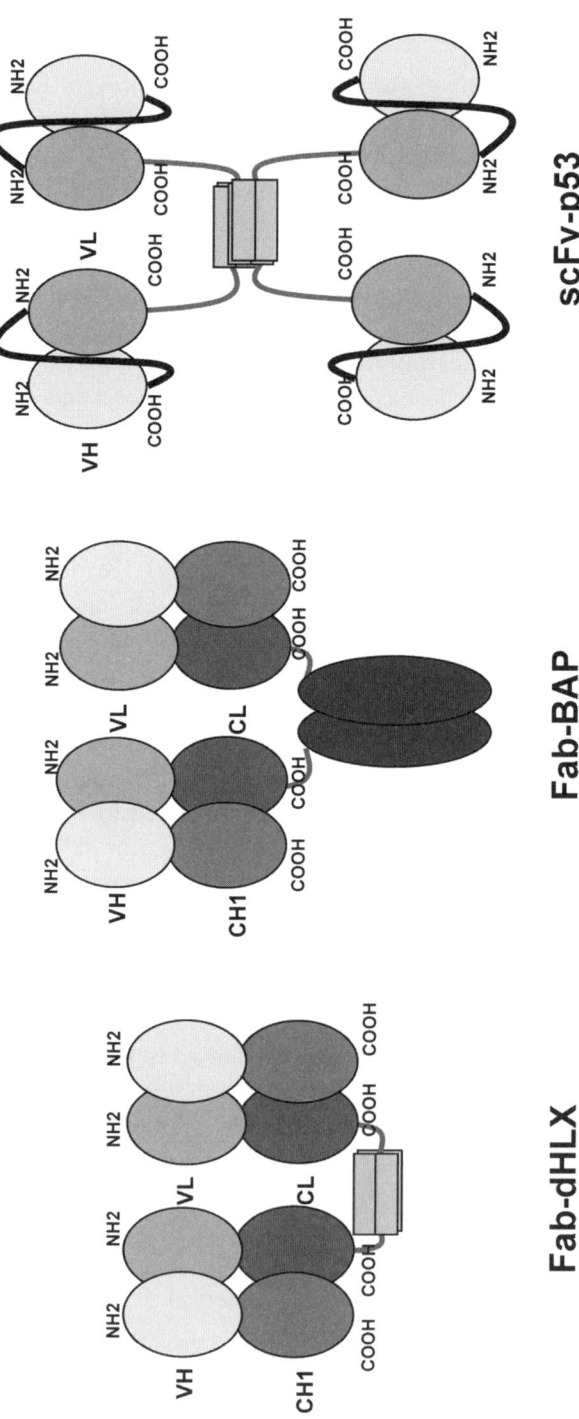

Fab-dHLX

Fab-BAP

scFv-p53

Fig. 4. Examples of multivalent antibody fragments obtained by genetic engineering. The Fab-dHLX fragment is dimerized by a self-assembling helix-turn-helix motif. The linker between the CH1 domain and the dimerization motif is derived from the mouse IgG3 upper hinge region. The Fab-bacterial alkaline phosphatase (BAP) format is obtained by fusing the bacterial *phoA* gene to the 3′-end of the heavy chain gene region. Because the BAP is a homodimeric molecule, the resulting antibodies are bivalent. The tetrameric scFv-p53 format is obtained by using the tetramerization domain of human p53. All these formats can be functionally expressed in *Escherichia coli*. Usually there are also peptide tags attached to the C-termini of the molecules, which are not shown here.

24

The following section will describe the use of recombinant antibody Fab fragments and derivatives in typical immunoassays such as Western blot, ELISA, and immunohistochemistry (IHC).

2. Materials (*see* Note 1)

1. Goat anti-human Fab (horseradish peroxidase [HRP]-conjugated and alkaline phosphatase [AP]-conjugated) from AbD Serotec, Oxford, UK.
2. Mouse anti-His-tag antibody (HRP-conjugated) from Roche Applied Science, Penzberg, Germany.
3. Recombinant antibodies have all been selected from the HuCAL® GOLD antibody library at MorphoSys AG, Martinsried, Germany.
4. ECL Plus or ECL Advance (GE Healthcare, Little Chalfont, UK) and AttoPhos (Roche).
5. Buffer antigen retrieval (Dako, Glostrup, Denmark).
6. Antibody-diluent (Dako, Glostrup, Denmark, cat. no. S 2022).
7. 3,3′-diaminobenzidine Chromogen and DAB substrate (DakoCytomation, cat. no. K 3468).
8. Hematoxylin (Sigma, St. Louis, USA, cat. no. MHS16-500ML).

3. Methods (*see* Note 2)

3.1. Western Blot (Fig. 5)

1. Run sodium dodecyl sulphate-polyacrylamide gel electrophoresis of your sample (*see* Note 3) and transfer to polyvinylidene fluoride (PVDF)-membrane. For initial testing, use 200 µg of cell lysate proteins or 300 ng of pure antigen.
2. Block membrane with 5% non-fat dry milk in TBST for 1 h on a shaker.
3. Rinse membrane with 20 mM Tris–HCl, pH 7.5, 0.5 mM NaCl, 0.5% Tween (TBST).
4. Add recombinant Fab antibody (5 µg/mL is recommended for initial experiments) to membrane in TBST with 1% non-fat dry milk, incubate 1 h at room temperature on a shaker.
5. Wash membrane three times for 5 min with TBST.
6. Add secondary antibody to membrane, for instance anti-human F(ab)$_2$ HRP-conjugate at 1:5000 dilution in TBST with 1% non-fat dry milk, shake for 1 h at room temperature.
7. Wash membrane three times for 5 min with TBST.
8. Develop membrane with ECL Plus or ECL Advance (Amersham) and use imager or X-ray films for detection.

3.2. ELISA (Fig. 6)

ELISA with recombinant antibodies can be done with the same protocols used for conventional polyclonal antibodies or MAbs as long as a suitable secondary antibody is used (*see* Notes). The indirect ELISA shown here is a

1   2

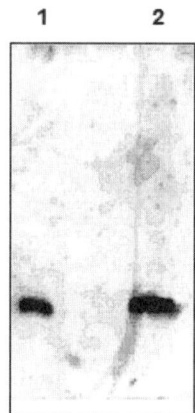

Fig. 5. Detection of human Cyclophilin A from HEK293 cell lysate by Western blot analysis, using a HuCAL® anti-Cyclophilin A antibody in the bivalent mini-antibody format. The antibody has been identified by standard selection on human Cyclophilin A antigen obtained by recombinant *Escherichia coli* expression. Human Cyclophilin A (lane 1: 5 ng of purified human Cyclophilin and lane 2: HEK293 lysate) was detected with 2 µg/mL HuCAL anti-Cyclophilin A antibody as primary antibody and anti-human F(ab')$_2$ horseradish peroxidase-conjugate as secondary antibody. The blot was developed using ECL Plus.

standard ELISA method in which the antigen is coated on the surface of a microtiter plate and detected by primary antibody followed by a secondary antibody. The secondary antibody is most frequently conjugated to an enzyme like AP or HRP and used together with a matching substrate for fluorescence detection.

1. Antigen coating: add 20 µL of antigen (5 µg/mL) in PBS to the wells of a 384-well Nunc Maxisorp™ microtiter plate.
2. Incubate overnight at 4°C.
3. Wash microtiter plate twice with phosphate buffered saline plus 0.05% tween (PBST).
4. Block microtiter plate with 100 µL/well 5% non-fat dry milk in PBST for 1–2 h at room temperature.
5. Wash microtiter plate twice with PBST.
6. Transfer 20 µL recombinant antibody to each well. The standard concentration is 2 µg/mL in PBS. For titrating the antibody, use a range of 10 µg/mL to 0.1 ng/mL. Incubate for 1 h at room temperature.
7. Wash microtiter plate five times with PBST.
8. Transfer 20 µL secondary antibody anti-human Fab AP-conjugate at 1:5000 dilution in PBS, incubate for 1 h at room temperature.
9. Wash microtiter plate five times with PBST.
10. Add 20 µL AttoPhos to each well and measure fluorescence after 10 min.

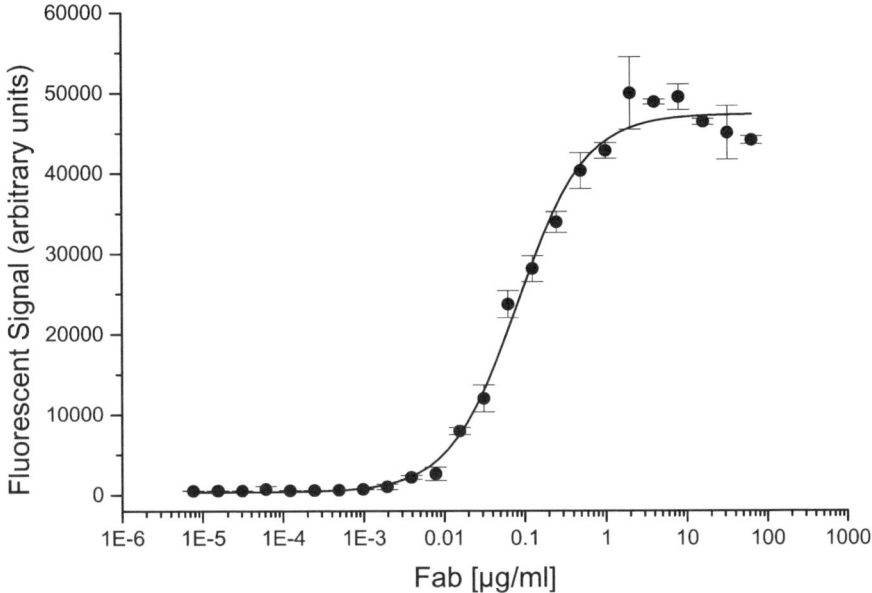

Fig. 6. A peptide containing the Ki-67 epitope "FKELF" was conjugated to a carrier protein and immobilized at 5 µg/mL in a microtiter plate. A HuCAL® antibody that had been identified by alternate selection on two peptides that both contained the FKELF motif but were otherwise different was titrated by an indirect ELISA method. Serial dilutions from 64 µg/mL to 8 pg/mL of the anti-pKi-67 antibody, followed by an anti-F(ab)$_2$ alkaline phosphates and detection with AttoPhos were used. Each data-point represents the mean of three independent measurements. Standard deviations are given as bars. The antibody shows 50% binding at a concentration of 80 ng/mL. Such titrations can be used to compare different antibodies to the same antigen.

3.3. IHC (Fig. 7)

MAbs are a valuable tool for IHC and are often preferred over polyclonal antibodies because of a usually much higher specificity. Recombinant antibodies are best used in a bivalent format to take advantage of avidity effects for localizing antigen in or on cells and tissues. The use of His-tagged recombinant antibodies allows direct detection with mouse HRP-conjugated anti-His-tag antibody (*see* **Notes 4–6**).

3.3.1. Deparaffinization and Rehydration

Deparaffinization and rehydration of paraffin-embedded tissue are required to assure access of the antibodies to the tissue antigen. Before deparaffinization with xylene, tissue sections should be dried for 1 h at 60°C to increase the adhesion of the tissue sections to the glass surface.

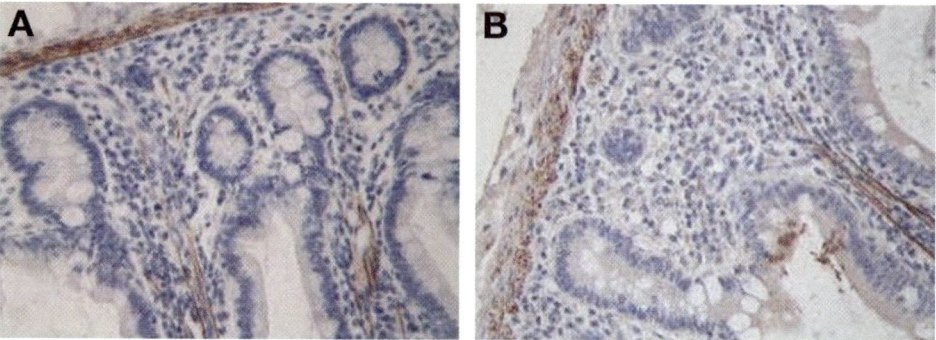

Fig. 7. Human formalin-fixed, paraffin-embedded small bowel tissue stained with either (**A**) a commercially available anti-Desmin antibody (DAKO, clone D33) that is known to work in immunohistochemistry, or (**B**) with an HuCAL® bivalent mini-antibody (Fab-dHLX) that had been selected against recombinant human Desmin. Both antibodies were used at a concentration of 10 μg/mL. The HuCAL antibody was detected by anti-His-tag antibody conjugated to horseradish peroxidase and DAB substrate. Counterstaining was performed with hematoxylin. Magnification ×400.

1. Fill the cuvets with xylene and incubate for 5 min with gentle shaking.
2. Transfer slides to a cuvet containing fresh xylene.
3. Incubate for 5 min, shake gently.
4. Repeat xylene washing steps for a total of four times for 5-min incubations.
5. Place the slides in 100% ethanol twice for 2 min.
6. Place the slides in 90% ethanol twice for 2 min.
7. Place the slides in 80% ethanol twice for 2 min.
8. Place the slides in 70% ethanol twice for 2 min.
9. Place the slides in 50% ethanol twice for 2 min.
10. Wash twice for 2 min with TBST.

3.3.2. Heat-Induced Epitope Pretreatment

The heat-induced epitope pretreatment results in increased staining intensity with many primary antibodies. Immersion of the tissue sections in preheated buffer solution and maintaining heat is supposed to break antigen cross-links and to retrieve the conformation of the antigen/epitope. Calcium ions are removed by citrate.

1. Preheat the buffer antigen retrieval with the slides in the microwave oven at 700–900 W until the boiling point is reached.
2. Boil slides for another 5–15 min at 300–700 W.
3. Replace evaporated water with ddH$_2$O.
4. Allow the sections to cool for 15 min in their retrieval buffer.
5. Wash the sections in TBST twice for 2 min.

3.3.3. Deparaffinize Heat-Induced Epitope Pretreatment Slides Following Protocol

1. Wash with TBST three times for 2 min.
2. Quench tissue peroxidase by incubating in 3% H_2O_2 in methanol for 10 min.
3. Wash with TBST three times for 2 min.
4. Perform protein blocking with 10% bovine serum albumin (BSA) in PBS for 15 min.
5. Tip excess blocking solution off sections.
6. Apply primary antibody (His-tagged) at 10 µg/mL in antibody diluent and incubate for 1 h.
7. Wash with TBST three times for 2 min.
8. Apply mouse-anti-His-tag antibody (HRP-conjugated) at 1:60 in antibody diluent and incubate for 30 min.
9. Wash with TBST three times for 2 min.
10. Add two drops (ca. 50 µL) DAB Chromogen per 1 mL of DAB substrate, mix by swirling, and apply to tissue. Incubate for 10 min.
11. Wash with TBST three times for 2 min.
12. For counterstaining apply hematoxylin for 1 min.
13. Apply tap water to the tissue to enhance blueing.
14. Rinse with ddH$_2$O.
15. Dehydrate with graded alcohol and cover permanent.

4. Notes

1. Recombinant antibody fragments do not contain the Fc part of full-length Ig molecules. Also, most recombinant antibodies are generated from human antibody libraries. Typical detection reagents like anti-mouse IgG can therefore not be used. For detection, anti-tag antibodies like anti-His or anti-Myc are a good choice. In case of human Fab antibodies, the use of a goat anti-human Fab secondary antibody is recommended because it gives higher sensitivity owing to signal amplification. Make sure the goat antiserum is directed against human Fab or F(ab')$_2$, and is preabsorbed on serum proteins from other mammals like mice.
2. Bi- or multivalent formats of recombinant antibody fragments are recommended for most applications like Western blot or IHC because the higher avidity usually gives a better sensitivity in these assays. The bivalent Fab fused to bacterial AP (Fab-BAP) is particularly valuable: detection can be first tried by using the AP activity. In case the sensitivity is not sufficient, a rabbit antibacterial AP-peroxidase-conjugated antibody can be applied, which usually gives a huge signal amplification effect. The Fab-BAP format has been successfully applied in ELISA, Western blotting, and IHC.
3. When performing Western blotting with cell lysates, the treatment of the lysate with ultrasound for a few seconds before loading it on the gel often reduces the background in the staining because of disruption of DNA.
4. For IHC, take care that the slides do not dry in any step of the heat retrieval procedure or the IHC. Optimal conditions for IHC detection must be determined for each individual situation.

5. In IHC, the use of His-tagged recombinant antibodies allows direct detection with mouse HRP-conjugated anti-His-tag antibody, and is therefore a quick but insensitive method because of low product yield. Because high concentrations of primary antibody are needed (10–25 μg/mL), background might become an issue. In this case, the use of a mouse anti-tag antibody plus a biotinylated anti-mouse antibody is recommended, followed by a streptavidin-HRP conjugate. Alternatively, the DAKO Envision system, which relies on an anti-mouse antibody bound to a HRP-labeled dextrane backbone can be used as well.

6. If IHC on murine tissue with low concentrations of primary antibody should be performed, the use of anti-mouse tertiary antibodies for detection will create high background staining. In this case, the use of tyramide-amplification systems is recommended. Here, the respective epitope of interest is marked with peroxidase via specific antibodies, and the labeled tissue is then incubated with biotinylated tyramide and H_2O_2. The peroxidase catalyzes a reaction resulting in "radicalized" tyramide, which then binds covalently to nearby tissue molecules. Finally, the biotin on the bound tyramide can easily be visualized by standard avidin biotinylated enzyme complex (ABC) techniques. This method needs only very low primary antibody concentration of 0.1–1 μg/mL.

Acknowledgments

The authors thank Dr. Ylera for providing us with **Fig. 5**, and Dr. Enzelberger for providing us with **Fig. 7**.

References

1. Nissim, A., Hoogenboom, H. R., Tomlinson, I. M., et al. (1994) Antibody fragments from a 'single pot' phage display library as immunochemical reagents. *EMBO J.* **13,** 692–698.
2. Knappik, A., Ge, L., Honegger, A., et al. (2000) Fully synthetic human combinatorial antibody libraries (HuCAL) based on modular consensus frameworks and CDRs randomized with trinucleotides. *J. Mol. Biol.* **296,** 57–86.
3. Soderlind, E., Strandberg, L., Jirholt, P., et al. (2000) Recombining germline-derived CDR sequences for creating diverse single-framework antibody libraries. *Nat. Biotechnol.* 18, 852–856.
4. Hoet, R. M., Cohen, E. H., Kent, R. B., et al. (2005) Generation of high-affinity human antibodies by combining donor-derived and synthetic complementarity-determining-region diversity. *Nat. Biotechnol.* 23, 344–348.
5. Hoogenboom, H. R., de Bruine, A. P., Hufton, S. E., Hoet, R. M. Arends, J. W., and Roovers, R. C. (1998) Antibody phage display technology and its applications. *Immunotechnology* **4,** 1–20.
6. Kretzschmar, T. and von Ruden, T. (2002) Antibody discovery: phage display. *Curr. Opin. Biotechnol.* **13,** 598–602.
7. Krebs, B., Rauchenberger, R., Reiffert, S., et al. (2001) High-throughput generation and engineering of recombinant human antibodies. *J. Immunol. Methods* **254,** 67–84.

8. Rauchenberger, R., Borges, E., Thomassen-Wolf, E., et al. (2003) Human combinatorial Fab library yielding specific and functional antibodies against the human fibroblast growth factor receptor 3. *J. Biol. Chem.* **278,** 38,194–38,205.

9. Rothlisberger, D., Pos, K. M., and Pluckthun, A. (2004) An antibody library for stabilizing and crystallizing membrane proteins: selecting binders to the citrate carrier CitS. *FEBS Lett.* **564,** 340–348.

10. Maynard, J. and Georgiou, G. (2000) Antibody engineering. *Annu. Rev. Biomed. Eng.* **2,** 339–376.

11. Hudson, P. J. and Kortt, A. A. (1999) High avidity scFv multimers; diabodies and triabodies. *J. Immunol. Methods.* **231,** 177–189.

12. Knappik, A. and Pluckthun, A. (1994) An improved affinity tag based on the FLAG peptide for the detection and purification of recombinant antibody fragments. *Biotechniques* **17,** 754–761.

13. Butler, J. E., Ni, L., Nessler, R., et al. (1992) The physical and functional behavior of capture antibodies adsorbed on polystyrene. *J. Immunol. Methods* **150,** 77–90.

14. Peluso, P., Wilson, D. S., Do, D., et al. (2003) Optimizing antibody immobilization strategies for the construction of protein microarrays. *Anal. Biochem.* **312,** 113–124.

15. Pluckthun, A. and Pack, P. (1997) New protein engineering approaches to multivalent and bispecific antibody fragments. *Immunotechnology* **3,** 83–105.

3

Soluble Fc Fusion Proteins for Biomedical Research

Meg L. Flanagan, Robyn S. Arias, Peisheng Hu, Leslie A. Khawli, and Alan L. Epstein

Summary

As a source of recombinant antigen, soluble constant fragment (Fc) fusion proteins have become valuable reagents for immunotherapy and laboratory investigations. Additional applications for these reagents include flow cytometry, immunohistochemistry, and in vitro activity assays. To aid investigators in the generation of these reagents, the materials and methods required for producing Fc fusion proteins are described. The investigator's protein moiety of interest is genetically linked to the N-terminus of murine Fc and subsequently expressed in large quantity using a mammalian cell expression system. The resulting Fc fusion proteins are purified on a protein A column and may be stored for at least one year at –20°C. The availability of easily purified, soluble Fc fusion proteins in such quantity can facilitate research in multiple fields of medicine and biotechnology.

Key Words: Antibody engineering; antibody production; soluble Fc; fusion protein; recombinant antigen; genetic engineering; protein expression; protein moiety; mammalian expression system.

1. Introduction

1.1. Introduction to Soluble Fc Fusion Proteins

The availability of soluble recombinant proteins has become a necessity of the modern research laboratory. Soluble Fc fusion proteins have a number of uses within the laboratory. As shown in **Table 1**, these Fc fusion proteins can be useful for in vitro as well as in vivo investigations. To facilitate the manufacture and testing of soluble Fc fusion proteins, this chapter will describe in detail the experimental methods and materials required for generating Fc fusion proteins containing a recombinant protein of interest.

A major advantage of generating Fc fusion proteins is the ability of the investigator to produce specific moieties of any protein. In order to generate

From: *Methods in Molecular Biology, vol. 378: Monoclonal Antibodies: Methods and Protocols*
Edited by: M. Albitar © Humana Press Inc., Totowa, NJ

Table 1
Summary of Fc Fusion Protein Applications

Field of interest	Application	Example	References
Biomedical research	Immunotherapy	Soluble P/Fc can be used in vivo to determine therapeutic outcome	*10*
	Immunization	Animals can be immunized with P/Fc to create polyclonal or monoclonal antibodies	*11,12*
	Pharmokinetics	Various clearance and half-life studies may be performed with soluble P/Fc fusion proteins	*10*
Biochemical applications	Flow cytometry and immunohistochemistry	Biotinylated P/Fc can be used to detect other proteins of interest	*13*
	Phage or yeast display	P/Fc may be used as a source of antigen (Ag) in order to generate fully human antibodies	*5,14–16*
	Domain specificity studies	Mutant proteins can be produced in order to study significant moieties within the protein	*17*
	In vitro assays	P/Fc can be used to antagonize or agonize cell surface receptor–ligand interactions	*18,19*

full-length Fc fusion proteins, the N-terminus of the protein of interest containing the biologically active site is linked to murine Fc (hinge-CH2-CH3). To describe the orientation of the protein linked to the N-terminus of murine Fc, it is designated as P/Fc. The purpose for fusing murine Fc to the protein of interest is that it allows for easy purification and also increases the half-life of the Fc fusion protein in vivo, which may be useful in immunotherapeutic applications.

Another major advantage of generating Fc fusion proteins using the method described here is that it allows the investigator to produce the Fc fusion protein in large scale (milligram-to-gram quantities). This provides the investigator with large amounts of stable protein sufficient for an extended period of time, which may aid the investigator in reproducing various datasets.

As shown in **Table 1**, a significant application of Fc fusion proteins is that they may be used as a source of antigen for the generation of either murine or fully human antibodies that may be too expensive to buy commercially, especially if animal studies are planned. Moreover, soluble Fc fusion proteins may be used for in vivo immunizations of mice in order to produce monoclonal antibodies using standard hybridoma techniques *(1–3)*. In addition, advancements in antibody (Ab) technology have led to the creation of synthetic libraries, which enable the investigator to generate fully human antibodies against any protein moiety of interest. For example, a recent advancement led to the construction of a yeast library comprised of yeast that express a wide repertoire of human Ab fragments on the cell surface *(4,5)*. The generation of soluble Fc fusion proteins allows the investigator to utilize such technology in order to quickly analyze and obtain human Ab fragments, which are specific for the protein moiety.

In addition, the investigator may use the soluble Fc fusion protein to detect other target proteins of interest. The Fc fusion proteins can easily be biotinylated for detection by streptavidin conjugates for either flow cytometry or immunohistochemistry. Also, obtaining a variety of biotinylated Fc fusion proteins would allow the investigator to detect many target proteins at the same time. Therefore, biotinylated Fc fusion proteins may substitute for an Ab that may not be commercially available to detect the target protein of interest.

1.2. Solubilizing Fc Fusion Proteins

The purpose of this chapter is to describe in depth how to genetically engineer, stably transfect, screen, produce, and purify Fc fusion proteins. A general outline of the following procedures is depicted in **Fig. 1**. Expression of soluble Fc fusion protein is entirely dependent on a mammalian expression system. The protein expression system described here involves the usage of an expression vector (pEE12) that is under the control of a strong viral promoter *(6)*. The viral promoter enables the coexpression of the Fc fusion protein with glutamine synthetase. Transfectants that maximally express the Fc fusion protein in addition to glutamine synthetase are positively selected using a murine myeloma cell line (NS0), which expresses insufficient amounts of glutamine *(7,8)*. Finally, utilizing a simple screening technique, such as enzyme-linked immunosorbent assay (ELISA), allows the investigator to identify productive transfectants, which can be grown in large-scale culture *(9)* for subsequent chromatographic purification. By these methods, the investigator is provided with a reliable and efficient method for solubilizing proteins of interest.

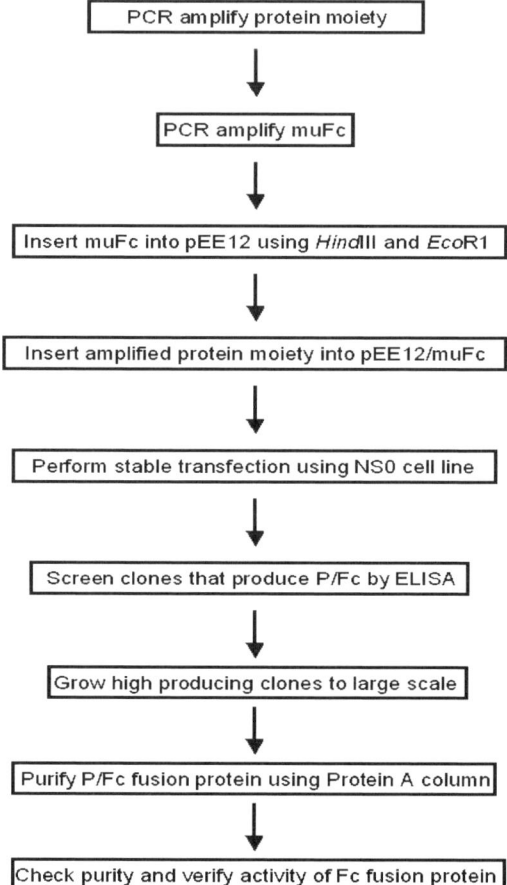

Fig. 1. Overview describing how Fc fusion protein is expressed and produced on a large scale. The final "transfection vector" is transfected for expression in the murine myeloma NS0 cell line. Expression of Fc fusion protein is verified by moiety-specific ELISA. The highest-producing clone is then grown to large scale for purification.

2. Materials

2.1. Cloning the Protein Moiety

1. cDNA encoding the protein of interest.
2. MacVector or DSGene DNA sequence analysis software (*see* **Note 1**).
3. Templates for designing target primers:

   FWD target:
   5′ CGT*AAGCTT*GCCGCCACCATGGGXXXXXXXXXXXXXXXXX (*Hind*III *site*; **Kozak sequence**; X_{17} = bp at 5′-end of target)

REV target:

5′ TAA*CGTACG*XXXXXXXXXXXXXXXXXXXXXXX (*Bsi*WI *site*; X_{21} = bp at 3′-end of target)

4. Thin-walled PCR tubes, autoclaved (Bio-Rad, cat. no. 223-9473).
5. 10 m*M* dNTP mix (Promega, cat. no. U151X).
6. 200 U Vent polymerase (10X PCR buffer included) (NEB, cat. no. M0254S).
7. Milli-Q deionized water (dH$_2$O), autoclaved.
8. PCR thermal cycler.
9. Tris-base (Trizma base, Sigma, cat. no. T1503).
10. Boric acid (Fisher, cat. no. BP168-1).
11. EDTA (Sigma, cat. no. E5134).
12. 0.5 *M* EDTA: dissolve 18.6 g in dH$_2$O, adding NaOH to dissolve. Adjust to pH 8.0; bring to 100 mL total volume with dH$_2$O.
13. 5X Tris-borate-EDTA (TBE) buffer: 54 g Tris base, 27.5 g boric acid, and 10 mL of 0.5 *M* EDTA, pH 8.0.
14. Glycerol (glycerin; Fisher, cat. no. G33-500).
15. Bromophenol blue (Bio-Rad, cat. no. 161-0404).
16. 6X Glycerol buffer: 7 mL of 0.5X TBE pH 8.0, 3 mL glycerol, and 25 mg bromophenol blue.
17. Agarose, molecular biology grade (Fisher, cat. no. BP1356-100).
18. Ethidium bromide (EtBr) prepared at 10 mg/mL (Sigma, cat. no. E8751) (*see* **Note 2**).
19. 1% Agarose gel: mix 0.5 g agarose + 50 mL of 0.5X TBE buffer in an Erlenmeyer flask, and boil in microwave until dissolved (≤1 min). When mixture reaches 60°C, add 2 µL EtBr, swirl to mix, and pour.
20. 100 bp DNA ladder (NEB, cat. no. N3231S).
21. Ultraviolet (UV) transilluminator (Fotodyne or similar).
22. Sterile scalpels (VWR, cat. no.100229-885).
23. QiaQuick PCR Gel Extraction Kit (Qiagen, cat. no. 28104).
24. Electrophoretic apparatus for resolving agarose gels (Owl Scientific or similar).

2.2. Generating the pEE12/muFc Master Expression Vector

1. pSK/muFc vector (obtained from the Epstein laboratory).
2. muFc primers:
   FWD muFc:
   5′CCCTAT*AAGCTT***CGTACG**GAGCCCAGAGGGCCCACAATC
   (*Hind*III *site*; ***Bsi*WI** *site*; <u>Hinge region</u>)
   REV muFc:
   5′ATCAAT*GAATTC*TCAC*GCGGCCGC*TTTACCCGGAGTCCGGGAGAA
   (*Eco*RI *site*; ***Not*I** *site*; <u>CH3 region</u>)
3. pEE12 GS expression vector (NS0 cells included; Lonza Biologics).
4. *Hind*III restriction enzyme (RE) (10X NEBuffer 2 included; NEB, cat. no. R0104S).
5. *Eco*RI RE (10X NEBuffer *Eco*RI included; NEB, cat. no. R0101S).

6. Montage PCR filter units (Millipore, cat. no. UFC7PCR50).
7. T4 DNA ligase (10X ligation buffer provided; NEB, cat. no. M0202S).
8. XL1-Blue *Escherichia coli* bacteria (Stratagene, cat. no. 200268).
9. SOC medium, sterile (Sigma, cat. no. S1797).
10. Bacterial shaker capable of 150 rpm.
11. Luria broth (LB), prepared according to manufacturer (Sigma, cat. no. L7658).
12. Ampicillin (Amp; Sigma, cat. no. A9518): prepare 25 mg/mL stock in sterile dH$_2$O.
13. LB plus Amp (LB/Amp): dilute Amp stock 1:250 in sterile LB.
14. LB agar plates plus Amp 100 µg/mL, prepared according to manufacturer (Sigma, cat. no. L7533).
15. Bacterial incubator, 37°C, nonhumidified.
16. Polypropylene round-bottom 14-mL tubes with caps (BD Falcon, cat. no. 352059).
17. Toothpicks, wooden, autoclaved.
18. Wizard Plus SV Miniprep kit (Promega, cat. no. A1330).
19. pSK/muFc vector map file (obtained via email from the Epstein laboratory).

2.3. Cloning the Protein Moiety Into pEE12/muFc

1. *Bsi*WI RE (10X NEBuffer 3 included; NEB, cat. no. R0553S).
2. *Not*I RE (100X bovine serum albumin [BSA] included; NEB, cat. no. R0189S).
3. Plasmid Maxi Kit (Qiagen, cat. no. 12163).

2.4. Expression and Screening of Soluble Fc Fusion Proteins

1. 1 L Hybridoma-SFM (serum-free medium) without L-glutamine (Life Technologies, cat. no. 93-0247-170).
2. Dialyzed fetal calf serum (FCS) (Hyclone, cat. no. SH30079.03).
3. 100X MEM nonessential amino acids solution (Cellgro, cat. no. 25-025-Cl).
4. 100X Penicillin-streptomycin (Pen-Strep) solution (Gemini BioProducts, cat. no. 400-109).
5. 50X GSEM (glutamine synthetase expression medium) supplement (Sigma, cat. no. G9785).
6. NS0 myeloma cells (included with pEE12 vector).
7. Characterized fetal bovine serum (FBS) (Hyclone, cat. no. SH30071.03).
8. 100X Glutamine/penicillin/streptomycin solution (Gemini, cat. no. 400-110).
9. Nonselective medium: 1-L bottle Hybridoma-SFM, 100 mL characterized fetal bovine serum, 10 mL glutamine/penicillin/streptomycin solution, and 12 mL MEM nonessential amino acids.
10. Selective medium: 1-L bottle Hybridoma-SFM, 22 mL GSEM supplement, 12 mL Pen-Strep, 12 mL MEM nonessential amino acids, and 100 mL dialyzed FCS.
11. *Sal*I RE (10X NEBuffer *Sal*I and 100X BSA included; NEB, cat. no. R0138S).
12. 0.4-cm Gene Pulser cuvet (Bio-Rad, cat. no. 165-2088).
13. Phosphate buffered saline, sterile, pH 7.4 (Invitrogen, cat. no. 10010-023).
14. 0.4% Trypan Blue solution (Sigma, cat. no. T8154).
15. Hemacytometer system (VWR, cat. no. 15170-168).

16. Gene Pulser II System (Bio-Rad).
17. Microtest 96-well plates, sterile (BD Falcon, cat. no. 353072).
18. Microplate aspiration manifold (from V&P Scientific or similar).
19. Reagent reservoir (VWR, cat. no. 53513-048).
20. Coating buffer: 25 mM sodium tetraborate decahydrate, pH 8.5 (Sigma, cat. no. S9640).
21. PBS: 0.15 M sodium chloride and 0.02 M sodium phosphate, pH 7.2 (nonsterile).
22. Blocking buffer: 1% BSA (Sigma, cat. no. A9647) in nonsterile PBS.
23. 96-Well flexible plates (BD Falcon, cat. no. 353912).
24. Microplate strip washer (BIO-TEK or similar).
25. PBST wash buffer: PBS and 0.1% Tween-20 (Fisher, cat. no. BP337-500).
26. Primary Ab: goat anti-mouse IgG, IgM (Caltag, cat. no. M30800).
27. Secondary Ab, Fc-specific: peroxidase-conjugated goat anti-mouse IgG (Sigma, cat. no. A9309).
28. Secondary Ab, protein moiety-specific: peroxidase-conjugated.
29. OPD peroxidase substrate (Sigma, cat. no. P9187).
30. ELX800 plate reader (BIO-TEK or similar).
31. RPMI complete: RPMI 1640 (Invitrogen, cat. no. 11875-093), 1X Pen-Strep, and 10% FCS.
32. DMSO (Sigma, cat. no. D5879).
33. Freezing medium: RPMI complete, 25% FCS and 10% DMSO.

2.5. Large-Scale Production of Fc Fusion Proteins

1. Selective medium (*see* recipe under **Subheading 2.4.**).
2. T25 sterile tissue culture flasks, vented caps (Corning, cat. no. 430639).
3. T225 sterile tissue culture flasks, vented caps (Corning Costar, cat. no. 3001).
4. AHB complete spinner flask (Bellco, cat. no. 1967-03000).
5. 3 L Air stone sparger assembly (Bellco, cat. no. 1965-45003).
6. Aquarium air pump 4000 (Profile 4000 or similar).
7. HEPA-CAP 36 disposable filter capsule (Whatman, cat. no. 6702-3600).
8. 0.2-μm Bottle-top filter unit (Corning, cat. no. 430015).
9. 1 L Glass bottles, autoclaved.

2.6. Purification of Fc Fusion Proteins

1. FPLC apparatus.
2. 5 mL HiTrap Protein A HP column (Amersham Biosciences, cat. no. 17-0403-01).
3. 1X Binding buffer: 0.15 M sodium chloride, 0.02 M citric acid in 1 L final vol, adjusted to pH 7.4 using HCl or NaOH.
4. 1X Elution buffer: 0.1 M sodium chloride, 0.02 M citric acid in 1 L final vol, adjusted to pH 3.0.
5. 1 L PBS (*see* **Subheading 2.4.** for recipe).
6. HiPrep 26/10 desalting column (Amersham Biosciences, cat. no. 17-5087-01).
7. 1 M Tris base, pH 9.0.
8. UV spectrophotometer.

2.7. Fc Fusion Protein Validation

1. 2-Mercaptoethanol (Sigma, cat. no. M7154).
2. Tris-HCl (Trizma; Sigma, cat. no. T5941): prepare 1 *M* solution, pH to 6.8.
3. Sodium dodecyl sulfate (SDS; EM Science, cat. no. 7910).
4. 2X Reducing buffer: each time a gel is run, add 50 µL of 2-mercaptoethanol (under fume hood) to 1 mL of buffer prepared as follows: 0.5 *M* Tris-HCl (10 ml), glycerol (8 ml), 10% SDS (16 ml), 0.05% bromophenol blue (5 ml), and dH$_2$O (37 ml).
5. 4–15% Tris-HCl gradient polyacrylamide gel (Bio-Rad, cat. no. 161-1104EDU).
6. Kaleidoscope prestained standard (Bio-Rad, cat. no. 161-0324).
7. Polyacrylamide Gel Electrophoresis (PAGE) apparatus (Bio-Rad Criterian Precast Gel System).

3. Methods

3.1. Cloning the Protein Moiety

Ideally, cDNA should be obtained from the laboratory that first cloned the protein of interest. Search the literature for the primary reference, and take note of the accession number reported. If cDNA cannot be readily obtained, consider obtaining it from a cDNA library made from an appropriate tissue and species. As a last resort, cDNA can be obtained from cell lines or animals (with or without a particular treatment) by reverse transcription of isolated RNA. SuperScript™ III First-Strand Synthesis System for RT-PCR (Invitrogen; www.invitrogen.com) is a comprehensive kit for cDNA synthesis from RNA templates.

3.1.1. Obtaining cDNA and Designing PCR Primers

1. Obtain cDNA encoding the protein of interest.
2. On the NCBI website (www.ncbi.nlm.nih.gov), search the "Nucleotide" database for the protein by entering the accession number. Download the sequence to MacVector or DSGene software (*see* **Note 1**).
3. Determine the sequence encoding the protein moiety to be included in the Fc fusion protein; this portion is referred to subsequently as the "target" (*see* **Note 3**).
4. To construct N-terminal fusion proteins, search the target sequence for *Hind*III (AAGCTT) and *Bsi*WI (CGTACG) restriction sites. If these restriction sites are absent from the target sequence, design PCR primers using the templates in **Subheading 2.1.** (*see* **Note 4**).
5. Order primers from an institutional core facility or online from IDT (www.idtdna.com). Resuspend primers at 10 pmol/µL.

3.1.2. Amplification and Purification of Target PCR Product

1. Assemble triplicate target PCR reactions in thin-walled tubes:

≤0.1 µg target cDNA	X µL
10 pmol FWD target primer	1 µL
10 pmol REV target primer	1 µL

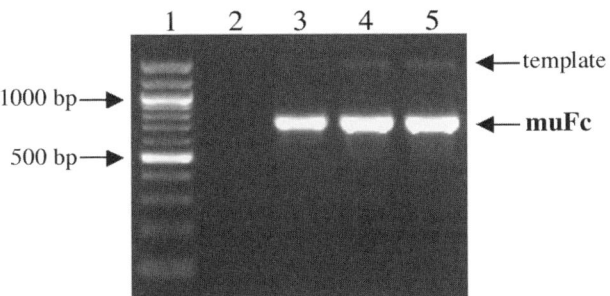

Fig. 2. Agarose gel electrophoresis of murine Fc (muFc) PCR product. Lane 1, 100-bp DNA ladder. Lane 2, negative control (without template). Lanes 3–5, triplicate muFc PCR reaction products ("**muFc**"), resolved as single bands approx 750 bp in length. The higher-MW pSK/muFc vector ("template") is faintly visible on the gel.

0.2 m*M* dNTP mix	1 µL
10X PCR buffer	5 µL
20 U Vent polymerase	1 µL
dH$_2$O	X µL
Total volume	50 µL

2. As a negative control, mix one tube containing all the previously listed components EXCEPT cDNA (*see* **Note 5**).
3. Place tubes in a thermal cycler programmed as follows: 5 min at 95°C; 30 cycles (30 s at 95°C, 30 s at 55°C, 30 s at 72°C); 7 min at 72°C.
4. Mix 10 µL from each PCR reaction with 2 µL 6X glycerol buffer, then load onto a 1% agarose gel in 0.5X TBE buffer and run at 100 V. Include 100 bp DNA ladder to verify PCR product size.
5. Clean the viewing surface of an UV transilluminator with 10% bleach; dry thoroughly. Visualize target PCR product (which should appear as a single band of correct molecular weight) and excise from gel using a sterile scalpel.
6. Purify target PCR product using QIAQuick Gel Extraction Kit. Store at –20°C.

3.2. Generating the pEE12/muFc Master Expression Vector

To amplify murine Fc, the FWD and REV muFc primers (**Subheading 2.2.**) must be ordered as in **Subheading 3.1.1.**, **step 5**. **Fig. 2** is an example of expected results when muFc PCR products are run on a 1% agarose gel. Ligation of the resulting muFc PCR product into the pEE12 expression vector is depicted in **Fig. 3**.

3.2.1. Amplifying Murine Fc and Cloning Into pEE12 GS Expression Vector

1. Amplify, isolate, and purify murine Fc PCR product from the pSK/muFc vector using FWD and REV muFc primers, as in **Subheading 3.1.2**.
2. Set up two restriction enzyme digests as follows; incubate tubes overnight in a 37°C water bath.

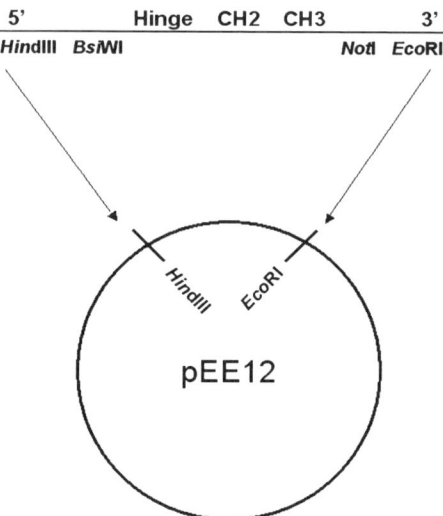

Fig. 3. Cloning schematic depicting the generation of pEE12 master vector. *Hind*III and *Eco*RI sites incorporated in the muFc primers are subsequently digested and used to ligate muFc (Hinge-CH2-CH3) into the pEE12 expression vector.

1 µg pEE12 vector	X µL		1 µg muFc PCR product	X µL
20 U *Hind*III	1 µL		20 U *Hind*III	1 µL
20 U *Eco*RI	1 µL		20 U *Eco*RI	1 µL
10X NEBuffer *Eco*RI	5 µL		10X NEBuffer *Eco*RI	5 µL
dH₂O	X µL		dH₂O	X µL
Total volume	50 µL		Total volume	50 µL

3. Purify digested DNA using Montage PCR filter units.
4. Prepare ligation reactions as follows. Mix DNA + dH$_2$O *first*, heat to 70°C for 3 min, let cool 2 min at room temperature, *then* add buffer and ligase. Incubate 1 h at room temperature.

	Tube 1	Tube 2	Tube 3
Digested pEE12 vector	1 µL	1 µL	1 µL
Digested muFc PCR product	1 µL	–	1 µL
dH₂O	7 µL	7 µL	6 µL
10X Ligation buffer	1 µL	1 µL	1 µL
T4 DNA ligase	–	1 µL	1 µL
Total volume	10 µL	10 µL	10 µL

5. Heat-inactivate ligase by incubating tubes 10 min at 65°C. The resulting ligation product will be referred to subsequently as "pEE12/muFc."

3.2.2. Bacterial Transformation and Amplification of pEE12/muFc

Transformation of pEE12/muFc into a bacterial host enables the user to amplify the vector for future use. This "master" vector can be used to generate additional Fc fusion proteins in less time because it already contains muFc DNA.

1. Thaw (on ice) 3×20 μL tubes of XL1-Blue *E. coli*.
2. Add 2 μL of ligation product from tube 1 to one tube of *E. coli*; repeat for tubes 2 and 3. Incubate 30 min on ice.
3. Warm 300 μL of SOC medium to 37°C.
4. Heat tubes at *exactly* 42°C for *exactly* 45 s. Transfer tubes to ice for 2 min.
5. Gently add 100 μL of warm SOC to each tube (avoid mixing). Incubate 1 h in a 37°C bacterial shaker set at 150–180 rpm.
6. Spread contents of each tube onto a fresh LB/ampicillin plate. Once dry, invert plates and incubate overnight.
7. Record the number of colonies appearing on each plate. Tube 1 should yield few or no colonies, whereas tube 3 should yield at least twice the number of colonies as tube 2 (*see* **Note 6**).
8. Aliquot 5 mL of LB/Amp into each of 11 capped round-bottom tubes.
9. Using a sterile toothpick, inoculate a tube of LB/Amp with bacteria from a single colony from the tube 3 plate. Repeat for an additional nine colonies. (Add no bacteria to the last tube; this negative control verifies that LB/Amp is sterile.) Tube caps should be loose, but secure.
10. Incubate tubes for 8 h in a bacterial shaker set to 37°C.
11. Shortly before retrieving bacterial cultures, prepare a master mix for PCR screening: 228 μL dH$_2$O, 30 μL buffer, 12 μL FWD muFc primer, 12 μL REV muFc primer, 12 μL dNTP mix, and 6 μL Vent polymerase. Aliquot 25 μL into each of 11 thin-walled PCR tubes. Keep on ice.
12. Pellet bacteria in culture tubes (spin 5 min at 2000g in a tabletop centrifuge).
13. Use a sterile pipet tip to inoculate PCR aliquots with pelleted bacteria from each culture. (The remaining PCR tube is a no-template control.) Repeat **Subheading 3.1.2.**, **steps 3–4**. The results should mirror those depicted in **Fig. 2**. Meanwhile, store bacterial pellets at 4°C.
14. Purify pEE12/muFc vector from muFc PCR-positive bacteria using Wizard Plus SV Miniprep kit. Discard bacterial pellets yielding no PCR products in biohazard waste.
15. Verify muFc sequence within the pEE12 vector: submit the required amount of purified plasmid plus FWD muFc primer to an institutional DNA sequencing facility or private sequencing company (e.g., SeqWright, Sequetech, or Genewiz). Use MacVector or DSGene to align the resulting sequencing data to the pSK/muFc vector map.

3.3. Cloning the Protein Moiety Into pEE12/muFc

At this final cloning stage, the target PCR product is inserted upstream (N-terminal) of the muFc, now present in the pEE12 expression vector. The final product will serve as the template for protein expression in NS0 cells. Ligation of the target PCR product into pEE12/muFc is depicted in **Fig. 4**.

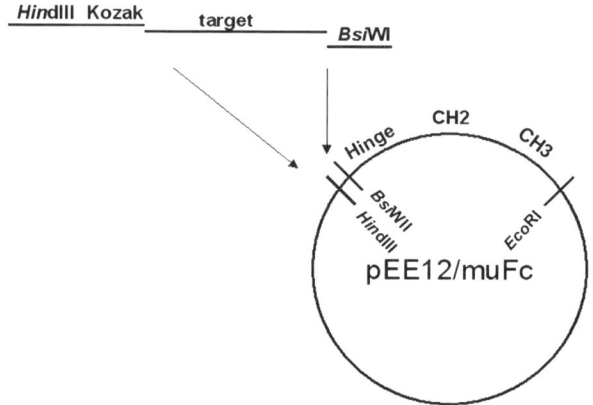

Fig. 4. The target PCR product is cloned upstream (N-terminal) of the muFc in the pEE12/muFc master vector, using the restriction enzyme sites *Hind*III and *Bsi*WI.

3.3.1. N-Terminal Fusion Construction

1. Set up the first of two sequential restriction enzyme digests as follows. Incubate overnight at 37°C. Use the target PCR product obtained in **Subheading 3.1.2.**, **step 6**.
   Step 1:

1 µg pEE12/muFc	X µL	1 µg target PCR product	X µL
20 U *Hind*III	1 µL	20 U *Hind*III	1 µL
10X NEBuffer 2	5 µL	10X NEBuffer 2	5 µL
dH₂O	X µL	dH₂O	X µL
Total volume	50 µL	Total volume	50 µL

2. Purify digested DNA using Microcon Centrifugal Filter Devices.
3. Using entire volumes of purified, *Hind*III-digested DNA, set up the second digest as follows. Incubate 2 h at 55°C.
   Step 2:

pEE12/muFc	20 µL	Target PCR product	20 µL
20 U *Bsi*WI	1 µL	20 U *Bsi*WI	1 µL
10X NEBuffer 3	5 µL	10X NEBuffer 3	5 µL
dH₂O	24 µL	dH₂O	24 µL
Total volume	50 µL	Total volume	50 µL

4. Purify double-digested DNA using Microcon Centrifugal Filter Devices.

3.3.2. Transformation and Screening of the Transfection Vector

1. Ligate double-digested pEE12/muFc and target, following **Subheading 3.2.1.**, **steps 4–5**.
2. Use the resulting ligation tubes to transform XL-1 *E. coli*, screen for positive colonies, and verify vector sequence following **Subheading 3.2.2.**, **steps 1–15**. Be sure to verify both target and muFc sequences.

3. Amplify bacteria harboring verified vector and purify using Qiagen Plasmid Maxi Kit. The resulting vector DNA will be used to transfect NS0 cells, and will be referred to subsequently as the "transfection vector."

3.4. Expression and Screening of Soluble Fc Fusion Proteins

For each transfection, 40 µg of transfection vector will be needed. It is helpful to obtain a high yield of pure transfection vector in case the transfection needs to be repeated in the future. In addition, one confluent T75 flask of NS0 cells is required per transfection. NS0 cells must be grown in nonselective medium prior to transfection. (Subculture three times per wk by splitting 1:5 in fresh nonselective medium.) All cell handling should be performed under a sterile hood to prevent contamination.

3.4.1. Stable Transfection of NS0 Cells

1. Digest transfection vector as follows. Incubate 4–16 h at 37°C (*see* **Note 7**).

40 µg Transfection vector	X µL
10X *Sal*I buffer	10 µL
100X BSA	1 µL
*Sal*I, 80 U	4 µL
dH$_2$O	X µL
Total volume	100 µL

2. Transfer entire digest volume to Gene Pulser cuvet. Keep on ice.
3. Prewarm 40 mL of *nonselective* medium at 37°C.
4. Obtain one confluent T75 tissue culture flask containing NS0 cells grown in nonselective medium.
5. Loosen NS0 cells by smacking flask against the palm of the hand.
6. Transfer entire volume of cells into a sterile 50-mL conical tube and centrifuge for 10 min at 300g with low brake.
7. Resuspend cell pellet in 5 mL of sterile PBS, then fill to 50 mL with sterile PBS. Repeat PBS wash.
8. Determine cell concentration using a hemacytometer.
9. Centrifuge cells again for 10 min at 300g with low-brake. Resuspend cell pellet in sterile PBS such that the cell concentration is 1.1×10^7 cells/mL (*see* **Note 8**).
10. Add 900 µL (or 1×10^7 cells) to the cuvet containing the digest. Gently mix cells by pipetting, being careful not to create excessive air bubbles.
11. Incubate on ice 5 min, then thoroughly dry metal sides of cuvet, which will come in contact with electrodes.
12. Place cuvet into electroporator and slide apparatus until there is contact between cuvet and electrodes. Adjust electroporator settings to 1.5 kV and 3.0 µF.
13. Pulse the cuvet by pressing the two red buttons. Repeat, then incubate cuvet on ice 5 min.
14. Pipet cuvet contents into prewarmed *selective* medium, invert several times to mix. Pour into a sterile reservoir, and with a multichannel pipettor, add 50 µL of cells per well to 8 sterile flat-bottom 96-well plates.

15. After 18–24 h, add 150 µL of prewarmed *selective* medium to all wells.
16. Three days later, remove medium from each well with aspiration manifold and add 150 µL of fresh *selective* medium to cells.
17. Incubate at 37°C for 3–4 wk (see **Note 9**), until colonies appear in wells and medium begins to turn yellow.

3.4.2. Screening Transfectants Using Fc-Specific ELISA

While preparing for the ELISA, make sure to have the appropriate positive and negative controls (*see* **Note 10**).

1. Coat plastic 96-well flexible plates with 100 µL of coating buffer containing 2–5 µg/mL of primary Ab (goat anti-mouse IgG and IgM). Cover plates with lid and incubate overnight at 4°C.
2. Wash plates three times with 200 µL of PBST using a microplate strip washer. Invert plates and tap to get rid of residual wash buffer in wells.
3. Add 50 µL of blocking buffer to all wells.
4. Add 50 µL of medium (1:2 dilution) from transfectant wells that contain colonies. Be careful not to disturb colonies at bottom of wells when removing medium. Incubate at 37°C for 1 h.
5. Repeat wash with PBST. Tap plate.
6. Make a 1:10,000 dilution of secondary Ab (peroxidase-conjugated goat anti-mouse IgG) in blocking buffer, then add 100 µL per well. Incubate at 37°C for 1 h.
7. Repeat wash with PBST. Tap plate.
8. Prepare OPD solution according to manufacturer's protocol; add 100 µL of fresh OPD solution to all wells. Incubate at room temperature for 30 min in the dark, or until brown color develops.
9. Read plate using a multiwell plate reader set to 450 nm, with a reference wavelength of 630 nm. The highest-producing clones are those with the highest OD reading.
10. Expand the highest-producing clones to a 24-well plate using selective medium. Grow cells until confluent to prepare for subcloning.

3.4.3. Subcloning of Highest-Producing Transfectants

1. Count cells from 24-well plate using a hemacytometer.
2. Subclone each transfectant as follows: remove a volume containing approximately 96 cells, add to 15 mL of prewarmed *selective* medium, then aliquot 150 µL per well in sterile 96-well plates, such that a 1 cell/well concentration is obtained (*see* **Note 11**).
3. Place plates in 37°C tissue culture incubator and allow to grow for 3–4 wk.

3.4.4. Screening Subclones Using ELISA Specific for the Protein Moiety

While the initial transfectants were screened with Fc-specific secondary Ab, it is important to subsequently screen subclones with an Ab specific for the protein moiety fused to murine Fc (*see* **Note 12**).

1. Coat flexible 96-well plates with 100 µL of coating buffer containing 2–5 µg/mL of primary Ab (goat anti-mouse IgG and IgM) to all wells. (One plate is needed for every 10 clones to be analyzed.) Cover plates with lid and incubate overnight at 4°C.
2. Wash plates three times with 200 µL of PBST using a microplate strip washer. Tap plates to get rid of excess wash buffer in wells.
3. Add 196 µL of blocking buffer to all wells in row A and 100 µL of blocking buffer to all remaining wells.
4. Remove 4 µL of supernatant from each subclone and add to well A1. Repeat for wells A2–A10 with supernatant from additional subclones. In well A11, add positive control protein of appropriate concentration. Add no medium to negative control well A12.
5. Using a multichannel pipettor, mix contents in row A and draw up 100 µL. Mix aliquots from row A with blocking buffer contained in row B. Continue with 1:2 dilutions for rows C–H (*see* **Note 13**).
6. Incubate plate at 37°C for 1 h. Wash plate three times with a microplate strip washer. Tap plate.
7. Dilute protein moiety-specific secondary Ab in blocking buffer at a ratio recommended by the manufacturer. Add 100 µL of secondary Ab to each well.
8. Incubate plate at 37°C for 1 h. Repeat wash.
9. Develop plate with OPD as in **Subheading 3.4.2.**, **step 8**. Read plate as in **Subheading 3.4.2.**, **step 9**.
10. Select the highest-producing clone (as determined by highest OD) for large-scale production. Freeze down four to five additional high-producing clones by resuspending each in 2 mL freezing medium; store at –80°C.

3.5. Large-Scale Production of Fc Fusion Proteins

For the following, prewarmed selective medium *must* be used in order to maintain the transfection vector in NS0 host cells. All incubations take place in a standard (37°C, 5% CO_2) humidified incubator for cell culture.

1. Grow highest-producing clone to confluency in a T75 flask with selective medium.
2. Expand cells to a T225 flask until confluent (4–5 d).
3. Add entire T225 culture into an autoclaved 3-L spinner flask, followed by 1 L of selective medium. Incubate 3–4 d with continuous stirring.
4. Bring culture volume to 3 L with selective medium, incubate another 3 d.
5. When concentration reaches 8×10^5 cells/mL, aerate medium via an autoclaved sparger assembly connected to an air pump. (Use HEPA-CAP filter to sterilize input air.) Incubate another 2–3 d.
6. Add 30 mL of 100X nonessential amino acids, 60 mL of 50X RPMI essential amino acids, 60 mL of GSEM supplement, and 30 mL of 100X glucose solution. Incubate aerated culture another 3 d.
7. Pellet cells by centrifugation: 10 min at 300g in a tabletop centrifuge at 4°C.
8. Filter supernatants through a 0.2-µm bottle-top filter unit into 1-L sterile bottles. The resulting filtered supernatant is ready for purification.

3.6. Purification of Fc Fusion Proteins

This section details the purification of Fc fusion proteins from filtered supernatant, as performed using the HPLC apparatus.

1. Wash protein A column with 60 mL dH$_2$O at a flow rate of 3 mL/min using a peristaltic pump. Wash no more than 2 h before use (*see* **Note 14**).
2. Equilibrate protein A column with 60 mL binding buffer at a flow rate of 3 mL/min.
3. Pump the supernatant collected from the highest producing clone through the protein A column at a flow rate of 3 mL/min (discard the effluent).
4. Wash protein A column with 60 mL of 1X binding buffer at a flow rate of 3 mL/min.
5. Pump elution buffer through the column at a flow rate of 3 mL/min. Measure the eluate using the UV monitor set to an absorbance of 280 nm. Begin to collect eluate when the A$_{280}$ of fractions rises to 0.3, and continue until it descends to 0.2.
6. If necessary, adjust pH of eluate to 7.2 with 1 *M* Tris buffer, pH 9.0.
7. Pool fractions collected. Follow manufacturer's protocol for using HiPrep 26/10 desalting column in order to change diluent to PBS.
8. Measure final Fc fusion protein concentration using an UV spectrophotometer set at 280 nm.

3.7. Fc Fusion Protein Validation

3.7.1. SDS-PAGE

1. In a 1.5-mL tube, mix 5 µg of fusion protein with 2X reducing buffer in the appropriate final volume. Boil 5 min, securing the tube's lid to prevent it from popping open.
2. Spin tube briefly to retrieve the entire sample, then load onto a 4–15% gradient Tris-HCl polyacrylamide gel. Load 10 µL of kaleidoscope prestained standard alongside the Fc fusion protein sample. Run gel at 100 V until standard is well resolved.
3. Compare predicted molecular weight of fusion protein (MW$_{moiety}$ plus MW$_{muFc}$) with molecular weight standard.

The predicted and actual molecular weight are often not identical, because muFc may be glycosylated. More important is resolution of a single band that approximates the predicted molecular weight. If the band is very thick, rerun less fusion protein (2 µg) to rule out doublet bands. **Fig. 5** is an example of Fc fusion proteins resolved by SDS-PAGE under reducing conditions.

3.7.2. ELISA

ELISA specific for the protein moiety of interest, as described in **Subheading 3.4.4.**, should be repeated to quantify purified Fc fusion proteins.

A   B   C

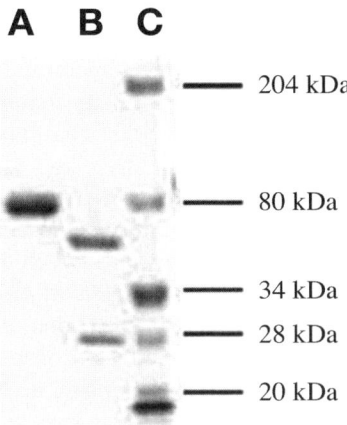

—— 204 kDa

—— 80 kDa

—— 34 kDa
—— 28 kDa

—— 20 kDa

Fig. 5. An example of SDS-PAGE electrophoretic analysis of a purified/Fc fusion protein (CD25/Fc). Lane A, Fc fusion protein run under reducing conditions. By contrast, a whole IgG antibody (Lane B) is resolved into two bands (heavy chains and light chains). Lane C, kaleidoscope prestained standard.

3.7.3. Activity Assay

Once the fusion protein has been detected by protein moiety-specific ELISA, the activity of the moiety must be verified. The appropriate activity assay will depend on the native activity of the protein, and must be one in which equimolar amounts of commercially available protein will yield positive results. Consult with the manufacturer to learn what assay is used to validate activity of their product. If replication of the manufacturer's assay is not possible, consult the primary literature or an appropriate volume of the *Current Protocols* series.

4. Notes

1. Sequence analysis programs MacVector (Macintosh platform) or DSGene (PC platform) can be purchased from Accelrys (www.accelrys.com). Analysis software is necessary in order to design PCR primers for the protein moiety, as well as to verify cloned sequences generated later in the protocol.
2. **Caution:** EtBr is a potent mutagen. When preparing EtBr solution, wear gloves, a dust mask, and eyewear to protect against particulate matter. Store solution in amber glass labeled with a clear warning. Always wear gloves when dispensing EtBr solution and handling gels to which EtBr has been added. Dispose of contaminated tips and used gels in accordance with institutional guidelines for the handling of mutagenic materials.

3. Depending on the application, the experimenter may choose the protein moiety to be genetically fused to murine Fc. However, any putative transmembrane regions must be excluded, as their inclusion will prevent soluble expression of the fusion protein by NS0 cells. It is reasonable to assume that a molecular weight limit exists, above which NS0 cells may yield insufficient amounts of recombinant protein.

4. The primer templates given were designed for the user's convenience, and represent the templates used in our laboratory in most cases. However, if the target contains *either* of the pertinent RE sites listed, then the user must redesign her target primers to replace that RE site with one that (1) appears in the multiple cloning site of the pEE12 expression vector, and (2) does *not* appear in the target sequence. The pEE12 vector map is obtainable from Lonza Biologics.

5. In the absence of the target cDNA template, no PCR product is expected. If the negative control tube yields PCR product, this suggests DNA contamination, and common reagents (dNTP, buffer, dH$_2$O, vent) should be replaced. If possible, assemble a positive control PCR tube, substituting unrelated cDNA and PCR primers known to yield product. This reaction will validate the dNTP, buffer, dH$_2$O, and Vent polymerase used.

6. Tube 3 should contain clones bearing the pEE12/muFc master vector, and thus should yield the most colonies. Tube 2 ("vector only") indicates the likelihood that the pEE12 vector was ligated to itself without inclusion of the muFc insert. If the number of colonies yielded by tube 2 approximates tube 3, then the likelihood of successful ligation is low, and litigation should be repeated. If subsequent tube 2 reaction yield numerous colonies, consider using calf intestinal alkaline phosphatase (CIP) to interfere with vector self-litigation (according to manufacturer's instruction). Tube 1 ("no ligase") should yield no colonies, though in practice may yield ≤10 clones; this tube indicates the extent to which pEE12 was successfully digested by *Hind*III and *Eco*RI. If tube 1 yields more than 10 colonies, the user should redigest vector and insert (**Subheading 3.2.1.**).

7. If necessary, less than 40 µg of transfection vector may be used to perform the stable transfection, but the number of NS0 cells and 96-well plates must be adjusted accordingly.

8. The maximum volume of the cuvet is 1 mL, which must contain the volume of transfection vector digest; NEB cat. no. M 0290S). 1×10^7 total NS0 cells. If the volume of the digest varies from the total 100 µL volume, adjust the volume of NS0 cells accordingly.

9. It is very important to not disturb the 96-well plates during this 3–4 wk incubation period. When the plates need to be checked for colonies, designate one plate that will be removed from the incubator to be checked from time to time.

10. For the Fc-specific ELISA, an appropriate positive control would be any murine Ab that is isotype IgG2a. Titer the positive control Ab so that an estimate of the user's Fc fusion protein can be made by comparing to known amounts of the positive control. For the negative control wells, add 50 µL of blocking buffer instead of 50 µL of transfectant medium.

11. In case the one cell/well subcloning is not successful, repeat subcloning at a concentration of two cells/well in an additional 96-well plate.
12. For protein moiety-specific ELISA, the appropriate positive control is the protein of interest. Only a small amount is needed (1–2 μg), and may be available from commercial sources or another laboratory. As in Fc-specific ELISA, blocking buffer is used in negative control wells.
13. One can make adjustments to the serial dilution factor used in the ELISA. According to the OD values obtained in the initial Fc-specific ELISA, serial dilutions may be adjusted to 1:4, 1:5, or 1:10. An optimal range of dilutions enables the user to best compare the expression of individual subclones.
14. Ensure that the protein A column is continually kept moist with buffer. If the column is left to dry out, it may affect the yield of purified Fc fusion protein obtained.

Acknowledgments

This work was supported in part by grants from the National Institutes of Health no. 5R41 CA1098884, the Philip Morris External Research Program and Cancer Therapeutics Laboratories (Los Angeles, CA).

References

1. Little, M., Kipriyanov, S. M., Le Gall, F., and Moldenhauer, G. (2000) Of mice and men: hybridoma and recombinant antibodies. *Immunol. Today* **21,** 364–370.
2. Kohler, G. and Milstein, C. (1975) Continuous cultures of fused cells secreting antibody of predefined specificity. *Nature* **256,** 495–497.
3. Kundu, P. K., Prasad, N. S., and Datta, D. (1998) Monoclonal antibody: high density culture of hybridoma cells and downstream processing for IgG recovery. *Indian J. Exp. Biol.* **36,** 125–135.
4. VanAntwerp, J. J. and Wittrup, K. D. (2000) Fine affinity discrimination by yeast surface display and flow cytometry. *Biotechnol. Prog.* **16,** 31–37.
5. Feldhaus, M. J., Siegel, R. W., Opresko, L. K., et al. (2003) Flow-cytometric isolation of human antibodies from a nonimmune *Saccharomyces cerevisiae* surface display library. *Nat. Biotechnol.* **21,** 163–170.
6. Tokushige, K., Moradpour, D., Wakita, T., Geissler, M., Hayashi, N., and Wands, J. R. (1997) Comparison between cytomegalovirus promoter and elongation factor-1 alpha promoter-driven constructs in the establishment of cell lines expressing hepatitis C virus core protein. *J. Virol. Methods* **64,** 73–80.
7. Bebbington, C. R., Renner, G., Thomson, S., King, D., Abrams, D., and Yarranton, G. T. (1992) High-level expression of a recombinant antibody from myeloma cells using a glutamine synthetase gene as an amplifiable selectable marker. *Biotechnology (N Y)* **10,** 169–175.
8. Bebbington, C. R. and Lambert, K. (1994) Genetic stability and product consistency of rDNA-derived biologicals from mammalian cells. *Dev. Biol. Stand.* **83,** 183–184.
9. Birch, J. R. and Froud, S. J. (1994) Mammalian cell culture systems for recombinant protein production. *Biologicals* **22,** 127–133.

10. Way, J. C., Lauder, S., Brunkhorst, B., et al. (2005) Improvement of Fc-erythro-poietin structure and pharmacokinetics by modification at a disulfide bond. *Protein Eng. Des. Sel.* **18,** 111–118.

11. Leenaars, M. and Hendriksen, C. F. (2005) Critical steps in the production of polyclonal and monoclonal antibodies: evaluation and recommendations. *Ilar. J.* **46,** 269–279.

12. Dinnis, D. M. and James, D. C. (2005) Engineering mammalian cell factories for improved recombinant monoclonal antibody production: lessons from nature? *Biotechnol. Bioeng.* **91,** 180–189.

13. Mathew, S. O., Kumaresan, P. R., Lee, J. K., Huynh, V. T., and Mathew, P. A. (2005) Mutational analysis of the human 2B4 (CD244)/CD48 interaction: Lys68 and Glu70 in the V domain of 2B4 are critical for CD48 binding and functional activation of NK cells. *J. Immunol.* **175,** 1005–1013.

14. Winter, G., Griffiths, A. D., Hawkins, R. E., and Hoogenboom, H. R. (1994) Making antibodies by phage display technology. *Annu. Rev. Immunol.* **12,** 433–455.

15. Hoogenboom, H. R., Henderikx, P., and de Haard, H. (1998) Creating and engineering human antibodies for immunotherapy. *Adv. Drug Deliv. Rev.* **31,** 5–31.

16. Feldhaus, J. M., Siegel, R. W., Feldhaus, J. M. and Wittrup, K. D. (2003) *Yeast Display scFv Antibody Library User's Manual Pacific Northwest National Laboratory.* pp. 1–44.

17. Hu, P., Mizokami, M., Ruoff, G., Khawli, L. A., and Epstein, A. L. (2003) Generation of low-toxicity interleukin-2 fusion proteins devoid of vasopermeability activity. *Blood* **101,** 4853–4861.

18. Ma, Q., DeMarte, L., Wang, Y., Stanners, C. P., and Junghans, R. P. (2004) Carcinoembryonic antigen-immunoglobulin Fc fusion protein (CEA-Fc) for identification and activation of anti-CEA immunoglobulin-T-cell receptor-modified T cells, representative of a new class of Ig fusion proteins. *Cancer Gene. Ther.* **11,** 297–306.

19. Ruocco, A., Nicole, O., Docagne, F., et al. (1999) A transforming growth factor-beta antagonist unmasks the neuroprotective role of this endogenous cytokine in excitotoxic and ischemic brain injury. *J. Cereb. Blood Flow Metab.* **19,** 1345–1353.

4

The Use of the Antibodies in the Diagnosis of Leukemia and Lymphoma by Flow Cytometry

Mohammad Reza Sheikholeslami, Iman Jilani, and Maher Albitar

Summary

Flow cytometry is an automated analysis of cells passing in the fluid suspension through a laser light beam, which react with monoclonal antibodies specific for a variety of cell surface antigens. A specimen of peripheral blood, bone marrow, or other cell suspension is incubated with fluorescent-labeled antibodies, which bind to target antigens on cell surfaces or—following cell permeabilization—to cytoplasmic and nuclear antigens. The analysis of surface antigens is performed on cells selected (gated) based on light-scatter properties. The expression of specific marker or confirmation of markers defines a specific cell population or the original of these cells. This in turn helps in diagnosis and classification of various hematological diseases and leads to choosing a specific therapy. Here, we describe a methodology for using flow cytometry with six colors for the analysis of various tissues for hematological diseases.

Key Words: Flow cytometry; leukemia; lymphoma; immunophenotyping; methodology.

1. Introduction

Antibodies are used in the diagnosis and monitoring of patients with various hematological diseases, in immunohistochemistry, and in flow cytometry (1–4).

Flow cytometry is an automated analysis of cells passing in the fluid suspension through a laser light beam. The cells are first reacted with monoclonal antibodies (MAb) specific for a variety of cell surface antigens. These antibodies are tagged with dyes (fluorochromes) that fluoresce when passed through the laser beam. As the cells pass sequentially through the laser beam, they absorb and scatter the light in forward and side (90°) angles. The forward-angle scatter is proportional to the size of the cell and the 90°-angle scatter is proportional to

From: *Methods in Molecular Biology, vol. 378: Monoclonal Antibodies: Methods and Protocols*
Edited by: M. Albitar © Humana Press Inc., Totowa, NJ

the internal structure (granularity) of the cell. Multiple fluorescent parameters may be analyzed simultaneously *(1,5–7)*.

A specimen of peripheral blood, bone marrow, or other cell suspension is incubated with fluorescent-labeled antibodies, which bind to target antigens on cell surfaces or—following cell permeabilization—to cytoplasmic and nuclear antigens. The labeled specimen then flows past laser beams, each of which excites a burst of light from a specific fluorescent label. The emitted light is captured by a camera, which records the occurrence of light emission (an "event"), its wavelength, and its intensity, a factor determined by the number of labeled antibodies bound to the target antigen. The antibody, the number of events, and the intensity of emitted light are recorded in the form of two-dimensional graphs or "dot plots" (also known as histograms). Examination of a series of dot plots permits cell enumeration and characterization, with the specific aim of identifying abnormal cell populations *(1,6)*.

The analysis of surface antigens is performed on cells selected (gated) based on light-scatter properties. Once the cells of interest are chosen, qualitative information may be obtained by measuring fluorescence intensity for each marker.

In the case of acute leukemia, leukemic blasts are assigned to B-lymphoid, T-lymphoid, or myeloid lineages. More rarely, leukemic blasts may be categorized as megakaryocytic precursors or erythroid precursors. MAb are used in six color combinations (all containing CD45) and analyzed using a technique that defines blasts by dim CD45 positivity and side scatter. The use of CD45 helps distinguish hematopoietic cells from nonhematopoietic cells (fibroblasts, epithelial, or endothelial cells) *(8,9)*.

In the case of chronic lymphocytic leukemia, common B-cell chronic lymphocytic leukemia (CD19+/CD5+) can be distinguished from T-cell proliferation. CD23 positivity and monoclonal expression of either κ- or λ-light chains are phenotypic features that are characteristically distinguish clonal from nonclonal B-cells *(9,10)*.

Non-Hodgkin's lymphoma typically shows expression of CD20 and bright expression of monoclonal light chain. CD10 is often expressed in follicular lymphomas *(9,10)*.

The expression of a specific marker or the confirmation of markers defines a specific cell population or the original of these cells. This in turn helps in diagnosis and classification of various hematological diseases and leads to choosing a specific therapy. Here, we describe a methodology for using flow cytometry with six colors for the analysis of various tissues for hematological diseases. The methodology described here is for the Beckton-Dichinson FACS Canto, also with sample prep associated II (SPA).

2. Materials

2.1. Specimen Integrity/Acceptability

Handling and transportation procedures must maintain the viability of the specimen. Specimen integrity is the composite product of anticoagulant, storage conditions (time and temperature), and sample preparation procedure *(5,7)*.

- If blood is hemolyzed or frozen, the specimen should not be analyzed. Hemolysis indicates that the blood was exposed to conditions that can cause erythrocyte lysis, which suggests that leukocytes may also be damaged.
- If clots are visible, the specimen should not be analyzed. Even a partial clot may cause selective loss or alteration of certain subpopulations.
- For some anticoagulants (i.e., ACD), a partially filled tube may produce hypertonic conditions that are deleterious to cells, especially if they are fragile neoplastic cells. Depending on the magnitude of the overfill, one may accept or reject the specimen.

1. Phosphate-buffered saline (PBS): 5.68 g sodium phosphate dibasic (0.01 *M*), 35.48 g sodium chloride (0.15 *M*), 2.8 g bovine albumin, 4.0 g sodium azide, Q.S. to 4 L with deionized water, pH to 7.4. Store at 2–8°C, stable for 1 yr.
2. Lysing agent: 33.04 g ammonium chloride, 4.0 g potassium bicarbonate, 0.148 g tetrasodium EDTA, Quantity Sufficient (Q.S.) with distilled water to 4 L, pH 7.2–7.4. Stable for 1 yr.
3. Flow sheath fluid: obtain from Becton Dickinson, Bioscience, San Jose, CA. Store at room temperature, stable for 1 yr.
4. Rabbit serum (nonimmunized). Store at 2–8°C.
5. RPMI Medium 1640 (Gibco Laboratories, cat. no. 380-6140AG). Store at 2–8°C, stable for 1 yr.
6. MAb (specific to leukemia/lymphoma panel). *See* **Table 1**.
7. Ficoll hypaque. Long-term storage at 2–8°C. Bring to room temperature prior to use. Stability is based on the manufacturer's recommendation.
8. Propidium iodide (PI) solution: 0.125 g PI and 250 mL flow PBS. Cover with aluminum foil. Store at 4°C; stable for 2 mo.
9. 22% Bovine albumin. Store at 2–8°C.
10. McFarland equivalence turbidity standard: 0.5 and 1.0. Store at room temperature
11. Antibodies (*see* **Table 1**).

2.2. Calibrators/Standards

Calibration of a flow cytometer is performed by service engineers upon installation and through annual preventative maintenance installation. Calibration is verified by setup beads on each daily shift (*see* proper manufacturer's instruction).

Table 1
Suggested Panel of Antibodies for Six-Color Antibody Configuration

Tube no.	FITC	PE	PerCPCy5.5	APC	PE Cy7	APC Cy7
1	IgG1 isotype control	IgG1 isotype control	IgG1 isotype control	IgG1 isotype control	IgG1 isotype control	CD45
2	CD2	CD3	CD4	CD8	CD56	CD45
3	CD20	CD19	CD5	CD11c	HLADR	CD45
4	CD38	CD13	CD19	CD23	CD34	CD45
5	CD7	CD64	CD33	CD117	CD34	CD45
6	IgG1 isotype control	IgG1 isotype control	IgG1 isotype control	IgG1 isotype control	IgG1 isotype control	CD45
7	Lambda	Kappa	CD5	CD19	CD10	CD45

2.3. Compensation Check, Positive and Negative Control

2.3.1. Compensation Check

The compensation of the six-color leukemia protocol should be verified daily. A normal whole blood sample is stained with six single-color isotypic controls. The matrix of this should be saved.

2.3.2. Positive and Negative Controls

2.3.2.1. ISOTYPIC NEGATIVE CONTROLS

1. Check reagent insert for corresponding isotypes of the MAb used for immuno-phenotyping *(5,7)*.
2. For each panel, tubes containing all isotypic controls for all six colors are set up to set the marker dividing positive fluorescence from negative.

2.3.2.2. NORMAL AND POSITIVE CONTROL FOR TESTING REAGENTS (ANTIBODY CONTROL)

1. A normal blood control is performed to check the working antibody.
2. The purpose of this control is to ensure the integrity of the antibodies used and the accuracy of the staining procedure. Record acceptable/not acceptable results. The staining pattern of the lymphocytes/monocytes/granulocytes should be appropriate for the population *(5,7)*.
   a. CD23, CD117, and CD34 are not normally expressed on a normal control. Positive control cells are added only if the positive control cells saved from a known positive patient is available.
   b. If any antibody does not perform as expected, make up a fresh working dilution and reset all relevant patient samples for that antibody with a new working dilution.

2.3.3. Parallel Testing of Reagents

1. Prior to putting new lot numbers of MAb in use, parallel testing with the old lot number is performed *(5,7)*.
2. Percent positivity using the new and old lot numbers is compared. The coefficient of variation must fall within the following limits:

%Positive	%CV
>50	<5%
20–50	<10%
<20	<20%

2.4. Instruments and Equipment

1. 12×75 mm Glass or plastic culture tubes.
2. Aluminum foil.
3. P200 (20–200 µL) or equivalent with disposable tips.
4. P1000 pipet (200–1000 µL) or equivalent with disposable pipet tips.
5. Eppendorf adjustable digital pipet (2–10 µL and 10–1000 µL).
6. Microscope slides.
7. Cover slips.
8. Disposable transfer pipets.
9. 15-mL Conical centrifuge tubes with caps.
10. Disposable plastic Petri dish.
11. Sterile scissors/blades and forceps.
12. Parafilm.
13. 53-µ*M* Mesh, cut into 1-in. squares.
14. Vortex (MaxiMix or equivalent).
15. Biosafety hood.
16. Microscope.
17. Centrifuge with swinging bucket rotor.
18. Safety lids for centrifuge buckets.
19. 37°C Incubator.
20. 2–8°C Refrigerator.
21. Flow cytometer (BD FACS Canto).
22. Sample Prep Assistant II (SPAII; BD).
23. Wash-Lyse Assistant (BD).

3. Methods

3.1. Preparation of Specimen for Testing

The goal of sample preparation is to process a specimen from a patient with suspected leukemia or lymphoma into a representative sample suitable for introduction into the flow cytometer for analysis *(5,7)*.

1. Always prepare slides with your sample for Wright stain preferably.
2. Prepare Wright stain touch imprints on tissue specimens.

3.1.1. Process Tissue Specimens

The goal of tissue preparation is to maximize the cellular yield while maintaining cell viability; therefore, rapid and gentle processing is imperative.

1. Place specimen between two pieces of 53-μM mesh in a Petri dish.
2. Cover with 3 mL of PBS.
3. *Gently* tease cells from tissue using the top of a 12 × 75-glass tube or the bottom of a syringe.
4. Filter cell suspension into a conical centrifuge tube.
5. Wash once with flow PBS.
6. Centrifuge at 804.2g for 5 min.
7. Aspirate supernatant carefully.
8. Resuspend in flow PBS, adjust to a 1+ cell suspension (turbidity standard). Proceed to **Subheading 3.1.2.**, **step 9**.

3.1.2. Process Fluid Specimens

1. Aliquot the fluids into 50-mL conical screw-cap centrifuge tubes.
2. Centrifuge at 800g for 10 min to obtain the cell pellet. (If the cell count is very low, process as much fluid as necessary to obtain enough cells to work with.)
3. Aspirate the supernatant and vortex the cell pellet.
4. Wash one time each with PBS as follows.
5. Centrifuge at 804.2g for 5 min.
6. Aspirate supernatant carefully.
7. Vortex the cell pellet vigorously.
8. Resuspend in flow PBS and adjust to a 1+ cell suspension.
9. Pipet 100 μL of cell suspension into all 9 (12 × 75 mm) test tubes prepared for each patient **Subheading 3.1.5**.
10. Mix tubes 1–10 thoroughly, and incubate at room temperature in the dark for 20–30 min.
11. Wash stained cells twice with PBS using the cell washer. Suspend cells in 500 μL PBS and analyze on Coulter XL. If excess red blood cell contamination is present lyse the cells before analysis (proceed to **Subheading 3.1.3.**, **step 3**).

3.1.3. Process Peripheral Blood

1. Count cells and if >10,000 cell/μL dilute with PBS and make sure that the sample contains no more than 10,000/μL.
2. Use SPA for preparing and staining as instructed.
3. Under reagent rack ID, change to "BD Basic Panel." This will display which antibody goes into which tube.

3.1.4. Processing Bone Marrow

This is the procedure for estimating total white blood count (WBC) for bone marrows. Obtain white cell count slide estimate as follows:

1. Scan the Wright-stained slide with low power first (either ×10 or ×20). Look for an area *most representative* of the total cellularity of the slide.
2. Switch to ×40 (high/dry) and count the number of WBCs per field.
3. Examine four to five fields and determine the average number of WBCs per field. *Do not* truncate. Include smudge cells and degenerated cells in your count. (If there is a significant number of nucleated red blood cells (NRBCs), these can also be noted separately.)
4. Determine WBC by multiplying the average number of WBC per field by 2000 (3000 if using ×50 magnification). Refer to sample volume and dilution guide to determine amount of sample to be used.

Follow the whole blood stain then the lyse procedure to stain the cells.

3.1.5. Mononuclear Cells Isolation From Peripheral Blood/Bone Marrow by Ficoll-Hypaque

Follow procedure as recommended by the manufacturer.

3.2. Viability Assessment

Cells that have lost plasma membrane integrity become permeable to external compounds, including dyes and enzymes, and are considered to be nonviable *(5,7)*.

PI is a DNA dye. When the membrane on a nonviable cell becomes permeable, PI will enter the cell and bind to DNA in the nucleus. The binding of PI to DNA is then analyzed by the flow cytometer.

Perform a viability assessment for each specimen. Cell viability assessment by PI:

1. Lyse an aliquot of blood (tube 14). For tissue/fluid cell suspension without excess red blood cell contamination proceed to the next step.
2. Wash twice with PBS, decant.
3. Add 500 µL PI and incubate at room temperature in the dark for 10 min.
4. Document result on face sheet. Optimal viability is ≥80%.
5. Viability of <80% indicates poor viability.

3.3. Data Reporting

1. Generally, the markers should be reported in percentages and as fluorescent intensities.
2. Microscopic review of the smear should be performed. The reviewer should approve or change gating and reporting results.

3.4. Interpretation

3.4.1. Interpretative Guidelines

1. Examine CD45 fluorescence patterns on each specimen histogram. Problems with lysis should not affect results as the CD45-gating strategy focuses on leukocyte populations as positive and other "noise" as negative.
2. Note any abnormal scattering characteristics for the particular panel (i.e., dim CD45 populations).

CD 45 versus side scatter/forward scatter
(Is there abnormal distribution or population of cells?)
Yes
No
Gate on this specific abnormal population and investigate for:
-Blasts or Lymphoma cells
-Plasma cells
-Hairy cell leukemia
Check for potential abnormalities in each cell population and investigate for:
-Chronic leukemia (Myeloid or lymphoid)
-Myelodysplastic syndrome
-Low-grade lymphomas

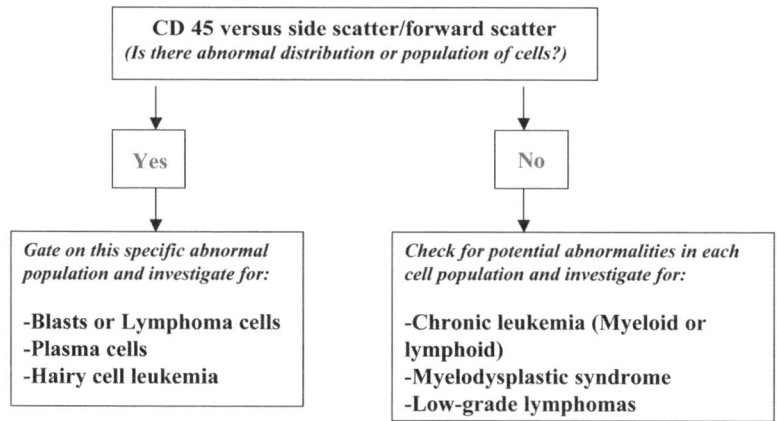

Fig. 1. Algorithm for screening for hematological abnormalities by flow cytometry.

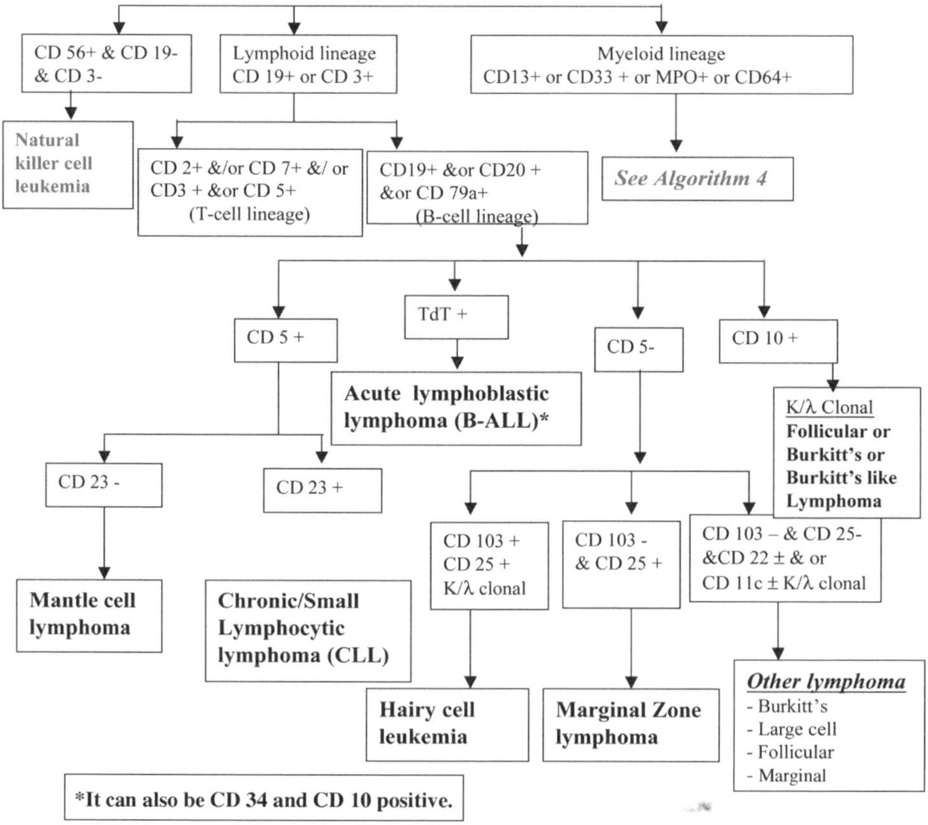

CD 56+ & CD 19- & CD 3-
Lymphoid lineage CD 19+ or CD 3+
Myeloid lineage CD13+ or CD33 + or MPO+ or CD64+
Natural killer cell leukemia
CD 2+ &/or CD 7+ &/ or CD3 + &or CD 5+ (T-cell lineage)
CD19+ &or CD20 + &or CD 79a+ (B-cell lineage)
See Algorithm 4
CD 5 +
TdT +
CD 5-
CD 10 +
Acute lymphoblastic lymphoma (B-ALL)*
K/λ Clonal
Follicular or Burkitt's or Burkitt's like Lymphoma
CD 23 -
CD 23 +
CD 103 + CD 25 + K/λ clonal
CD 103 - & CD 25 +
CD 103 – & CD 25- &CD 22 ± & or CD 11c ± K/λ clonal
Mantle cell lymphoma
Chronic/Small Lymphocytic lymphoma (CLL)
Hairy cell leukemia
Marginal Zone lymphoma
Other lymphoma
- Burkitt's
- Large cell
- Follicular
- Marginal
*It can also be CD 34 and CD 10 positive.

Fig. 2. Algorithm for the analysis of an abnormal population.

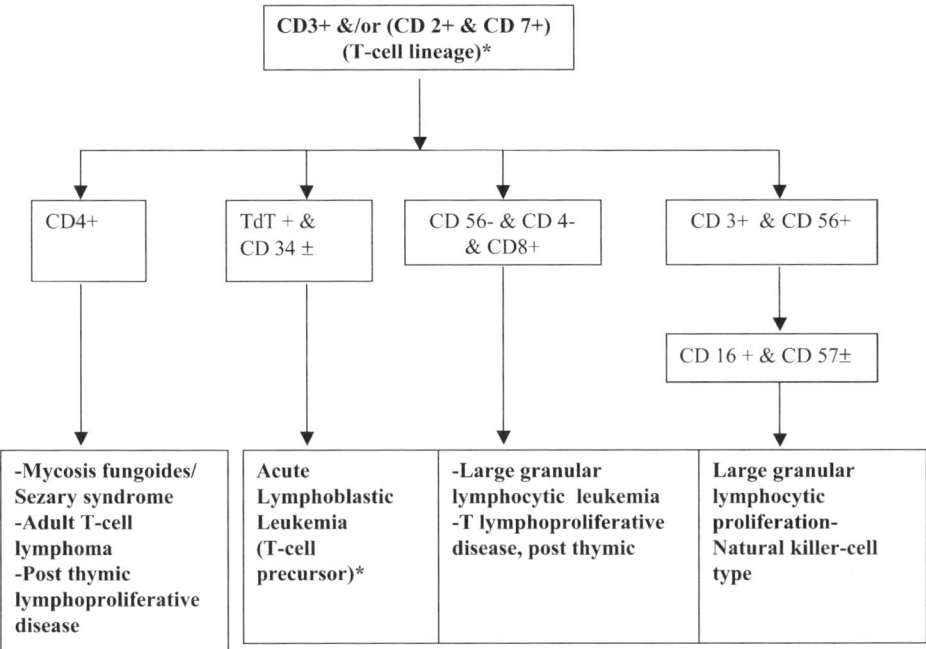

Fig. 3. The analysis and diagnosis of T-cell neoplasms.

3. Note any abnormal marking characteristics that may not be appropriate for the particular population selected or which may indicate additional testing to aid in diagnostic interpretation.
4. Always correlate flow cytometric results with morphology review. Any discrepancies should be investigated.

3.4.2. Interpreting Data

Record percent positive (include double marking) with respect to specific markers tested. Each completed specimen protocol sheet with history, viability, differential, fluorescent marking characteristics, and related histograms should be reviewed. Positivity and negativity for certain markers are characteristics for specific differentiation and growth of hematopoietic cells. Specific diagnosis can be rendered based on these characteristics. The following is an algorithm that can be used for the differential diagnosis of various hematopoietic neoplasma. However, final diagnosis should be based on integrating information from clinical history, histological and morphological evaluation, other laboratory data, and clinical history *(1,6,8–10,12–19)*.

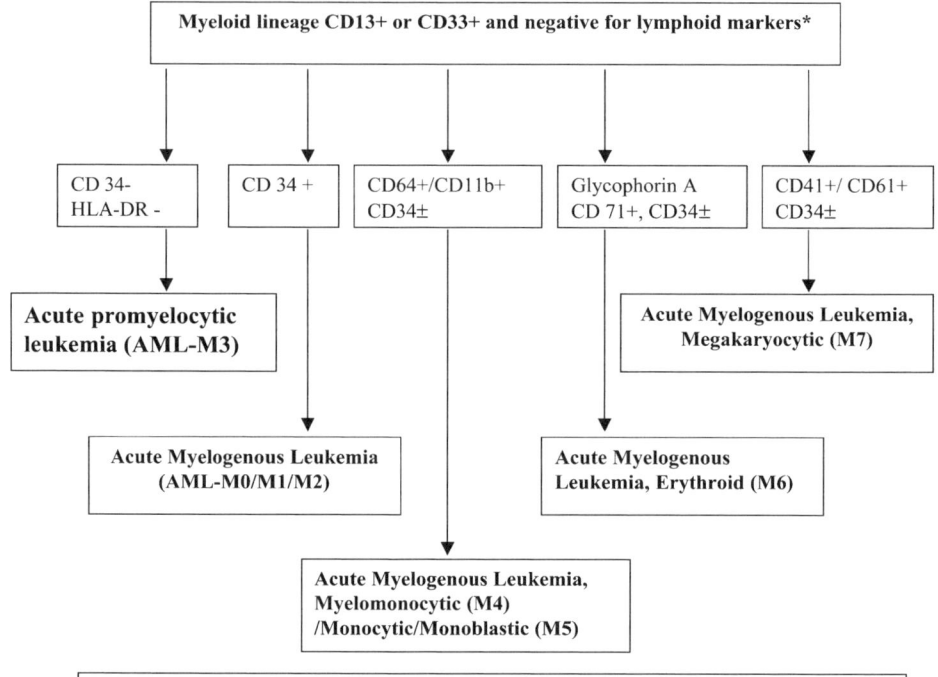

Fig. 4. The analysis and diagnosis of myeloid neoplasms.

References

1. Bauer, K. D., Duque, R. E., and Shankey, T. V. (1993) *Clinical Flow Cytometry: Principles and Applications*, Williams and Wilkins Baltimore, MD USA.
2. Bowman, G. P., Neame, P. B., and Soambonsrup, P. (1986) The contribution of cytochemistry and immunophenotyping to the reproducibility of the FAB classification in acute leukemia. *Blood* **68,** 900–905.
3. Falini, B., Pileri, S., and Martelli, M. F. (1989) Histologic and immunohistological analysis of human lymphomas. *Crit. Rev. Oncol. Hematol.* **9,** 351–419.
4. Harrington, D. S., Masih, A., and Duggan, M. (1991) Immunohistochemical diagnosis of lymphoproliferative diseases. *Crit. Rev. Oncol. Hematol.* **11,** 137–164.
5. Borowitz, M., Duque, R., Bauer, K., et al. (1998) *Clinical Applications of Flow Cytometry: Quality Assurance and Immunophenotyping of Lymphocytes.* National Committe for Clinical Laboratory Standards.
6. Keren, D. F. (2005) *Flow Cytometry in Clinical Diagnosis.* ASCP, Chicago, IL.
7. National Committe for Clinical Laboratory Standards document H43-A. (1998) *Clinical Applications of Flow Cytometry: Immunophenotyping of Leukemic Cells; Proposed Guideline.* National Committee for Clinical Laboratory Standards.

8. Sobol, R.E., Bloomfield, C.D., and Royston, I. (1988) Immunophenotyping in the diagnosis and classification of Acute Lymphoblastic Leukemia. In Clinics in Laboratory Medicine; classification, diagnosis, and molecular biology of Lymphoproliferative disorder. Vol 8, 151–162. W. B. Saunders Company, Philadelphia, PA.

9. Nadler, L. M. and Freedman, A. S. (1987) Cell surface markers in hematologic malignancies. *Semin. Oncol.* **14,** 193–212.

10. Ricker, L. J., Weiss, L. M., Medeiros, L. J., Wood, G. S., and Warnke, R. A. (1987) Immunophenotypic criteria for the diagnosis of non-Hodgkin's lymphoma. *Am. J. Pathol.* **128,** 181–201.

11. Braylan, R. C., Orfao, A., Borowitz, M. J., et al. (2001) Optimal number of reagents required to evaluate hematolymphoid neoplasias: results of an international consensus meeting. *Cytometry* **46,** 23–27.

12. Shapiro, H. M. (2003) *Practical Flowcytometry.* Wiley-Liss, New York.

13. Foon, K. A., and Todd, R. R. III. (1986) Immunologic classification of leukemia and lymphoma. *Blood* **68,** 1–31.

14. Griffin, J. D., Mayer, R. J., Weinstern, J. J., et al. (1983) Surface marker analysis of acute (myeloblastic leukemia) identification of differentiation-associated phenotypes. *Blood* **62,** 557–563

15. Nguyen, D. T., Diamond, L. W., and Braylan, R. C. (2003) *Flow Cytometry in Hematopathology: A Visual Approach to Data Analysis and Interpretation.* Humana Press, Totowa, NJ.

16. Borowitz, M. J., Guenther, K. L., Shults, K. E., et al. (1993) Immunophenotyping of acute leukemia by flow cytometric analysis. Use of CD45 and right-angle light scatter to gate on leukemic blasts in three-color analysis. *Am. J. Clin. Pathol.* **100,** 534–540.

17. Dworzak, M. N. and Panzer-Grumayer, E. R. (2003) Flow cytometric detection of minimal residual disease in acute lymphoblastic leukemia. *Leuk. Lymphoma* **44,** 1445–1455.

18. Riley, R. S., Massey, D., Jackson-Cook, C., et al. (2002) Immunophenotypic analysis of acute lymphocytic leukemia. *Hematol. Oncol. Clin. North Am.* **16,** 245–299.

19. Venditti, A., Maurillo, L., Buccisano, F., et al. (2003) Multidimensional flow cytometry for detection of minimal residual disease in acute myeloid leukemia. *Leuk. Lymphoma* **44,** 445–450.

5

Quantification of Surface Antigens and Quantitative Flow Cytometry

Huai En Huang Chan, Iman Jilani, Richard Chang, and Maher Albitar

Summary

Measuring expression levels of cell surface antigens is important for the diagnosis of diseases such as B-cell chronic lymphocytic leukemia and the monitoring of targeted therapy, particularly antibody-based therapy. In some cases, the number of antigens that the therapeutic antibodies bind on the cell surface may reflect the efficacy of therapy. Thus, quantitating the number of molecules on the surface of cells before, during, and after therapy would provide important information for monitoring antibody-based therapy and potentially can be used to adjust dosing. We describe a quantitative flow cytometry approach to measuring levels of the CD20 surface antigen, the molecular target of rituximab.

Key Words: CD20; surface antigen; quantitative flow cytometry; antibody therapy.

1. Introduction

One of the most well-characterized therapeutic monoclonal antibodies is rituximab (Rituxan®, Genentech, South San Francisco, CA; Biogen Idec, Cambridge, MA), a chimeric anti-CD20 antibody. CD20 is a 33–36-kDa transmembrane phosphoprotein expressed on the surface of mature B-cells and the majority of immature B-cells *(1,2)*. It is involved in proliferation, most likely by regulating transmembrane calcium conductance *(3)*. Rituximab induces apoptosis through complement fixation and antibody-dependent, cell-mediated cytotoxicity *(4–6)*. Immunotherapy with rituximab has been successful both alone and in combination with chemotherapy in treating B-cell lymphoproliferative diseases *(7–10)* with high response rates in various non-Hodgkin's lymphomas and chronic B-Chronic Lymphocytic Leukemia (CLL) *(10–12)*.

Quantitative flow cytometry can be applied to measure cell surface antigens such as CD20. Measuring levels of surface antigens would provide valuable

From: *Methods in Molecular Biology, vol. 378: Monoclonal Antibodies: Methods and Protocols*
Edited by: M. Albitar © Humana Press Inc., Totowa, NJ

insight to optimal dosing and scheduling of therapy. It has been observed that CD20 antigen cannot be detected by flow cytometry on the surface of B-cells in patients treated with rituximab because of the masking effect of rituximab on CD20 itself *(13)*. Hence, monitoring levels of CD20 delineates the efficacy of rituximab therapy. We describe a three-color flow cytometry immuno-phenotyping procedure to assess the expression of CD20 on specific cellular populations such as B-cells. CD20 is labeled with phycoerythrin (PE) in a 1:1 fluorescence-to-protein ratio. This methodology would be beneficial for monitoring response in patients treated with rituximab and can also be applied to other cell surface markers.

2. Materials

2.1. Surface Marker Staining

1. Flow PBS: prepare with 5.6 g sodium phosphate dibasic anhydrous, 35.48 g sodium chloride, 2.8 g albumin-bovine, and 4.0 g sodium azide. Add deionized water to 4 L and adjust to pH 7.4.
2. Red blood cell lysing reagent: 8.26 g ammonium chloride, 1.0 g potassium bicarbonate, and 0.037 g tetrasodium EDTA. Add deionized water to 1 L and adjust to pH 7.2–7.4.
3. Isotype controls: IgG1 PE, IgG1 FITC, and IgG1 APC (BD Biosciences, San Jose, CA).
4. Surface markers: CD20-PE, CD19 FITC, and CD3 APC (BD Biosciences).
5. Sorvall Cell Washer 2 (Thermo Electron Corporation, Asheville, NC).

2.2. Flow Cytometric Analysis

1. FACSCalibur™ flow cytometer (BD Biosciences).
2. QuantiBRITE™ PE beads (BD Biosciences).
3. Cell Quest Pro™ acquisition and analysis software (BD Biosciences).
4. FlowJO™ analysis software (Treestar, Ashland OR).
5. CaliBRITE™ 3 beads (BD Biosciences).
6. APC beads (BD Biosciences).

3. Methods

This is a three-color immunophenotyping assay to assess the expression of CD20 on B-cells. We use QuantiBRITE PE beads to establish a fluorescence standard for each experiment. Each of the four bead populations has a calibrated mean number of bound PE molecules/bead. Samples are stained with antibodies that have PE conjugated at a 1:1 ratio. The number of bound PE-conjugated antibodies/cell in the sample is extrapolated using the PE beads as a standard. Thus, PE molecules bound per cell is equivalent to the number of antibodies bound to the cell. This in turn is equivalent to the number of molecules of target protein in each cell.

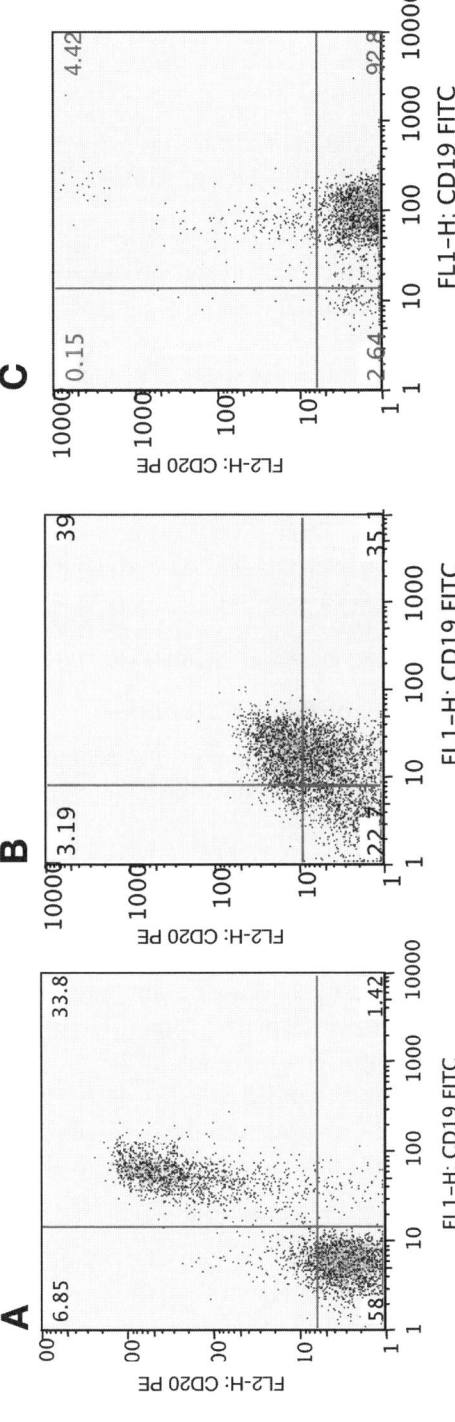

Fig. 1. Dot plots representing examples of CD20 expression in B-cells (CD19+) pre- (**A**) and post-treatment with rituximab (**B**,**C**). The antibody-binding capacity is 1367, 780, and 0 for **A**, **B**, and **C**, respectively.

3.1. Instrument Setup

1. Calibration should be performed according to the manufacturer's protocol using CaliBRITE 3 beads with addition of APC beads every time the cytometer is used.
2. QuatiBRITE PE beads are reconstituted by addition of 1 mL flow PBS and vortexing.
3. CellQuest Pro software is launched and the appropriate acquisition template and instrument settings are selected. 5000 events are captured.

3.2. Surface Marker Staining

1. Each sample is represented in two tubes: one stained with the isotype controls and the other stained with specific markers.
2. The appropriate volume of adjusted cells (equivalent to 1×10^6 cells) is pipetted into each of the two 12×75-mm flow tubes.
3. The control tube is incubated with 5 µL of IgG1 FITC, IgG1 PerCP, and IgG1 APC. The markers tube is incubated with 10 µL of CD19 FITC, CD20-PE, and CD3-APC. Incubations take place for 15 min at room temperature in the dark.
4. The samples are then incubated with 2 mL lysing reagent for 10 min at room temperature in the dark.
5. The samples are washed and resuspended in 500 µL flow PBS for analysis.

3.3. Acquisition of Samples on Flow Cytometer

1. The samples are acquired up to 5000 events. An example of the results is shown in **Fig. 1**.

3.4. Discussion

We describe a simple and quantitative approach to the measurement of cell surface antigens using CD20 as an example. Though it is believed that effective treatment with rituximab will mask CD20 expression, quantitation of levels of CD20 may help in determining efficacy of therapy and give insight on the optimal dosage and scheduling of therapy. Patients without complete masking may not have received adequate dosing. This method can be modified to detect surface antigens in plasma and can be expanded to other antibody-based therapies such as alemtuzumab (anti-CD52; CamPath®, Berlex, Montville, NJ) *(14)* and gemtuzumab ozogamicin (anti-CD33; Mylotarg®, Wyeth Ayerst, Madison, NJ) *(15)*.

References

1. Stashenko, P., Nadler, L. M., Hardy, R., and Schlossman, S. F. (1980) Characterization of a human b lymphocyte-specific antigen. *J. Immunol.* **125,** 1678–1685.
2. Andeson, K. C., Bates, M. P., Slaughenhoup, B. L., Pinkus, G. S., Schlossman, S. F., and Nadler, L. M. (1984) Expression of human B cell-associated antigens on leukemias and lymphomas: a model of human B cell differentiation. *Blood* **63,** 1424–1433.

3. Bubien, J. K., Zhou, L. J., Bell, P. D., Frizzell, R. A., and Tedder, T. F. (1993) Transfection of the CD20 cell surface molecule into ectopic cell types generates a Ca2+ conductance found constitutively in B-lymphocytes. *J. Cell Biol.* **121,** 1121–1132.

4. Demidem, A., Lam, T., Alas, S., Hariharan, K., Hanna, N., and Bonavida, B. (1997) Chimeric anti-CD20 (IDEC-C2B8) monoclonal antibody sensitizes a B cell lymphoma cell line to cell killing by cytotoxic drugs. *Cancer Biother. Radiopharm.* **12,** 177–186.

5. Shan, D., Ledbetter, J. A., and Press, O. W. (2000) Signaling events involved in anti-CD20-induced apoptosis of malignant human B cells. *Cancer Immunol. Immunother.* **48,** 673–683.

6. Hofmeister, J. K., Cooney, D., and Coggeshall, K. M. (2000) Clustered CD20 induced apoptosis: src-family of kinase, the proximal regulator of tyrosine phosphorylation, calcium influx, and caspase 3-dependent apoptosis. *Blood Cells Mol. Dis.* **26,** 133–143.

7. McLaughlin, P. (2001) Rituximab: perspective on single agent experience, and future directions in combinational trials. *Crit. Rev. Oncol. Hematol.* **40,** 3–16.

8. Schulz, H., Winkler, U., Staak, J. O., and Engert, A. (2000) The monoclonal antibodies Campath-1H and rituximab in the therapy of chronic lymphocytic leukemia. *Onkologie* **23,** 526–532.

9. Czuczman, M. S., Fallon, A., and Mohr, A. (2002) Rituximab in combination with CHOP or fludarabine in low grade lymphoma. *Semin. Oncol.* **18,** 3135–3143.

10. Maloney, D. G., Liles, T. M., and Czerwinski, D. K. (1994) Phase I clinical trials using escalating single-dose infusion of chimeric anti-CD20 monoclonal antibody (IDEC-C2B8) in patients with recurrent B-cell lymphoma. *Blood* **84,** 2457–2466.

11. Piro, L. D., White, C. A., Grillo-Lopez, A. J., et al. (1999) Extended rituximab (anti-CD20 monoclonal antibody) therapy for relapsed or refractory low-grade or follicular non-Hodgkin's lymphoma. *Ann. Oncol.* **10,** 655–661.

12. Coiffer, B., Haioun, C., and Ketterer, N. (1998) Rituximab (anti-CD20 monoclonal antibody) for the treatment of patients with relapsing or refractory aggressive lymphoma: a multi-center phase II study. *Blood* **92,** 1927–1932.

13. Davis, T. A., Czerwinski, D. K., and Levy, R. (1999) Therapy of B-cell lymphoma with anti-CD20 antibodies can result in the loss of CD20 antigen expression. *Clin. Cancer Res.* **5,** 611–615.

14. Flynn, J. M. and Byrd, J. C. (2000) Campath-1H monoclonal antibody therapy. *Curr. Opin. Oncol.* **12,** 574–581.

15. van Der Velden, V. H., te Marvelde, J. G., and Hoogeveen, P. G. et al. (2001) Targeting of the CD33-calicheamicin immunoconjugate Mylotarg (CMA-676) in acute myeloid leukemia: in vivo and in vitro saturation and internalization by leukemic and normal myeloid cells. *Blood* **97,** 3197–3204.

6

CD13 and CD10 Expression of Granulocytes as Markers for the Functioning of the Immune System

Quantification of the Expression of Membrane Molecules Using 1:1 Labeled Monoclonal Antibodies and Flow Cytometry

Patrick Schroeter, Arnim Sablotzki, and Dagmar Riemann

Summary

HLA-DR expression on monocytes as a marker for the functioning of the immune system is known to be severely depressed in immunodeficiency. Up to now, other markers for the function of the immune system are scarce. In the peripheral blood of patients with open heart surgery the expression of the membrane peptidases neprilysin/CD10 and aminopeptidase N/CD13, was determined on granulocytes in comparison to the monocytic HLA-DR expression. We used the QuantiBRITE™ flow cytometry system, which yields an absolute antigen expression value (antibodies bound per cell) and may be useful in standardizing surface antigen expression analysis. This system makes use of a highly purified phycoerythrin-labeled antibody with a 1:1 fluorochrome-to-protein ratio, and multilevel calibrated beads with known absolute phycoerythrin fluorescence. Our results show that both membrane peptidases on granulocytes show a similar time-course of expression after heart surgery as do HLA-DR molecules on monocytes, with a decrease from days one to three and a subsequent recovery to normal values. In future analyses a possible relationship between the immunodeficiency of patients and a diminished expression of both membrane peptidases on granulocytes has to be investigated.

Key Words: Flow cytometry; monocytes; granulocytes; heart surgery; HLA-DR; CD13; CD10; antibodies bound per cell; ABC.

1. Introduction

Flow cytometers are instruments that can quantify fluorescence intensity data and provide unique information about cell populations. Fluorescence intensity calibration allows the establishment of a comparable window of analysis across different times and laboratories. Significant advances have been made

From: *Methods in Molecular Biology, vol. 378: Monoclonal Antibodies: Methods and Protocols*
Edited by: M. Albitar © Humana Press Inc., Totowa, NJ

in terms of calibration reagents, standardized sample preparation, and data analysis to ensure interlaboratory comparability and reproducibility. The design and use of calibration beads labeled with predefined amounts of dye allows instrument-independent expression of fluorescence intensity in units of molecules of equivalent soluble fluorochrome *(1)*. This method was refined by the combined use of such standards with monoclonal antibodies (MAb) conjugated 1/1 with phycoerythrin (PE), allowing translation of fluorescence intensity into numbers of antibodies bound per cell (ABC) *(2)*. Commercially available 1:1 labeled MAb have been used in patient diagnostics for several years now. In HIV infection, for example, antigen density changes in CD38 expression of CD8-positive T-cells may be an important indicator of disease progression *(3)*.

In an earlier study, we quantitatively determined the simultaneous expression of HLA-DR and aminopeptidase N/CD13 on peripheral blood monocytes of patients suffering major trauma *(4)*. Trauma patients are known to have an early onset depression of the overall cellular immune response, which is associated with a high rate of infection and mortality. Several investigators have shown that the expression of monocyte HLA-DR as a marker for their antigen-presenting capacity is severely impaired and correlates with the outcome of patients *(5,6)*. The mechanisms involved in the regulation of HLA-DR include shedding of HLA-DR from the cell surface and regulation of HLA-DR gene transcription *(7)*. We described that the recovery of the attenuated monocytic HLA-DR expression after trauma was accompanied by a strong increase in the membrane enzyme aminopeptidase N/CD13 on monocytes *(4)*. Fourteen days after trauma, the monocytic expression of CD13 was still much higher than in normal volunteers used as a control group. Membrane peptidases are multifunctional molecules. Not only do these enzymes hydrolyse small peptide mediators, resulting in activation or inactivation; they also function as receptors and as molecules participating in cell motility and in adhesion to extracellular matrix *(8)*. Therefore, the expression of these antigens on leukocytes could be useful for characterizing the function of the immune system. We investigated the expression of two membrane peptidases on granulocytes in patients undergoing open heart surgery. Using quantitative immunofluorescence and flow cytometry, we showed a similar time-course both of the expression of HLA-DR on monocytes and of the membrane peptidases Aminopeptidase N/CD13 and neprilysin/CD10 on granulocytes.

2. Materials

2.1. Specimen Requirements

EDTA anticoagulated whole blood is the required specimen. After collection, keep blood at room temperature. Staining and cell fixation must be completed within 4 h of blood draw in the case of HLA-DR quantification of monocytes (*see* **Note 1**). For other leukocyte surface molecules, the stability of antigen expression has to be investigated.

2.2. Patients

Fifty–four patients (mean age of 64 ± 7.5 yr, 72% were men) undergoing open heart surgery owing to coronary heart disease or heart valve replacement were prospectively enrolled in this study, which was performed with the approval of the ethics committee of the University Halle-Wittenberg. Informed consent was obtained from the patients. The patients spent an average of 3.4 ± 1.2 d in intensive care. Patient's mean white blood cell counts ranged from 8.3 to 13.7×10^3 cells/mm^3 with a peak on day 1. Preoperatively, as well as on days 1, 3, 7, and 10, 2.7 mL EDTA-treated venous blood was obtained. Fourteen healthy, age-matched individuals served as controls.

2.3. Reagents

1. BD FACS™ Lysing Solution (BD Biosciences, San Jose, CA).
2. Phosphate-buffered saline (PBS): prepare 10X stock with 1.37 M NaCl, 27 mM KCl, 100 mM Na$_2$HPO$_4$, 18 mM KH$_2$PO$_4$ (adjust to pH 7.4 with HCl if necessary), and filtrate before storage at 4°C. Prepare working solution by dilution of one part with nine parts of filtrated water.
3. QuantiBRITE™ PE beads (BD Biosciences), a set of four precalibrated bead levels in the form of lyophilized pellet to calibrate the fluorescence (FL)2 axis in terms of numbers of PE molecules.
4. HLA-DR 1/1 PE (clone L243)/anti CD14 PerCP-Cy5.5 MAb (BD Biosciences, cat. no. 340827).
5. CD13 1/1 PE (clone L138; prepared as a customer service, BD Biosciences, cat. no. 347830).
6. CD10 1/1 PE (clone HI10a; prepared as a customer service, BD Biosciences).

3. Methods

3.1. Principle of the Test

PE-labeled beads are commercially available in a kit, which contains one tube with a mixture of beads with four different predefined levels of PE. The PE-labeled antibodies used for staining of surface antigens on blood cells are at a 1:1 fluorochrome-to-antibody ratio. This allows determination of the ABC when beads are run under the same photomultiplier and compensation settings as blood cells (*see* **Notes 2** and **3**).

All samples were analyzed on a FACS Calibur (BD Biosciences) using the software CellQuest™. The monocytes and granulocytes were separated on the basis of their forward scatter and side scatter patterns, and the staining with CD14 was used to check the identification of the monocytes. At least 3000 monocytes were analyzed per sample. Additionally, 10,000 events in the granulocyte gate were counted. The PE fluorescence within the gates was measured as specific geometric mean fluorescence intensity of the whole population of cells (*see* **Note 4**). QuantiQuest is a quantitative calibration feature within the CellQuest acquisition software that calculates the linear function relating fluorescence to PE molecules. So with help of the Microsoft Excel™-spreadsheet, geometric mean fluorescence was converted into the term ABC.

3.2. Monoclonal Antibody Staining

1. Pipet 50 µL of whole blood into each of (three) 5-mL tubes (*see* **Note 5**). Add 20 µL of the HLA-DR/CD14 MAb mixture to tube 1 (*see* **Note 6**). Add 10 µL of CD13 MAb to tube 2 and 10 µL of CD10 MAb to tube 3.
2. Incubate for 30 min in the dark at 4°C (*see* **Note 7**).
3. Add 2 mL of FACS Lyse (*see* **Note 8**), mix, and incubate for 30 min in the dark at 4°C.
4. Centrifuge for 5 min at 300*g* and decant supernatant (*see* **Note 9**).
5. Analyze cells in 0.5 mL PBS. Store at 4°C in the dark until measurement.

3.3. Acquisition and Analysis

All samples were analyzed on a FACS Calibur™ using the software CellQuest (BD Biosciences). After launching the acquisition software, all instrument parameters have to be adjusted for the cells you want to analyze. One has to make sure that the instrument is compensated properly (*see* **Note 10**).

The PE-stained beads are run first, at least 10,000 events should be acquired. Place an active gate on the bead singlet population using forward scatter (FSC) and side scatter (SSC). The instrument setting should remain unchanged with respect to fluorescence once the beads have been run. The analysis of the samples should be performed using the same settings.

3.3.1. Beads

1. Reconstitute one tube of QuantiBRITE beads with 0.5 mL of PBS and vortex. Run the QuantiBRITE bead tube thresholding on FSC or SSC and collect 10,000 events. Display a FSC vs SSC dot plot and adjust the gate around the singlet bead population.
2. Display a FL-2 histogram and adjust markers around the four bead populations. View histogram statistics (make sure geometric means are displayed).
3. Click the "Copy means" button to copy the geometric means of the four bead peaks from the histogram statistics window.
4. Select histogram statistics view and choose quantitative calibration from the "Acquire" menu. Enter the lot-specific PE/bead values from the flyer in the kit.
5. Click "Calibrate" for CellQuest to perform regression analysis and to display the slope, intercept, and correlation coefficient. Save the document.
6. Do not adjust photomultipliers or compensation after acquiring these events.

3.3.2. Acquisition and Analysis of Patient Samples

1. Display a FL-1 vs FL-3 dot plot and gate on monocytes (**Fig. 1A**). Count at least 3000 gated events in each sample (*see* **Note 11**).
2. Display a FL-2 histogram of the monocytes. The geometric mean of the entire monocyte population is then used to determine the ABC.
3. Granulocytes were recognized in the forward vs sideward scatter diagram (**Fig. 1B**).

3.4. Calculations

The measurement of multilevel calibrated QuantiBRITE fluorescent beads enables the construction of a standard curve for antigen quantification. Using a Microsoft Excel-spreadsheet referring to CellQuest, provided by BD Biosciences, the sample fluorescence measured can be converted into the term ABC as shown in **Fig. 1C** for the expression of neprilysin/CD10 on granulocytes. QuantiCALC™ (BD Biosciences) is an automated quantitation analysis software, which automatically converts the FL2 axis to PE molecules per cell and reports statistics in PE molecules per cell. Without these tools a manual analysis can be performed:

1. On a statistics spreadsheet, enter the geometric means from the histogram statistics view for the four beads.
2. Enter the lot specific values for PE molecules per bead from the flyer in the kit.
3. Calculate the $\log_{10}$ for each FL-2 geometric mean and for the PE molecules per bead.
4. Plot a liner regression of $\log_{10}$ PE molecules per bead against $\log_{10}$ fluorescence using the equation $y = mx + c$.
5. Determine the ABC values for the PE-stained samples by substituting the log FL2 geometric mean of that population and solving for the log ABC (the antilog of this number is the ABC value).

3.5. Results and Discussion

We used a standardized immune monitoring program based on recent advances in flow cytometry (exact quantification of surface marker expression) to investigate 54 patients with open heart surgery. All patients showed postoperative immunodepression, documented by decreased monocytic HLA-DR. During the postoperative follow-up, all markers investigated tended to recover.

One day after open heart surgery, monocytic HLA-DR expression revealed a marked attenuation compared with values determined preoperatively (9437 ± 854 ABC vs 30,644 ± 2868 ABC; **Fig. 2A**), as already described for patients after cardiopulmonary bypass surgery *(10)*. Thereafter, expression of HLA-DR on monocytes slowly increased within 10 d to reach normal values in most of the patients. The time-course of the expression of both the membrane peptidases

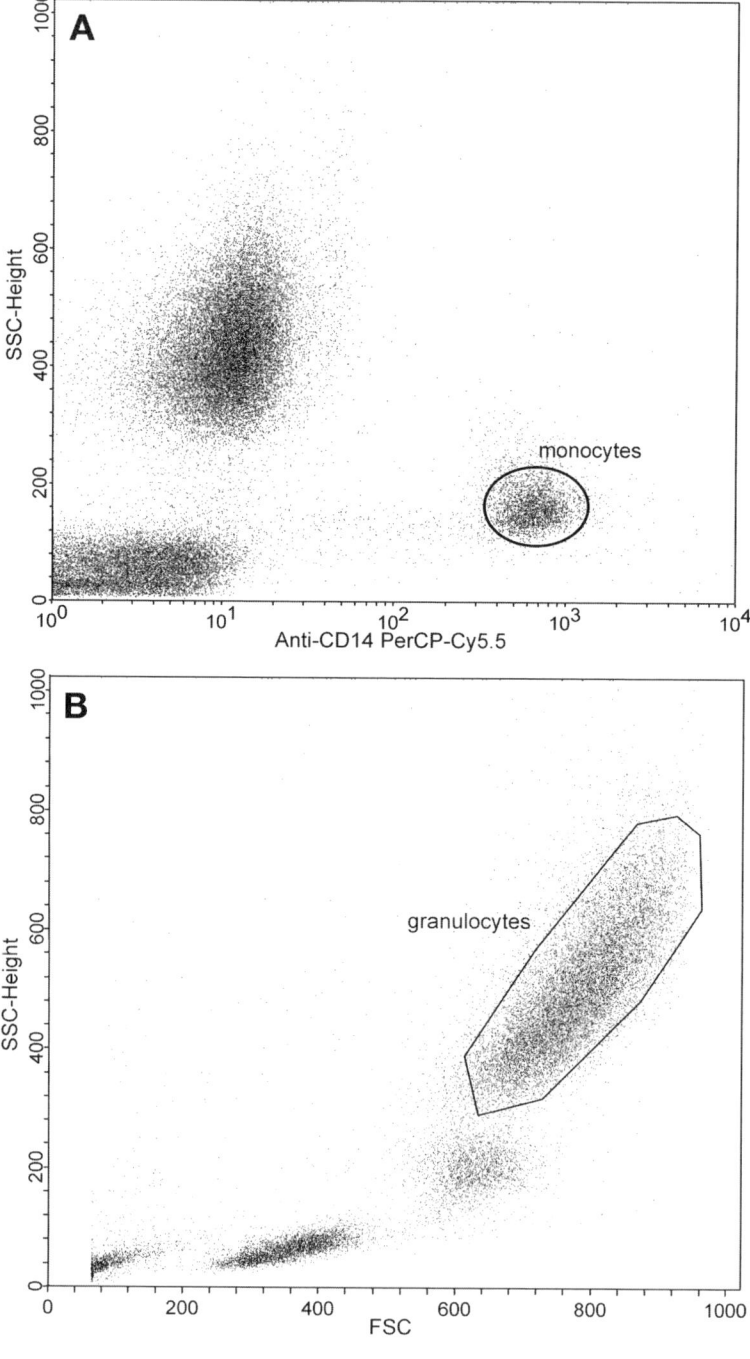

Fig. 1. (*Continued*)

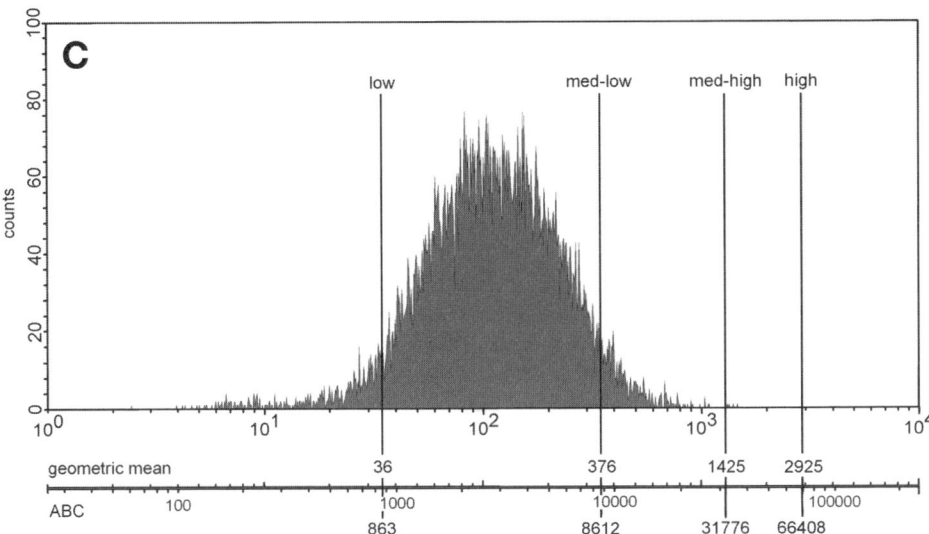

Fig. 1. Gating on the monocytes for determination of HLA-DR (**A**), and on the neutrophil granulocytes (**B**) for determination of neprilysin/CD10 and aminopeptidase N/CD13. (**C**) The estimation of the granulocytic expression of neprilysin/CD10 is shown in a FL2 histogram. The lines on the *x*-axis represent the geometric mean values of the beads measured that are related to molecules per cell. In this particular case, the patient's granulocytes expressed, on average, 2644 neprilysin/CD10 molecules per cell.

aminopeptidase N/CD13 and neprilysin/CD10 on granulocytes showed a similar behavior with a decrease, especially on day one after heart operation, and a return to values of healthy volunteers within 7 d after open heart surgery (**Fig. 2B,C**). Neutrophils are a key component of the innate immune system because they represent the first line of defense the body has upon invasion by a foreign micro-organism. These cells do not express major histocompatibility complex (MHC) class II molecules. However, quantification of Fcγ receptor I/CD64 has been found to be a useful indicator of granulocytic activation in septic patients (*11*). Now, we report that the expression of membrane peptidases could be a useful marker for the immunomonitoring of patients undergoing open heart surgery. In future analyses, a possible relationship between an immunodeficiency of patients and the diminished expression of both membrane peptidases on granulocytes has to be investigated.

4. Notes

QuantiBRITE PE beads provide a useful tool for standardized analysis across labs. When used in conjunction with 1:1 conjugates of PE-to-MAb, the QuantiBRITE PE beads provide a simple yet robust means of quantitating

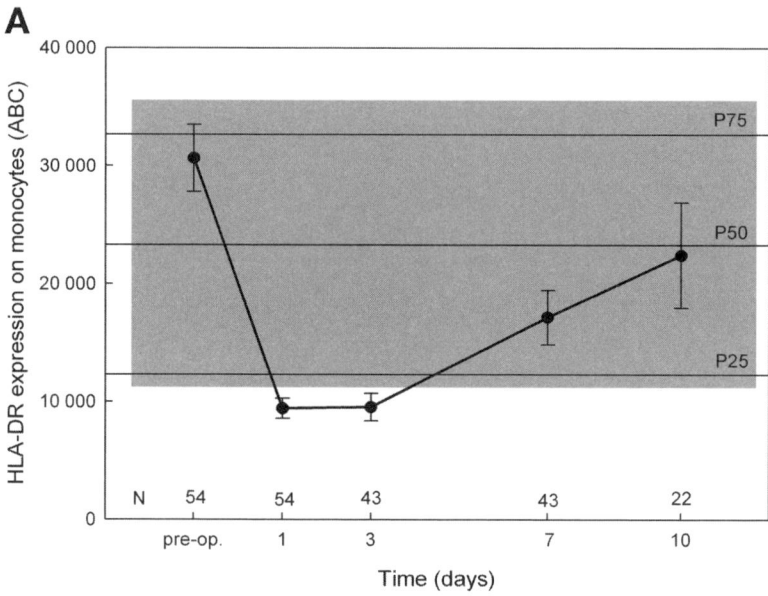

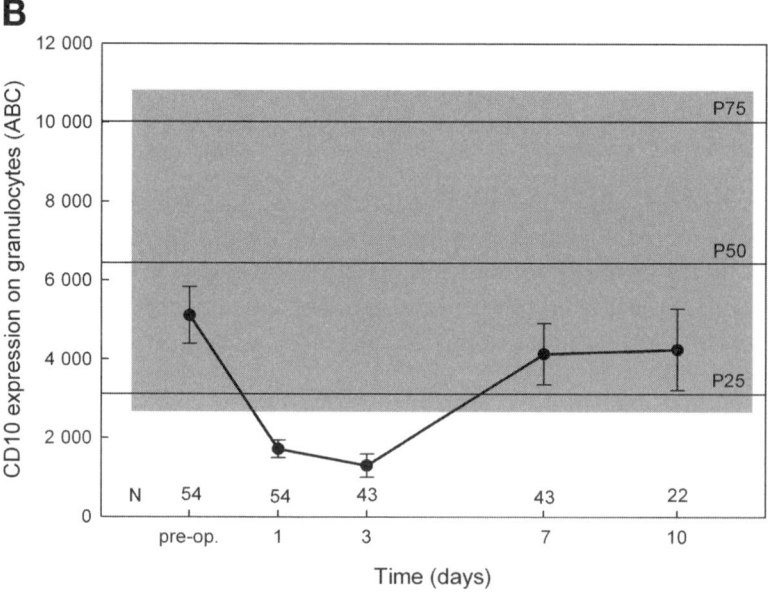

Fig. 2. (*Continued*)

expression levels in terms of ABC *(2)*. However, a number of variables are critical for standardized quantitative flow cytometry. Time of analysis, method of fixation, lysing method, the pH value of the buffers used, and other factors may all influence the quantitative values obtained with this procedure. As

C

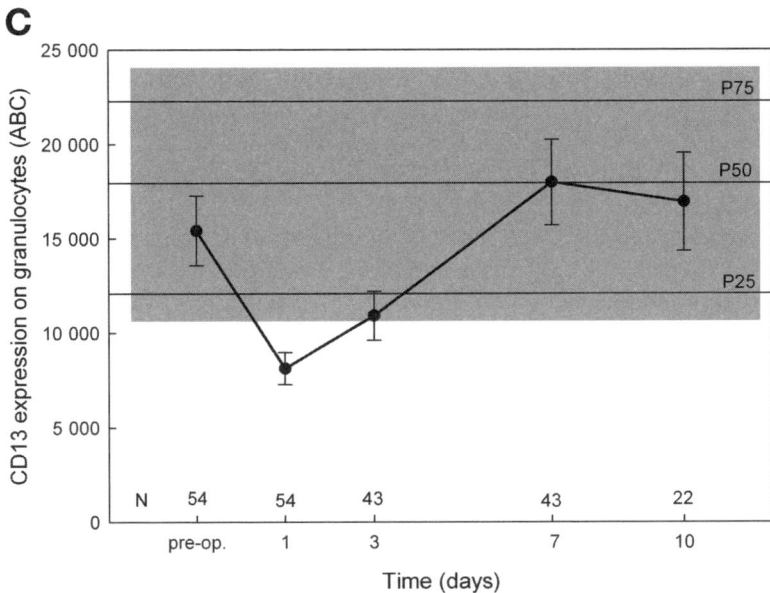

Fig. 2. Changes in antigen expression of monocytes and granulocytes in 54 patients undergoing open heart surgery compared with healthy volunteers (hatched area). All results are expressed as antibodies bound per cell (ABC; mean ± SEM). Percentiles are indicated for healthy volunteers with P25 (25th percentile), P50 and P75. One day after surgery, all patients showed a diminished expression of the markers investigated compared to reference values. N = number of patients. (**A**) Monocytic HLA-DR of patients started preoperatively in the range of the 75th percentile of the control group and revealed a marked attenuation from day one to three after surgery. Thereafter, expression slowly increased within 10 d, reaching normal values in most of the patients. (**B**) Neprilysin/CD10 expression on granulocytes paralleled the decrease in monocytic HLA-DR expression with values less than those of the control group on days one to three after surgery and a normalization by day seven. (**C**) Similarly, expression of aminopeptidase N/CD13 on neutrophils revealed a sharp decrease 1 d after surgery. Recovery to normal values already started on day three.

such, the protocol must be precisely followed to assure comparability between laboratories.

1. Our own observations show that storage of blood at room temperature for longer then 4 h results in a time-dependent increase in the expression of HLA-DR on monocytes. One reason for this effect might be that the decrease in monocytic HLA-DR expression could be the result of an intracellular accumulation of HLA-DR molecules caused by an incomplete posttranslational processing (*7*). Keep blood specimen on ice after collection if you cannot finish staining procedure within 4 h.
2. BD claims that it is not necessary to subtract the cell blank (negative cell population) from the positive cell population because in the first decade the fluorescence

of the bead alone is very similar to that of the negative cell population. To subtract the isotype control value it would be necessary to order a PE-labeled isotype control antibody with the same 1:1 fluorochrome-to-protein ratio.

3. The specific number of PE molecules per bead varies from lot to lot, with low fluorescence intensity in the range of approx 800 and high fluorescence intensity in the range of approx 70,000 PE molecules per bead. Only within this range is the linearity of ABC values guaranteed.

4. The arithmetic mean is well suited to the analysis of data that is collected on a linear scale, whereas as a general rule, the geometric mean is better suited for use with data collected with a logarithmic amplifier. The geometric mean is calculated by multiplying the individual values of a group together, thus obtaining the nth root of the product.

5. The MAb for the labeling of blood cells have to be applied at saturating amounts. Therefore, a white blood cell count must be performed before processing, and the cell concentration adjusted accordingly. One should aim at a cell concentration of 1×10^6/test tube. Samples with a leukocytosis may need to be diluted.

6. The same reagent (single batch) from the same company and in the same dilution should be used throughout the experiment.

7. The mechanisms involved in the decrease of HLA-DR in sepsis include shedding of HLA-DR from the cell surface of monocytes *(7)*. MHC molecules are known to be shedded very easily, e.g., after treatment of cell with interferon *(9)*. To prevent shedding by antibody ligation, the staining procedure of MHC molecules should be carried out at 4°C. We observed no differences between results of labeling of membrane peptidases at 4°C or at room temperature. For reason of simplicity we used 4°C for all antibody incubation steps.

8. In an earlier study authors noted that erythrocyte-lysing reagents cause varying and sometimes substantial reduction in the fluorescence intensity of cells stained directly with CD34 MAb conjugates *(1)*. Therefore, do not change the lysing solution within your study.

9. No-wash protocols and methods using washing steps can clearly differ in their results. We often observed that higher ABC values are obtained in no-wash procedures. Because most investigators in the field of quantitative flow cytometry use at least one washing step, we opted for this method.

10. Flow cytometers should be calibrated according to each laboratory's standard operating procedure. Compensation is a very important point that can affect interlaboratory comparability and reproducibility. In your assay it is useful to avoid multicolor staining with fluorescent dyes that bleach into the PE channel.

11. Two thousand events are a 95% guarantee that the result is within 2% of the "true" value (binomial sampling). This sample mode assumes that the variability of determining replicates is <2%.

References

1. Serke, S., van Lessen, A., and Huhn, D. (1998) Quantitative fluorescence flow cytometry: a comparison of the three techniques for direct and indirect immunofluorescence. *Cytometry* **33,** 179–187.

2. Pannu, K. K., Joe, E. T., and Iyer, S. B. (2001) Performance evaluation of QuantiBRITE phycoerythrin beads. *Cytometry* **45,** 250–258.
3. Schmitz, J. L., Czerniewski, M. A., Edinger, M., et al. (2000) Multisite comparison of methods for the quantitation of the surface expression of CD38 on CD8(+) T lymphocytes. The ACTG Advanced Flow Cytometry Focus Group. *Cytometry* **42,** 174–179.
4. Huschak, G., Zur Nieden, K., Stuttmann, R., and Riemann, D. (2003) Changes in monocytic expression of aminopeptidase N/CD13 after major trauma. *Clin. Exp. Immunol.* **134,** 491–496.
5. Volk, H. D. (2002) Immunodepression in the surgical patient and increased susceptibility to infection. *Crit. Care* **6,** 279–281.
6. Hershman, M. J., Cheadle, W. G., Wellhausen, S. R., Davidson, P. F., and Polk, H. C., Jr. (1990) Monocyte HLA-DR antigen expression characterizes clinical outcome in the trauma patient. *Br. J. Surg.* **77,** 204–207.
7. Perry, S. E., Mostafa, S. M., Wenstone, R., Shenkin, A., and McLaughlin, P. J. (2004) HLA-DR regulation and the influence of GM-CSF on transcription, surface expression and shedding. *Int. J. Med. Sci.* **1,** 126–136.
8. Riemann, D., Blosz, T., Wulfaenger J., Langner, J., and Navarrete Santos, A. (2002) Signal transduction via membrane peptidases. In: *Ectopeptidases,* (Langner, J. and Ansorge, S., eds.), Kluwer Academic/Plenum Publishers, New York, pp. 141–170.
9. Gershon, H. E., Kuang, Y. D., Scala, G., and Oppenheim, J. J. (1985) Effects of recombinant interferon-gamma on HLA-DR antigen shedding by human peripheral blood adherent mononuclear cells. *J. Leukoc. Biol.* **38,** 279–291.
10. Strohmeyer, J. C., Blume, C., Meisel, C., et al. (2003) Standardized immune monitoring for the prediction of infections after cardiopulmonary bypass surgery in risk patients. *Cytometry B Clin. Cytom.* **53,** 54–62.
11. Davis, B. H., Bigelow, N. C., Curnutte, J. T., and Ornvold, K. (1995) Neutrophil CD64 expression: Potential diagnostic indicator of acute inflammation and therapeutic monitor of interferon-γ therapy. *Lab. Hem.* **1,** 3–12.

7

Monitoring Cell Signaling Pathways by Quantitative Flow Cytometry

Huai En Huang Chan, Iman Jilani, Richard Chang, and Maher Albitar

Summary

As the signaling pathways involved in leukemogenesis are being elucidated, several proteins have emerged as potential targets for therapy. Downstream from those targets are numerous intracellular factors that are constantly modulated. Monitoring those factors could provide insight into the potential efficacy of therapies by predicting which patients will respond to them and by determining the optimal dosage that will inhibit the target protein. We describe a flow cytometry method for quantitation of total and phosphorylated intracellular proteins. Compared with Western blot analysis, this technique dramatically decreases time and labor while providing multiparameter information on specific cell populations. As an example, total and phosphorylated CRKL is quantitated. The methodology has the potential for widespread application in the monitoring of targeted therapy.

Key Words: Targeted therapy; quantitative flow cytometry; CML; BCR-ABL; cell-signaling.

1. Introduction

Dysregulation of the factors downstream of the BCR-ABL fusion protein contributes to evasion of programmed cell death and uncontrolled proliferation. Such dysregulation and has been regarded as the driving force for the development of chronic myelogenous leukemia (CML) *(1)*. Though the tyrosine kinase inhibitor imatinib mesylate (Gleevec) has achieved clinical success in the targeting of the BCR-ABL fusion product *(2–4)*, a significant subset of patients has developed resistance to it as a result of mutations affecting the *ABL* kinase domain *(5)*. Thus, several more specific tyrosine kinase inhibitors are being

From: *Methods in Molecular Biology, vol. 378: Monoclonal Antibodies: Methods and Protocols*
Edited by: M. Albitar © Humana Press Inc., Totowa, NJ

developed. A simple and reliable test adaptable for clinical laboratories is needed to monitor BCR-ABL activity and its subsequent inhibition. Measuring the large and unstable BCR-ABL fusion protein itself is difficult (*see* **Note 1**). Thus, the activity of BCR-ABL has been monitored by Western blot analysis of downstream effectors such as CRKL, an adaptor protein that is directly phosphorylated by the BCR-ABL fusion protein in CML and plays a central role in propagating the kinase signal to downstream effectors (*6–8*). Here, we describe a flow cytometry approach that can quantitate intracellular proteins and their phosphorylated forms.

Our approach is based on the permeabilization of viable cells, antibody staining of specific intracellular proteins, and quantification of the stained protein molecules in each cell. The costaining of each cell with surface and intracellular protein markers allows measurement of the number of molecules in specific cell populations. The monitoring of changes in response to therapy is possible owing to protein-specific modifications (for example, phosphorylation). In the following sections, we describe how quantitative flow cytometry can be applied to monitoring levels of total and phosphorylated CRKL in clinical samples and cell lines. We also describe ex vivo drug manipulation of a cell line to ensure antibody specificity and provide a positive control for the assay. For example, exposing K562 (a BCR-ABL–positive blast crisis CML cell line) to imatinib mesylate down–regulates levels of CRKL phosphorylation.

2. Materials

2.1. Fixation and Permeabilization

1. Intraprep permeabilization reagent (Beckman Coulter, Miami, FL).
2. Phosphate-buffered saline (flow PBS): prepare with 5.6 g sodium phosphate dibasic anhydrous, 35.48 g sodium chloride, 2.8 g bovine albumin, and 4 g sodium azide. Add water to 4 L and adjust to pH 7.4 with HCl.
3. Fluorochrome-labeled surface markers: CD3-FITC, CD19-PerCP, and CD34-APC (BD Bioscience, San Jose, CA).
4. Fluorochrome-labeled isotype controls: IgG-FITC, IgG-PerCP, and IgG-APC (BD Bioscience).
5. Primary monoclonal mouse antibody: CRKL (32H4) (Cell Signaling Technology, Beverly, MA).
6. Primary polyclonal rabbit antibodies: phospho CRKL (Tyr 207) (Cell Signaling Technology).
7. Secondary antibodies: goat anti-rabbit conjugated to phycoerythrin (PE) fluorochrome (Santa Cruz Biotechnology, Santa Cruz, CA) and goat anti-mouse conjugated to PE fluorochrome (Jackson ImmunoResearch Laboratories, West Grove, PA).
8. Sorvall cell washer 2 (Thermo Electron Corporation, Asheville, NC).
9. Imatinib mesylate (Gleevec) (Novartis, East Hanover, NJ).

2.2. Flow Cytometric Analysis

1. FACs Calibur flow cytometer (BD Bioscience).
2. CaliBRITE 3 beads (BD Bioscience).
3. CaliBRITE APC beads (BD Bioscience).
4. QuantiBRITE PE beads (BD Bioscience).
5. Cell Quest Pro acquisiton and analysis software (BD Bioscience).
6. FlowJO analysis software (Treestar, Ashland, OR).

3. Methods

Our methodology enables the analysis of specific cell populations by quantitating the number of binding sites (epitopes or molecules) per cell. This is achieved by the use of calibrated bead populations that bind a quantifiable amount of antibody (antibody-binding capacity [ABC]), generating a standard curve that converts channels of mean fluorescence intensity into molecular equivalents of soluble fluorochrome. Specifically, we use QuantiBRITE PE beads (BD Biosciences), where each of the four bead populations has a calibrated mean number of bound PE molecules/bead, which establishes a fluorescence standard for each experiment. Samples are stained with antibodies that are conjugated with PE at a 1:1 ratio. The number of bound PE-conjugated antibodies/cell in the sample is extrapolated using PE beads as a standard. Thus, PE molecules bound/cell is equivalent to the number of antibodies bound to the cell. This, in turn, is equivalent to the number of molecules of target protein in each cell.

3.1. Instrument Setup

1. Calibration is performed prior to each acquisition with CaliBRITE 3 beads and addition of CaliBRITE APC beads, according to the manufacturer's protocol.
2. FACSCalibur is prepared for acquisition by the launching of Cell Quest Pro software. After the flow sheath and waste levels are checked (recommended), the appropriate acquisition template and instrument settings are selected.
3. Before acquisition of samples, standardization is performed with QuantiBRITE PE beads, which are reconstituted with 1 mL of flow PBS. Five thousand events are acquired on the FACSCalibur. An example of a result is shown in **Fig. 1**.

3.2. Specimen and Reagent Preparation for Quantitative Flow Cytometry

1. To quantitate CRKL, label four 12×75-mm flow tubes—one tube each for total and phosphorylated primary CRKL antibodies and one tube each for each primary antibody's isotype controls (*see* **Note 2**).
2. Pipet the appropriate volume of peripheral blood (equivalent to 1×10^6 cells) into each of the four flow tubes and incubate in the presence of either 10 µL surface markers or 5 µL isotype controls for each fluorochrome for 15 min at room temperature in the dark.

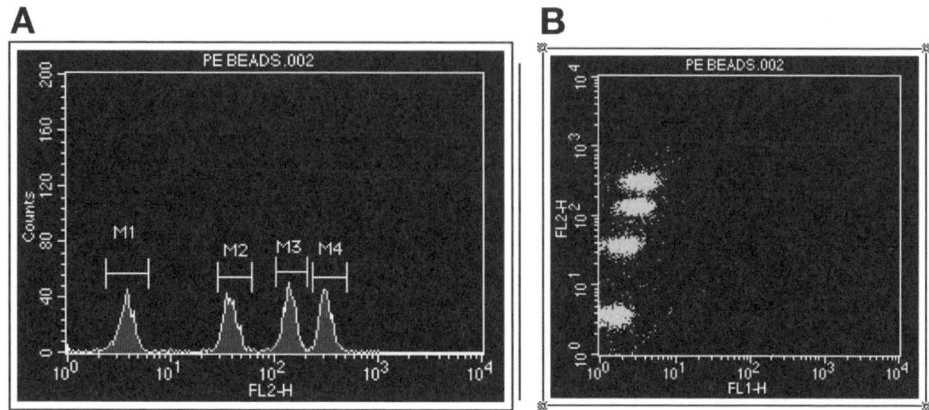

Fig. 1. Histograms (**A**) and dot plot (**B**) representing QuantiBRITE phycoerythrin (PE) beads. QuantiBRITE PE beads are a set of four beads with known levels of PE conjugated on them. These are acquired in every experiment and used as a fluorescence standard to convert molecular equivalents of soluble fluorochrome to antibody-binding capacity.

3.3. Fixation and Permeabilization

1. Fix cells in 100 µL Intraprep reagent 1 for 15 min at room temperature in the dark, and then wash in the cell washer with flow PBS (*see* **Note 3**).
2. Vortex to ensure full resuspension of the cell pellet, then permeabilize cells with 100 µL Intraprep reagent 2 for 5 min at room temperature in the dark.
3. Incubate cells in the presence of 1 µg IgG isotype control or primary antibody (CRKL [32H4] or phospho-CRKL [Tyr 207]) for 15 min at room temperature in the dark.
4. Wash cells in the cell washer and resuspend them in 50 µL flow PBS.
5. Incubate the cells in the presence of 0.75 µg PE-conjugated secondary antibody for 15 min at room temperature in the dark.
6. Wash cells in the cell washer and resuspend in flow PBS for analysis (keep samples in the dark until ready to acquire).

3.4. Acquisition and Analysis

1. 5000 events are acquired for every sample (*see* **Note 4**). Flow cytometry output is in the form of FCS files.
2. Analysis gates are placed around cellular populations of interest for the evaluation of the percentage of cells stained with antibodies relative to cells stained with isotype controls. An example of a result is shown in **Fig. 2**.
3. Flow cytometry output is converted in terms of ABC of CD3+, CD19+, or CD34+ cells using PE labeled with antibodies in a 1:1 ratio.
4. Though several data analysis programs are commercially available, we use FlowJO software.

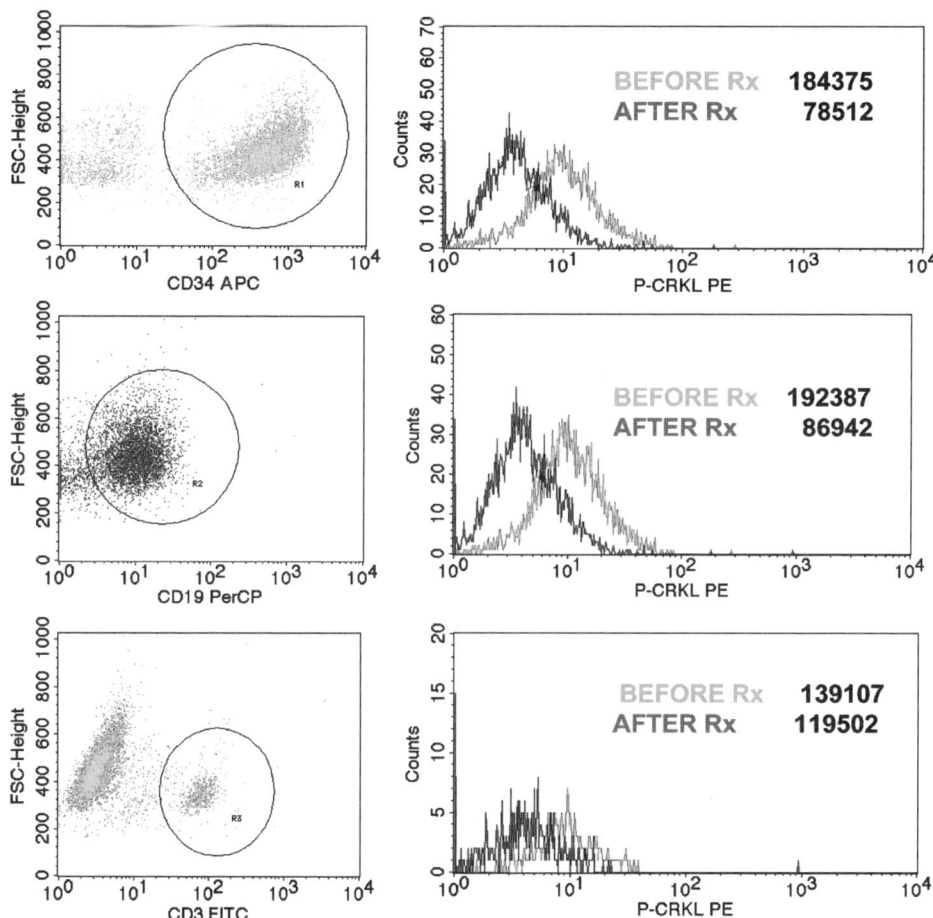

Fig. 2. Dot plots and histograms representing cells from a chronic myelogenous leukemia patient in lymphoid blast crisis before and after treatment with a tyrosine kinase inhibitor. Cells were fixed and stained with antibodies specific for phospho-CRKL at Tyr 207 residue (0.05 mg/50 μL). The left column shows dot plots of a sample before treatment. The *x*- and *y*-axis correspond to CD surface marker and phospho-CRKL PE, respectively. Analysis gates (R1-3) were placed around CD34+, CD19+, and CD3+ cell populations. The right column shows histograms based on cellular populations delineated by analysis gates before and after treatment. In each histogram, the *y*-axis represents cell count while the *x*-axis represents phycoerythrin shift. Index values of cells are noted pre- and post-therapy.

5. For each sample, each cellular population generates the percentage positivity and ABC, which, when multiplied together, generate the index value (*see* **Note 5**).

3.5. Procedure for Culturing and Drug Treatment of the K562 Cell Line

1. K562 cells are maintained in RPMI-1640 supplemented with 10% fetal bovine serum and antibiotics.
2. 1×10^6 K562 cells are plated in a six-well tissue culture plate and treated with dimethyl sulfoxide alone or 0.5 μM imatinib. Cells are incubated 18 h at 37°C in 5% CO_2.
3. Cells are then washed two times with 1X PBS followed by lysing and permeabilization according to the protocol, starting with **Subheading 3.3.** An example of a result is shown in **Fig. 3**.

3.6. Discussion

We describe a rapid and reliable procedure for quantitation of intracellular proteins modulated by targeted therapy. The approach presents several advantages over conventional Western blot analysis. Costaining specific cell populations with surface markers allows monitoring of total and phosphorylated intracellular protein levels for each subpopulation. Quantitative multiparameter information is generated for each sample per analyte for every 100 cells. Technically, this approach requires much less sample volume and minimal manipulation of sample, maintaining the integrity of the proteins of interest.

The modulation of intracellular proteins can be manifested as changes in cellular positivity or fluorescence intensity. Combining the two factors into an index value provides a unit for measuring changes in total and phosphorylation levels of proteins. The ratio of phosphorylated-to-total protein changes could provide insight on drug efficacy.

The same approach can be used to monitor intracellular protein modulation other than phosphorylation. For example, histone acetylation can be quantitated in patients undergoing treatment with histone deacetylase (HDAC) inhibitors. Monitoring levels of these downstream factors may provide a means of customizing therapy by predicting which patients will respond to a given treatment and determining optimal dosage.

4. Notes

1. A novel bead-based approach to the direct and quantitative measurement of fusion proteins such as BCR-ABL is described in Chapter 12.
2. When available, rabbit and mouse isotype controls are used. Nonstaining cell populations within the sample can be used as negative controls.
3. Several other fixation and permeabilization reagents also available.
4. Though it is preferable to acquire 5000 events, depending on the sample, a smaller number may provide adequate quantitative information.
5. The index is derived by multiplying the percentage positivity by the ABC. This takes into account both changes.

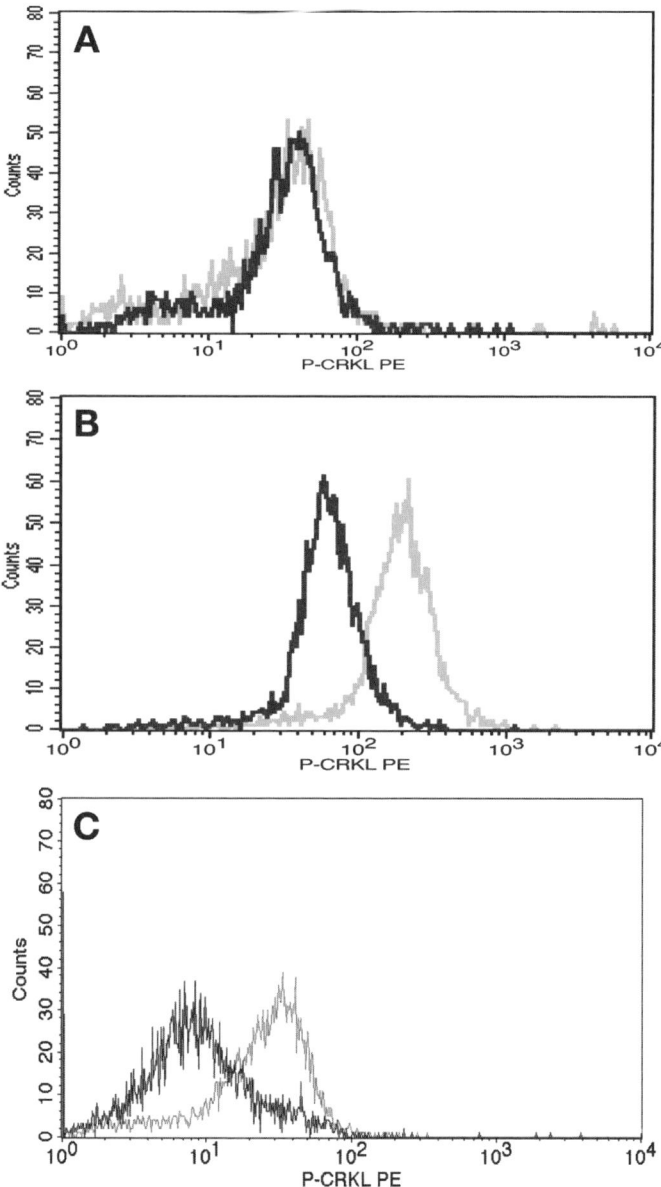

Fig. 3. Histograms representing the effect of an imatinib mesylate on drug insensitive cell lines **(A)**, a drug-sensitive BCR-ABL positive cell line **(B)** and CD34+ blast
cells from a chronic myelogenous leukemia patient **(C)**. Cells were fixed and stained
with phospho-CRKL (0.05 mg/50 μL). The grey (pretherapy) and black (posttherapy)
lines denote immunofluorescence before and after treatment, respectively. Index values
of cells are noted pre- and posttherapy.

References

1. Chopra, R., Pu, Q. Q., and Elefanty, A .G. (1999) Biology of BCR-ABL. *Blood Rev.* **13,** 211–229.
2. Kantarjian, H. M., Talpaz, M., Cortes J., et al. (2003) Quantitative polymerase chain reaction monitoring of BCR-ABL during therapy with imatinib mesylate (STI571; Gleevec) in chronic-phase chronic myelogenous leukemia. *Clin. Cancer Res.* **9,** 160–166.
3. O'Brien, S. G., Guilhot, F., Larson, R. A., et al. (2003) Imatinib compared with interferon and low-dose cytarabine for newly diagnosed chronic-phase chronic myeloid leukemia. *N. Engl. J. Med.* **348,** 994–1004.
4. Deininger, M., Buchdunger, E., and Druker, B. J. (2003) The development of imatinib as a therapeutic agent for chronic myeloid leukemia. *Blood* **105,** 1321–1331.
5. Gorre, M. E., Mohammed, M., Ellwood, K., et al. (2001) Clinical resistance to STI-571 cancer therapy caused by BCR-ABL gene mutation or amplification. *Science* **293,** 876–880.
6. ten Hoeve, J., Arlinghaus, R. B., Guo, J. Q., Heisterkamp, N., and Groffen, J. (1994) Tyrosine phosphorylation of CRKL in Philadelphia+ leukemia. *Blood* **84,** 1731–1736.
7. Oda, T., Heaney, C., Hagopian, J. R., Okuda, K., Griffin, J. D., and Druker, B. J. (1994) Crkl is the major tyrosine-phophorylated protein in neutrophils from patients with chronic myelogenous leukemia. *J. Biol. Chem.* **269,** 22,925–22,928.
8. Nichols, G. L., Raines, M. A., Vera, J. C., Lacomis, L., Tempst, P., anf Golde, D. W. (1994) Identification of CRKL as the constitutively phosphorylated 39-kD tyrosine phosphoprotein in chronic myelogenous leukemia cells. *Blood* **84,** 2912–2918.

8

Antibodies and Immunohistochemical Evaluation for the Diagnosis of Hematological Malignancies

An Overview

Dennis P. O'Malley and Attilio Orazi

Summary

The immunohistochemical evaluation of hematopoietic tissues has expanded our knowledge of both the function and pathological processes in a wide range of lymph nodal, extranodal tissues, and bone marrow. It is impossible to cover in detail the full range of immunohistochemical markers, which are available to study hematopoietic cells and their malignant counterparts. This chapter attempts to provide an overview of the antibodies, which are commonly used in studying the hematopoietic and lymphoid tissues and to diagnose hematological disorders. In addition, an immunohistology-based diagnostic approach to identify specific neoplastic entities is described in some length.

Key Words: Bone marrow; lymph node; spleen immunohistochemistry; leukemia; lymphoma; diagnosis.

1. Introduction

The immunohistochemical evaluation has expanded our knowledge of both the function and pathological processes in a wide range of lymph nodal, extranodal tissues, and bone marrow (BM). It is impossible to consider the full range of immunohistochemical markers available for studying hematopoietic tissues as well as the wide variety of ways to approach the evaluation of lymph node, extranodal tissues, or BM.

Without a doubt, immunohistochemistry (IHC) is more extensively used in hematopathology than in any other subspecialty area of pathology. In parallel with our understanding of phenotypical and immunological composition of the hematopoietic system, our armamentarium of paraffin section-reactive markers has grown as well. In some cases, it could be said that we have "too many

From: *Methods in Molecular Biology, vol. 378: Monoclonal Antibodies: Methods and Protocols*
Edited by: M. Albitar © Humana Press Inc., Totowa, NJ

markers," leading to confusion and challenges in choosing and interpreting them wisely.

It is important to recognize that fundament for IHC interpretation is a careful histological analysis of a thin, well-stained H&E section. Simply having the best histology possible can avoid a variety of problems. Too often, poor quality is replaced by a battery of IHC stains. This is unfortunate, not cost effective, and ultimately is poor patient care. Rather than try to make a difficult diagnosis on suboptimal material, it may be best to simply obtain another better quality specimen. Among the technical factors that plague interpretation of IHC are thickness of section, folds or wrinkles in section, interference by fixative (i.e., B5, Bouin's), inadequate blocking of endogenous peroxidase (especially liver or peroxidase-rich cells), ineffective counterstaining (hematoxylin, fast green), and over/understaining *(1–4)*.

Especially when dealing with small biopsy samples, it is crucial to order up front, in addition to the H&E-stained sections, an adequate number of unstained slides, as an insurance policy for the potential need for additional stains. Proper selection of immunostains requires a preliminary differential diagnosis. A careful microscopic interpretation is as important for IHC as it is for conventionally stained sections *(5)*. It is important to know the expected reaction pattern of the immunostain being used because the cellular and tissue localization of the stain reaction is often a critical factor in its interpretation. Surface staining may be especially difficult to evaluate, particularly when numerous cells are closely crowded together. Cytoplasmic staining tends to be easier to interpret. Golgi staining is often very specific (e.g., seen with CD30, CD15), but is seen only in selected cases. Nuclear staining can be also very specific, in the right context, particularly in stains that are expected to have exclusive nuclear reactivity (such as TdT, cyclin D1, and so on). "Edge artifact" is common, resulting in intensification of staining along section edges. Its cause is not fully understood, but it can hamper adequate interpretation.

2. IHC of Bone Marrow

2.1. Bone Marrow

A comprehensive evaluation of BM involves examination of both marrow smears and tissue sections; each is complementary to the other. With the growing battery of paraffin-reactive immunohistological reagents, coupled with newer techniques of antigen retrieval, new vistas have opened in the study of BM biopsies (BMB) *(6)*.

Normal BM consists of a heterogeneous population of cells proceeding along various differentiation pathways. Although most cell types can be easily distinguished on BM aspirate smears and biopsy sections, IHC is valuable in identifying specific cell subsets.

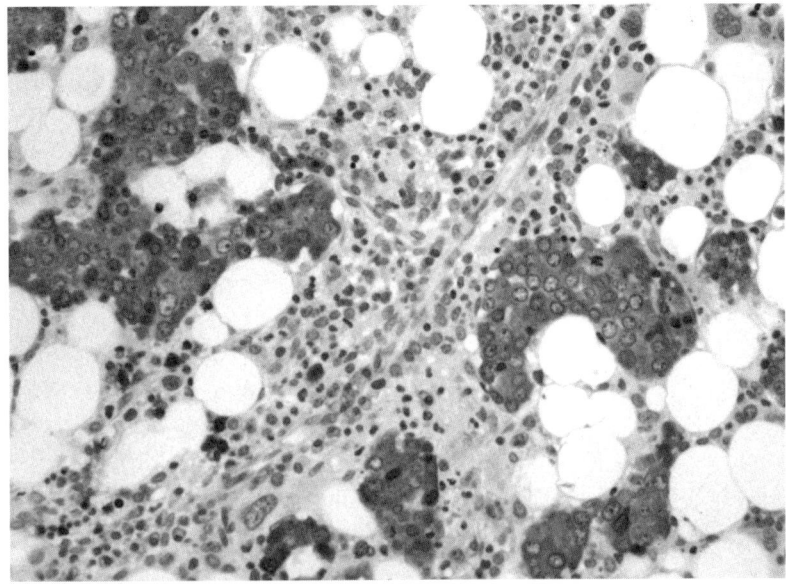

Fig. 1. Antihemoglobin stain highlighting erythroid precursors in bone marrow with megaloblastic leukemia.

2.1.1. Erythroid

Erythroid cells account for 5–38% of the nucleated cells in normal BM. Antibodies reactive with hemoglobin (**Fig. 1**) or glycophorin A can be used to identify the erythroid cells in BMB.

2.1.2. Granulocytes and Monocytes

Myeloid cells account for 23–85% of the nucleated cells in the normal BM and can be effectively identified by using an anti-myeloperoxidase (MPO) antibody *(7)*. MPO is expressed in cells of to the neutrophilic and eosinophilic series, as well as by some monocytes (**Fig. 2**). Other antibodies that can be useful in selected cases include CD15, CD45RO, and CD43. The KP-1 epitope of CD68 and lysozyme (**Fig. 3**) react with both myeloid and monocytes/macrophages cells, the PG-M1 epitope is mostly restricted to latter cells *(8)*.

2.1.3. Megakaryocytes

Megakaryocytes can be identified in tissue sections by their positivity with factor VIII, CD42b, CD61, CD31, and anti-LAT. Although these markers are more strongly expressed in mature megakaryocytes, they can also be used to identify immature cells of the megakaryocytic lineage *(9)*.

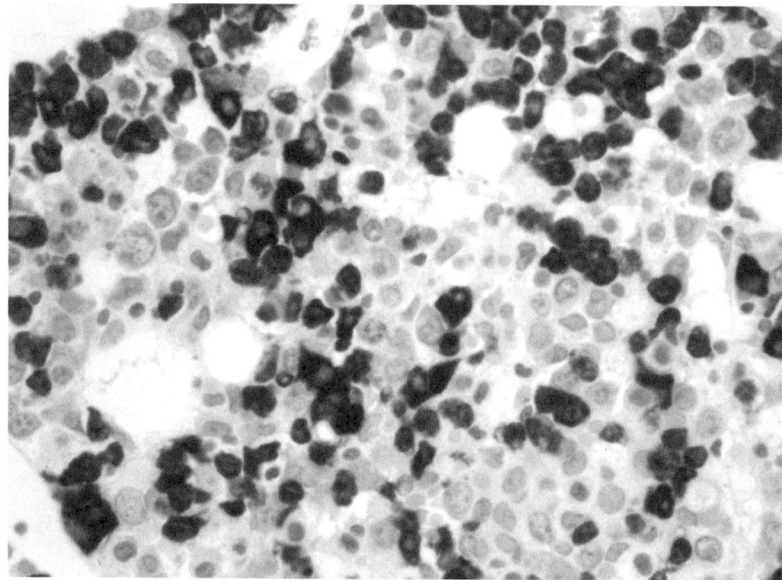

Fig. 2. Myeloperoxidase stain in bone marrow, which highlights granulocytic cells and some monocytes.

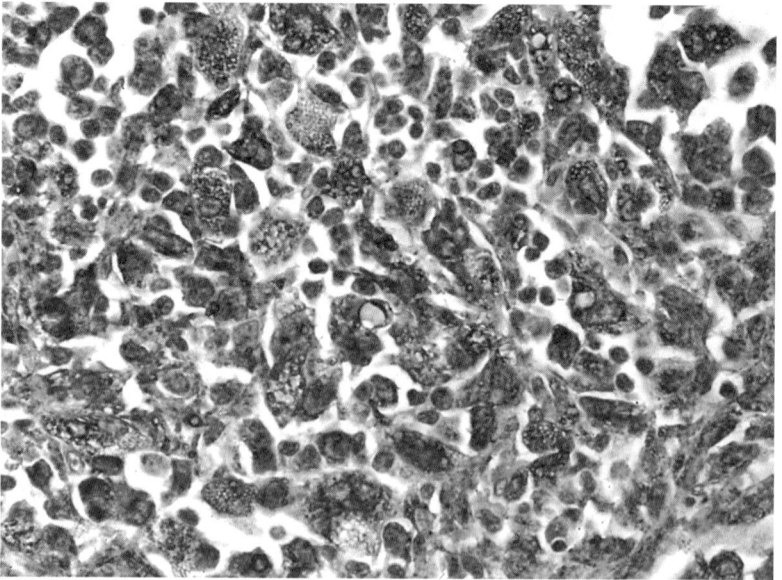

Fig. 3. Lysozyme immunohistochemical stain, highlighting numerous granulocytes, monocytic elements, and macrophages in this bone marrow.

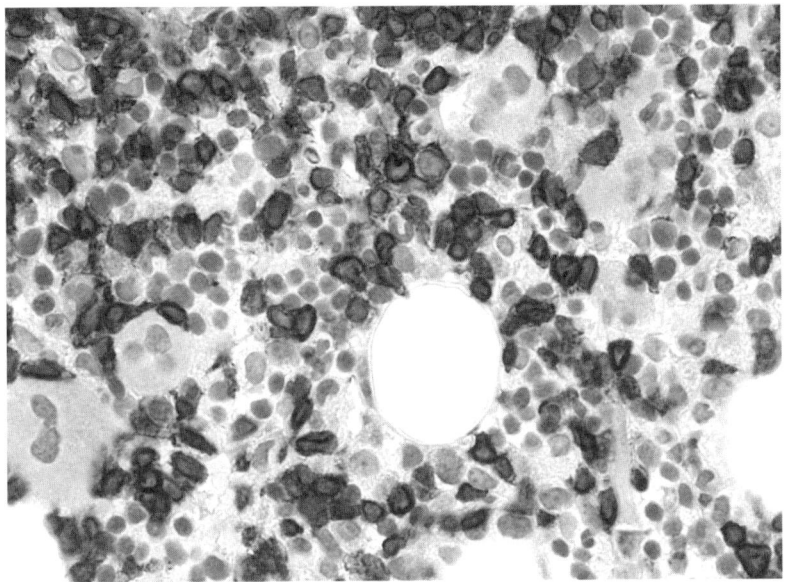

Fig. 4. A CD3 stain showing infiltration of bone marrow by numerous T-cells in this case of T-cell large granular lymphocytic leukemia.

2.1.4. Lymphoid Cells

Lymphocytes typically account for 1–5% of the nucleated cells in the normal BM. Lymphoid follicles may also be observed, especially after the age of 50. There are a wide variety of antibodies available for identification of benign and malignant lymphoid cells in BM. The most useful of these are CD20 (B-cells) and CD3 (T-cells) (**Fig. 4**).

2.1.5. Precursor Cells

TdT-, CD10-, and CD79a-positive early B-cell precursors (also termed hematogones) are normally present in small number in the adult marrow, whereas they are more numerous in the pediatric ages. Hematogones are occasionally difficult to distinguish from acute lymphoblastic leukemia (ALL). In ALL, the blasts are usually uniformly positive for CD34 and TdT, and hematogones are less uniformly positive for CD34. In both pediatric and adult BM, CD34-positive cells, which may be either myeloid or lymphoid precursors, are present singly and account for less than 5% of the nucleated cells *(10)*.

2.2. Acute Leukemias

Immunophenotypical features of leukemic cells are an integral component of the current World Health Organization classification of hematological

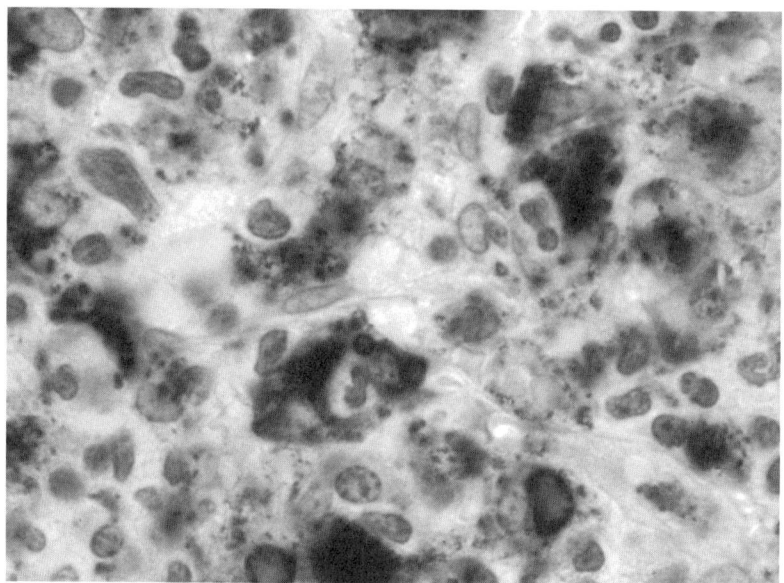

Fig. 5. CD68 (PG-M1) expression in macrophages in this case of hemophagocytic syndrome.

malignancies. Immunophenotypical information by IHC is of particular value when interpreting BMB in patients where marrow aspirates are unavailable (e.g., owing to myelofibrosis).

CD34, TdT, CD117 markers, which are only expressed by immature cells, can be of particular value in assessing the proportion of blasts present in a BMB *(11,12)*. This might be particularly valuable in highlighting small numbers of residual blasts in posttreatment samples (minimal residual disease).

Acute myeloid leukemias (AML) are a group of neoplastic proliferations of BM precursor cells ("blasts") of granulocytic, monocytic, erythroid, or mega-karyocytic lineages *(7)*. Using an appropriate battery of lineage- and differenti-ation-associated immunostains, the nature of the blasts can often be correctly identified.

MPO is positive in blasts of both neutrophilic and eosinophilic lineages. Cells of monocytic derivation are weakly positive or nonreactive. MPO immunostaining is more sensitive than cytochemistry performed on BM aspi-rates in recognizing minimally and poorly differentiated AML *(13)*. Lysozyme represents a useful "back up" pan-myeloid antibody.

CD68 is expressed throughout the monocytic differentiation, usually more intensely in macrophages than in monocytes (**Fig. 5**). In BMB, CD68 antibod-ies are used to identify cases of AML with a monocytic component; the CD68/

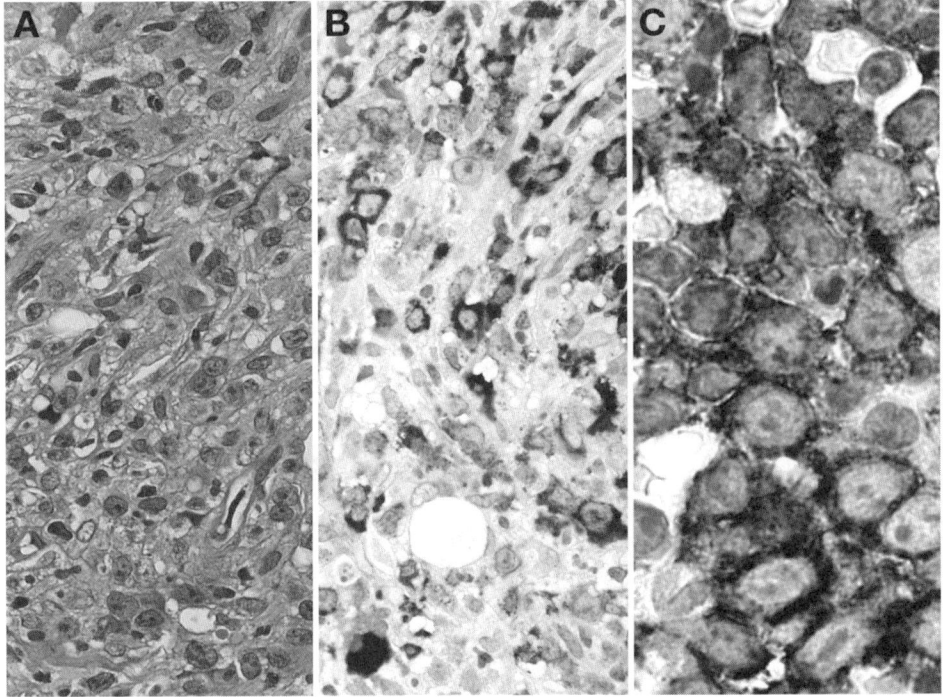

Fig. 6. Staining a case of acute megakaryoblastic leukemia. (**A**) H&E. (**B**) Factor VIII antigen (von Willebrand factor). (**C**) Anti-LAT antibody expression in megakaryoblasts.

PG-M1 epitope being preferred *(8)*. CD163 represents another useful marker, which has recently become available *(14)*.

Acute erythroleukemia can be identified by the antihemoglobin (or anti-glycophorin A) immunostain. The stain(s) can also be used to confirm the erythroid nature of the "worrisome looking" proerythroblasts observed in patients with megaloblastic anemia.

Identification of megakaryocytes is typically not difficult by morphology, although several immunohistochemical stains are available including factor VIII, CD42b, CD61, CD31, and anti-LAT (**Figs. 6** and **7**) *(9)*. Megakaryoblastic leukemia is typically associated with extensive marrow fibrosis, which usually precludes the possibility of employing marrow aspirate-based diagnostic techniques. Immunoperoxidase staining of BMB is often the crucial diagnostic step in these patients. All antibodies stain normal megakaryocytes in biopsy sections but only a proportion of cases of acute megakaryoblastic leukemia. Often, a panel of antibodies is necessary to achieve a correct identification. Of the antibodies previously listed, CD31 is the least specific and factor VIII the one associated highest nonspecific background. Identification of micromegakaryocytes

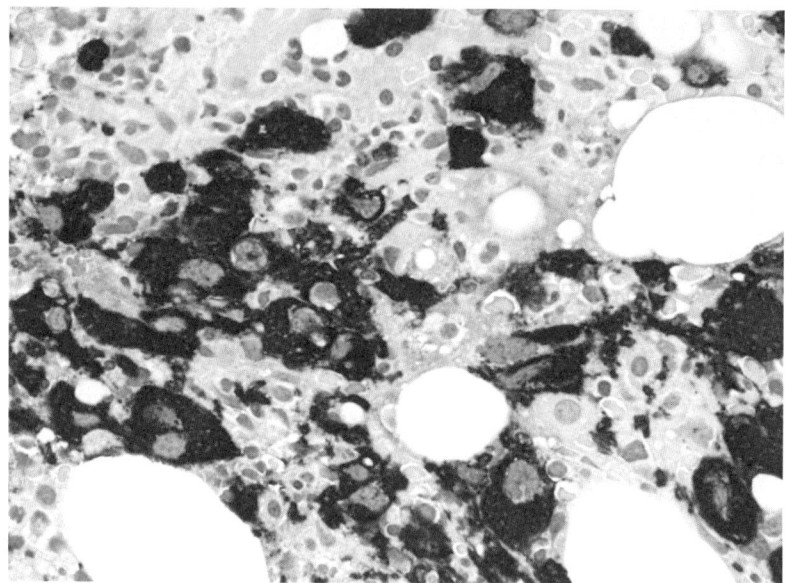

Fig. 7. CD42b expression in large, abnormal megakaryocytes and megakaryoblasts in a case of acute panmyelosis with myelofibrosis.

is useful in confirming acute panmyelosis with myelofibrosis and myelodysplastic syndromes with fibrosis (MDS-f).

ALL is one of the most common malignancies seen in pediatric patients. Although flow cytometry and cytogenetics retain their dominant role in the evaluation of ALL, paraffin IHC may provide important adjunct information. TdT, CD34, and CD99 positivity is used to confirm the precursor status of the leukemic cells (**Fig. 8**) *(15)*. TdT is positive in almost all T- and most B-cell ALLs *(11)*. CD79a is more frequently positive than is CD20 in precursor B-ALL. CD10 is positive in the majority of cases of precursor B-cell ALL, and, less frequently (40%), in T-ALL; TdT and CD99 are usually negative in mature B-cell ALL; in these CD10 and CD20 are strongly expressed. CD3 is employed, in conjunction with TdT, to identify cases of T-cell ALL. Other T-cell antibodies CD2, CD5, CD7, and CD1a can also be useful in selected cases.

2.3. Myelodysplastic Syndromes, Myeloproliferative Disorders, and Aplastic Anemia

Myelodysplastic syndromes (MDS) are a heterogeneous group of clonal hematopoietic disorders that are divided into diagnostic categories primarily based on the percentage of blast cells, the presence of ringed sideroblasts, and the cell lineage affected by dysplasia.

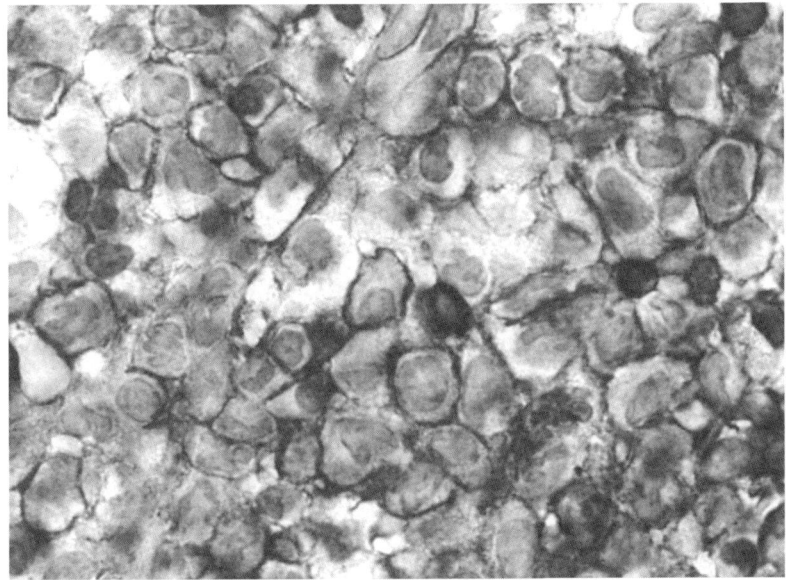

Fig. 8. CD99 expression in blasts of an acute leukemia.

In MDS, the presence of clusters of blasts in nonparatrabecular or perivascular location (also termed abnormal localization of immature precursors) are associated with a poor prognosis. CD34 can be used to highlight the presence of abnormal localization of immature precursors (**Fig. 9**) *(12,16,17)*. This finding, as well as an increase in the percentage of CD34-positive cells, is associated with a higher frequency of leukemic transformation and short survival in MDS cases. The occurrence of large sheets of CD34-positive blasts confirms transformation AML. Similar findings may be associated with transformation of CML to acute leukemia *(18)*. Immunostaining for CD34 is especially important in two subsets of patients with MDS: MDS with fibrosis and MDS with hypocellular marrow (MDS-h). MDS-f is characterized by the presence of significant degrees of marrow fibrosis, which preclude aspiration for either flow cytometric or cytogenetic analysis. In these cases, the presence of increased CD34 expression in the marrow is often helpful in the diagnosis (most cases of MDS-f have an excess of blasts). In MDS-h, CD34 can be used to distinguish hypoplastic MDS from acquired aplastic anemia (**Fig. 10**). The former disorder is characterized by higher CD34 counts as compared with aplastic anemia *(19)*.

3. IHC of Lymphoid Tissues

One useful approach to the evaluation of lymphoid tissues is to examine it in terms of "functional" compartments. Using lymph node as the archetype, the

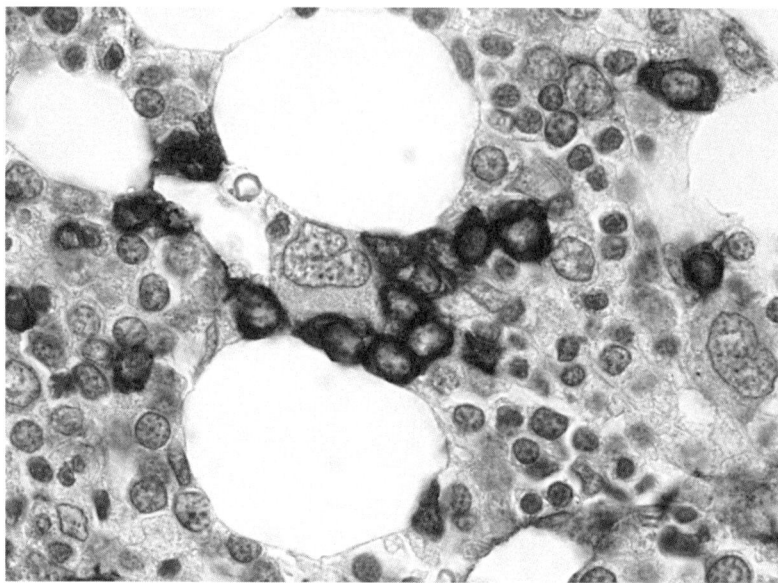

Fig. 9. CD34 expression in a cluster of cells, highlighting abnormal localization of immature precursors in a case of myelodysplastic syndrome.

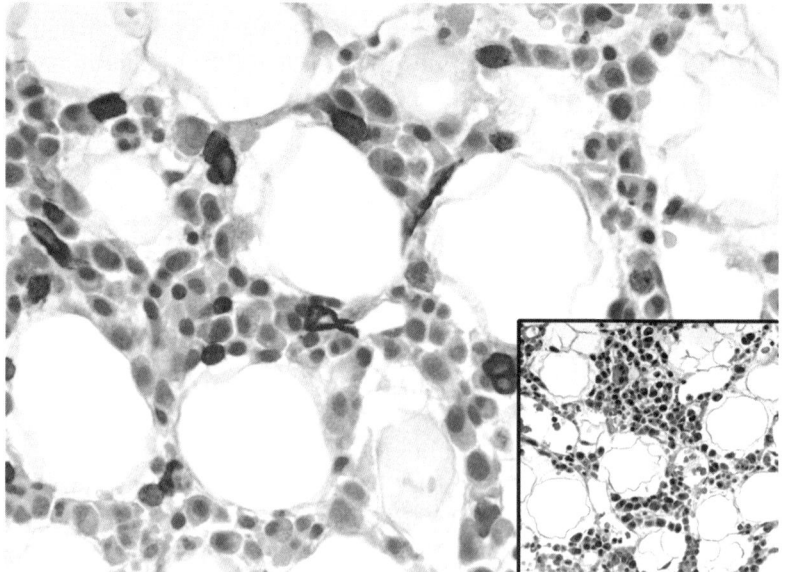

Fig. 10. Hypoplastic myelodysplastic syndrome with increased CD34 expression in blasts. Inset: H&E section of same case.

lymphoid tissue can be divided into several components. The first of these is the lymphoid follicle, which is predominantly composed of B-cells. Additionally, there is the interfollicular compartment, composed of a mixture of both B- and T-cells, with predominance of the latter. Then, there are the lymphoid sinuses, other distinctive components of the lymph node include the medullary cords, the stromal framework, and other functional areas.

3.1. B-Cells

Evaluation of B- cells in general is facilitated by a wide variety of antibodies *(20,21)*. The most commonly used antibody is CD20, an antibody directed at the surface molecule of B- cells involved in activation, proliferation, and differentiation. This antibody is robust in its technical performance and in its sensitivity and specificity for identification of B-cells. CD20 expression is limited in B-cell development; it is not expressed on the earliest B-lymphoid precursors (e.g., precursor B-cell ALL), and is also not expressed in plasma cells. New treatments based on monoclonal antibodies directed against CD20 molecule are regularly used in the treatment of B-cell lymphomas. Because of this, it is likely that many recurrences of lymphomas will downregulate the expression of CD20, lessening the usefulness of this IHC for this antibody in certain circumstances.

There are other B-cells antibodies that are also quite useful. CD79a is a molecule that has a functional role in supporting and maintaining the surface immunoglobulin receptors on the surface of B-cells. It is expressed throughout the entire lifespan of B-cells, from the stage of early, committed B-cell lymphoblasts, through immature and mature B-cells, as well as plasma cells. PAX-5, CD22, CD74, LN1/LN2 are other antibodies that are preferentially expressed on B cells, both benign and malignant (**Fig. 11**) *(22–24)*. Plasma cell neoplasms are identified with great specificity and sensitivity by using CD138 (**Fig. 12**) *(25)*.

3.1.1. Lymphoid Follicles

The follicles of the lymph node are home to the B-cell component of the immune response. Follicle composition, morphology, and cellular composition are affected by the state of the immune response.

Several antibodies are selectively expressed on germinal center B-cells *(26–29)*. Bcl-6 is preferentially expressed in B-cells of follicle center derivation. Besides normal secondary follicles/germinal centers, Bcl-6 is also expressed in neoplasms of follicle center cell derivation including follicular lymphoma, subsets of diffuse large B-cell lymphomas (DLBCL), and Burkitt lymphoma. Bcl-6 expression is not seen in other B-cell lymphomas, such as mantle cell lymphoma or marginal zone lymphoma. Bcl-6 is a nuclear protein and the pattern of immunohistochemical expression is that of distinct nuclear positivity. CD10 is also expressed on cells of follicle center derivation (**Fig. 13**). Besides

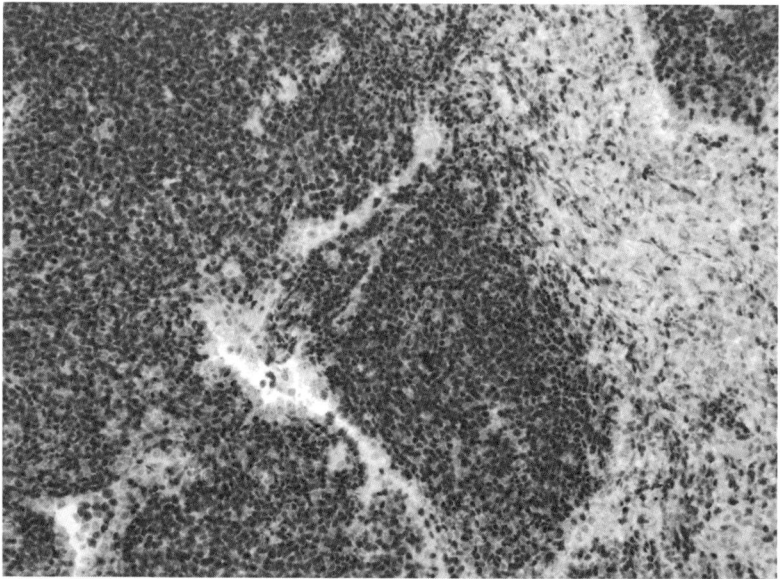

Fig. 11. Diffuse, nuclear expression of PAX-5 in this small B-cell lymphoma.

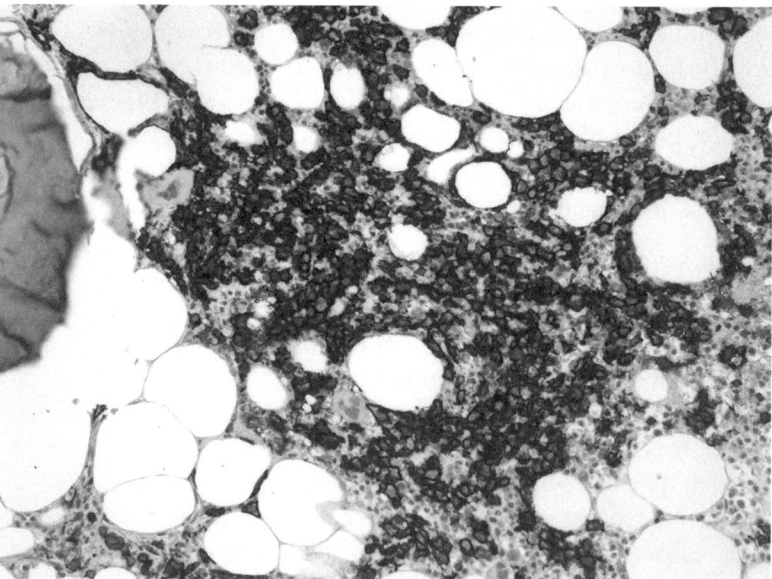

Fig. 12. CD138 strongly stains plasma cells in this case of plasma cell myeloma in the bone marrow.

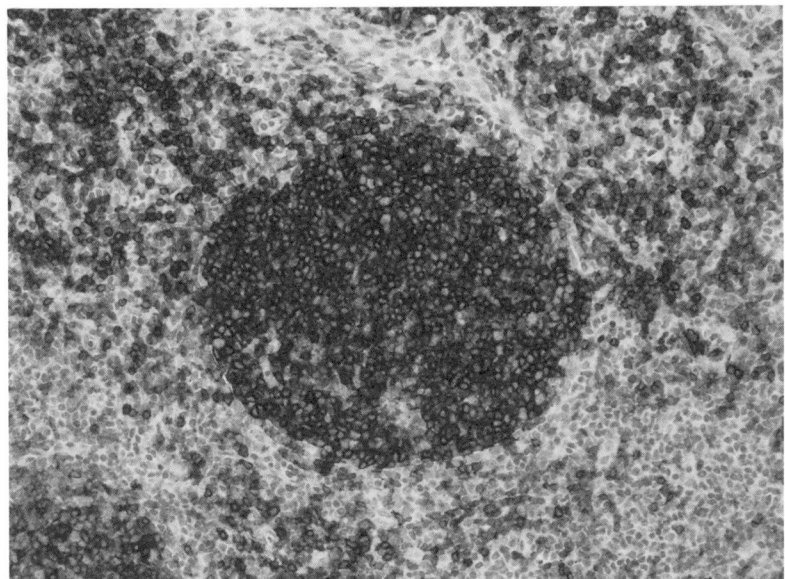

Fig. 13. A follicular lymphoma showing strong CD10 expression in the neoplastic cells.

follicle center cells, it is also expressed on a subset of ALL, DLBCL, and Burkitt lymphoma. A proportion of the malignant cells in angioimmunoblastic T-cell lymphoma coexpress CD10 and T-cell antigens.

3.2. T-Cells

Numerous antibodies reactive with T-cells have become available during the last decade. Among these, CD3 and CD2 are widely used as pan T-cell markers because they are expressed throughout the entire lifespan of T-cells, from the stage of early T-cell precursor lymphoblasts, through immature and mature CD4 or CD8 positive T-cells. CD45RO and CD43 antibodies, which were previously used extensively as pan T-cell markers, lack specificity and should not be considered as "first line" T-cell markers. Other paraffin-reactive antibodies frequently used to characterize T-cell lymphoid malignancy include TdT, CD1a, CD5, CD4, CD8, CD7, CD30, Alk-1, CD56, and TIA-1.

T-cell lymphomas are relatively rare and account for only about 10% of lymphomas in North America. T-cell lymphomas consist of a wide range of different clinical entities; however, most are classified in the general category of peripheral T-cell lymphoma unspecified.

Diagnosis of T-cell lymphomas is dependent on finding a proliferation of abnormal T- cells. Although simply the presence of large numerical increases (e.g., >80% of cellularity), in T-cells is suspicious it is not diagnostic. The most

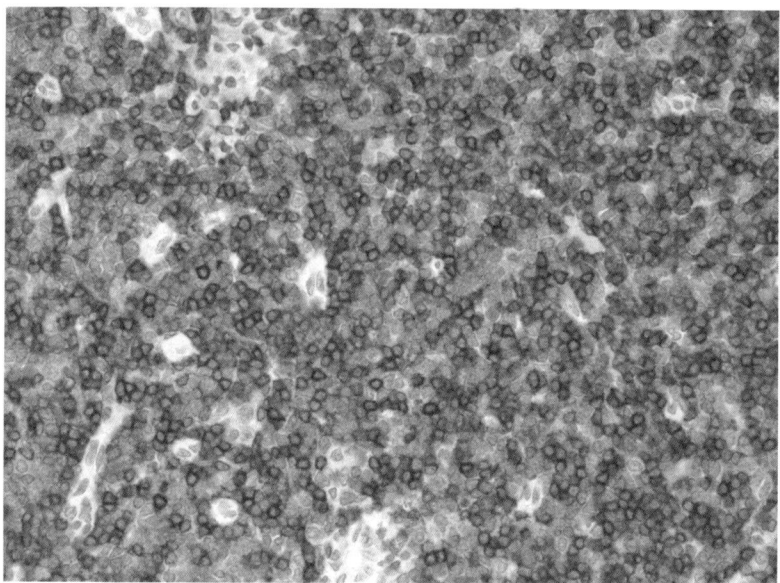

Fig. 14. T-cell lymphoblastic lymphoma with CD1a expression. CD1a expression is not seen in normal, mature T-cells.

supportive findings of T-cell lymphomas are, in order of importance: the presence of T-cell clonality by molecular techniques, an aberrant T-cell immunophenotype (e.g., selective loss of T-cell antigen expression), a large numerical preponderance of a specific subtype of T-cells (either CD4 or CD8) or expression of CD1a or TdT (**Fig. 14**). Although each of these criteria is important, there are circumstances where each may be seen in nonneoplastic conditions, so individual features should be taken in the general clinical context.

Precursor T-cell immunophenotype is decidedly abnormal except in very limited circumstances. Namely, they are normally found in the thymus. They are also found in thymoma. Precursor T-cell lymphoblastic lymphoma will often have expression of immature T-cell immunophenotype *(11,30)*. This includes expression of TdT and often CD1a. The lack of CD4 and CD8 expression (e.g., seen in hepatosplenic T-cell lymphoma) or coexpression of CD4 and CD8 (e.g., T-cell prolymphocytic leukemia) are occasionally helpful in the differential diagnosis of T-cell lymphomas.

3.2.1. Lymphoid Sinuses

As a compartment, the sinuses of a lymph node are often inapparent. Occasionally, when there is a reactive process, there may be dilation of the sinuses because of the presence of an increased number of lymphocytes. An increased number of intrasinusoidal macrophages are also often seen in reactive

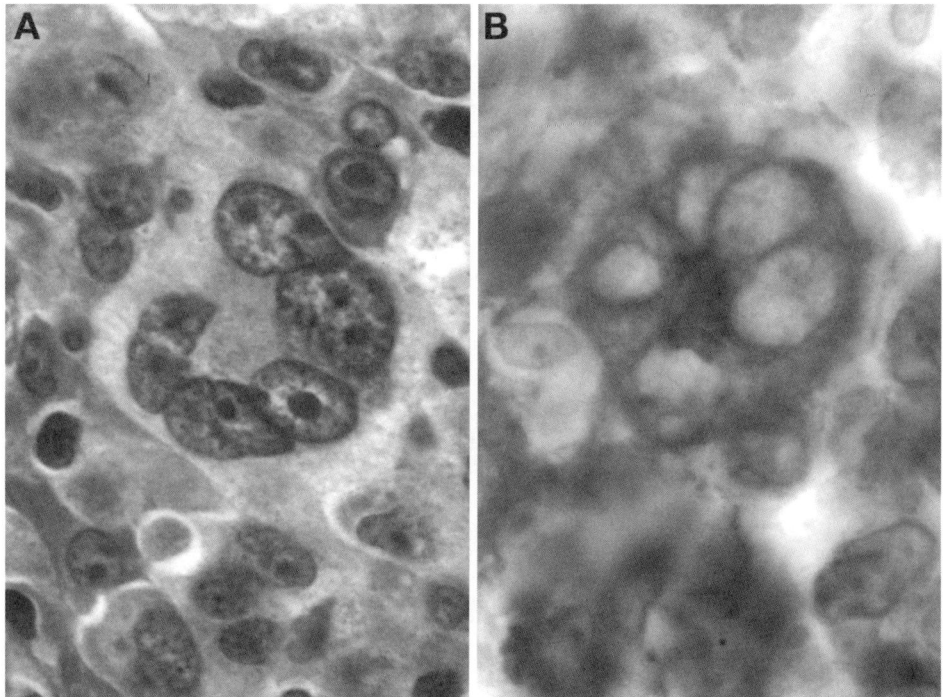

Fig. 15. (A) H&E of a "hallmark" cell of anaplastic large cell lymphoma with (B) CD30 expression. Note the strong staining of the Golgi zone in this case.

conditions (sinus histiocytosis). Malignancies that have a significant leukemic spread (e.g., leukemic disorders such as chronic lymphocytic leukemia) often cause an expansion of the sinus compartment as well as of the interfollicular areas. Other neoplasms with a sinusoidal tropism include lymphoplasmacytic lymphoma, anaplastic large cell lymphoma (ALCL), and metastatic carcinoma.

ALCL often, at least initially, involves lymph nodes in a sinusoidal pattern, which may simulate the appearance of metastatic carcinoma. ALCL is usually identified at least initially by its positivity for CD30. The staining is often membranous and cytoplasmic, sometimes with a Golgi pattern (**Fig. 15**). Although of T-cell derivation, ALCL only occasionally expresses a full complement of T-cell antigens. It is only positive for CD3 in about 50% of cases. They are most often positive for CD4, CD43, and TIA-1 *(31)*.

3.2.2. Proliferation

Although not required for diagnostic evaluation, the assessment of proliferative and apoptotic activities can occasionally be of value in diagnosing lymphomas and in providing prognostic information *(32–34)*.

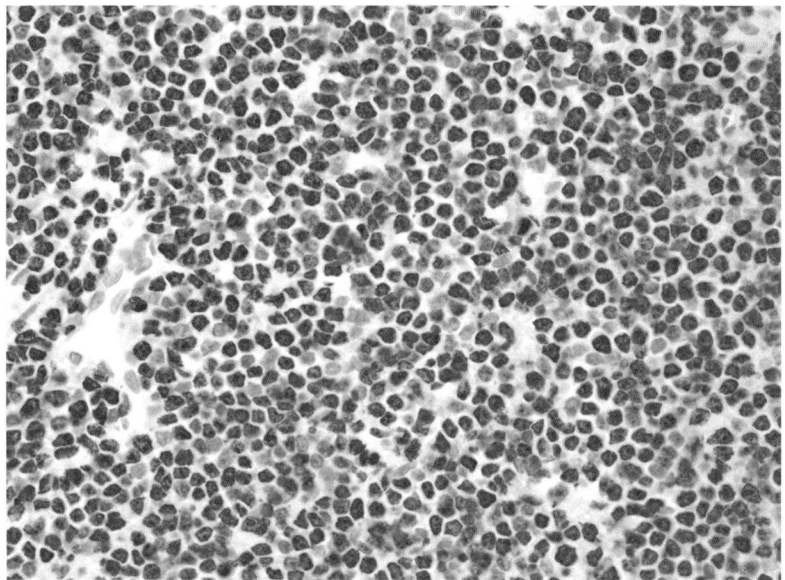

Fig. 16. Ki-67 expression in a case of Burkitt lymphoma. The near 100% prolifera-tion rate helps to confirm a diagnosis of Burkitt lymphoma.

By far, the most commonly used antibody to evaluate proliferation is Ki-67; also known by one of its more common epitope names, MIB-1. Ki-67 is a protein that is associated with cells in S-phase. As a diagnostic tool in lymphoma, Ki-67s use is relatively limited in routine practice. In the appropriate context, a prolif-eration rate of near 100% supports a diagnosis of Burkitt lymphoma (**Fig. 16**). Ki-67 can also be used to evaluate other types of lymphomas, which have char-acteristic patterns of proliferation. Examples include foci of high proliferation in a background of diffuse, low proliferation can be indicative of a diagnosis of small lymphocytic lymphoma with proliferation centers. Likewise, the differential diagnosis of follicular hyperplasia would be supported by a high proliferation rate, whereas a low proliferation rate in follicles would be seen in low-grade follicular lymphomas (**Fig. 17**).

3.3. Specific Antibodies and Their Diagnostic Combinations

Because of the multitude of IHC stains available to characterize lymphoid neoplastic processes, a preliminary differential diagnosis based on the histo-logical assessment typically drives the selection of markers to be applied in a particular case. Next, several specific antibodies and their combinations are discussed in the context of lymphoid proliferations, as well as specific diagnoses.

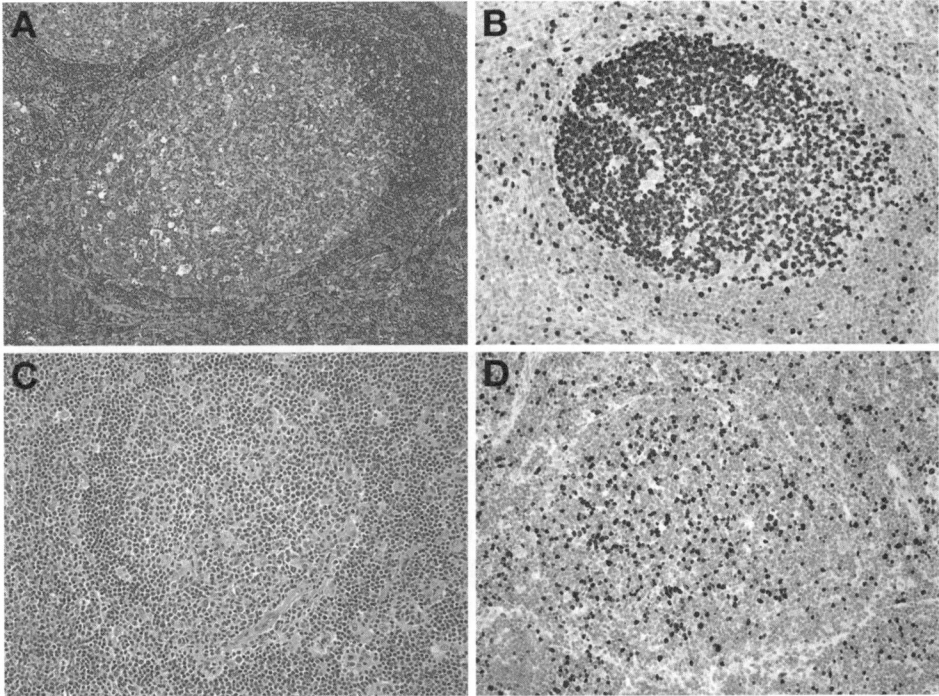

Fig. 17. Comparison of follicular hyperplasia and follicular lymphoma. (**A**) H&E and (**B**) Ki-67 proliferation rate of follicular hyperplasia. This contrasts with (**C**) H&E and (**D**) Ki-67 in a case of low-grade follicular lymphoma.

3.3.1. CD3/CD20

In lymphoid lesions, CD3 and CD20 immunostains should always be used in concert. This allows assessment of number and distribution of B- and T-cells. It is important not to order only a CD20 stain alone, because the number of T-cells can be significantly underestimated. Additional immunostains can be used to identify B-cells. These are particularly helpful in cases in which the neoplastic cells do not express CD20, or express it only weakly, such as chronic lymphocytic leukemia/small lymphocytic lymphoma (CLL/SLL), B-ALL, or HIV-associated B-cell lymphomas. In these cases, the most useful antibodies are CD79a and PAX-5, which are both pan-B-cell antigens. Another antibody used occasionally is CD74 (LN2).

3.3.2. CD45

Besides confirming the hematological nature of a poorly differentiated neoplasm, the use of CD45 is somewhat limited. If lymphoma is reasonable certain, the first step is to use the CD3/CD20 combination, as mentioned previously (*see* **Subheading 3.3.1.**). If other hematopoietic lesions (i.e., myeloid sarcoma, plasmacytoma) are being considered, then specific stains (or CD43; *see* **Subheading 3.3.3.**) should be used. CD45 is most useful in the context of classical Hodgkin lymphoma (CHL) as a negative finding.

3.3.3. CD43

It is important to remember that CD43 (and the formerly used pan-T-cell marker CD45RO) is not a true T-specific marker, as it will stain other hematopoietic elements, myeloid cells in particular. In cases where the expression of CD43 (and CD45RO) is greater than that of CD3, there are often macrophages or granulocytes present. However, in spite of its lack of specificity, the addition of CD43 to the CD3/CD20 combination adds considerable value to the diagnostic algorithm *(20,34,35)*. CD43 is expressed on a variety of normal hematopoietic cells including: normal T-cells, most marrow-derived cells, and macrophages/histiocytes. It is not typically coexpressed on normal B-cells. It is often expressed by malignant B-cells, including several of the small cell types of lymphoma. CD43 is almost always expressed on mantle cell lymphoma (MCL) and SLL/CLL. It is expressed in a subset of marginal zone lymphoma (MZL) (20–40%) and is essentially never expressed in follicular lymphoma (FL). It is occasionally positive in cases of T-cell rich/histiocyte rich B-cell lymphomas, which may be helpful in its differential diagnosis with CHL. Moreover, CD43 may also provide additional useful information in several instances: (1) if positive in B-cells, then it is almost always lymphoma; (2) it is a confirmatory stain for T-cells and should parallel CD3 staining; and (3) it can help identify hematopoietic neoplasms that are CD3 negative and CD20 negative, such as myeloid sarcoma, mast cell disease, and plasma cell neoplasms.

3.3.4. CD15/CD30/CD45

This combination of immunostains is valuable in evaluating lymphoid neoplasms in which CHL is part of the differential diagnosis. CD45 positivity in large abnormally neoplastic cells greatly decreases the likelihood of CHL and favors other diagnostic considerations *(37,38)*.

Conversely, CD15 positivity in large abnormally nucleolated cells is fairly specific and sensitive for CHL. Of course, there are rare exceptions, and no individual stain should be considered as absolutely diagnostic. CD15, however, is not always expressed in cases of CHL; even when it is positive, it may be only weak and in a few cells. Thus, a careful examination of Hodgkin/Reed–Sternberg cells for even weak positivity is recommended. CD15 will stain granulocytes, sometimes strongly, and so confirmation of the positive cell size and type is important. If a case is otherwise perfect for CHL, lack of CD15 should not prevent a diagnosis.

Table 1
Immunohistochemical Evaluation of Classical Hodgkin Lymphoma, Nodular Lymphocyte-Predominant Hodgkin Lymphoma, and T-Cell-Rich/Histiocyte-Rich Large B-Cell Lymphoma and Anaplastic Large Cell Lymphoma

Large neoplastic cells	CHL	NLPHL	TCRBCL	ALCL
CD30	+	–/+ (10%)	–/+ (30%)	+
CD15	+/– (75%)	–	–	–
CD45	–	+	+	+/– (40–50%)
CD3	–	–	–	–/+ (25%)
CD20	–/+ (20–40%; weak, variable staining)	+	+	–
CD79a	–	–/+ (10–30%)	+/–	–
Bcl-6	+/– (50%)	+	+/–	–
EMA	–	+ (30%)	–/+	+/–[a]
EBV-LMP	–/+[b] (40%)	–	–/+ (10%)	–
ALK-1	–	–	–	+/– (60–85%)
BOB.1	–/+	+	+	–
Oct-2	–/+	+	+	–
Vimentin	+	–	–	+/–

[a]EMA staining often parallels ALK-1 staining.
[b]More often positive in mixed cellularity subtype.

CD30 is always positive in the malignant cells of CHL. However, other lymphoma entities may be positive as well. Besides ALCL (*see* **Subheading 3.2.1.**) examples include cases of T-cell rich/histiocyte rich B-cell lymphoma, and rarely, nodular lymphocyte predominant Hodgkin lymphoma (**Table 1**). This may lead to confusion in their differential diagnosis with CHL. In addition, many nonhematopoietic neoplasms stain for CD30. CD30 staining in reactive lymph nodes is often over interpreted. Both T and B immunoblasts/transformed cells can be positive. Plasma cells can be positive, as well. ALCL, a subtype of T-cell lymphoma, consistently expresses CD30 but it may lack staining for many T-cell antigens including CD3. Occasionally the differential diagnosis with cases of CHL (particularly CD15 negative) may be difficult. The expression of CD30 is also seen in rare cases of DLBCL associated with an anaplastic morphology. Invariably, these stain for some B-cell markers (i.e., CD20, CD79a, CD22, PAX-5) and lack T-cell markers. Because of a significant difference in prognosis and differences in biology, the distinction is important.

A subset of ALCL express anaplastic lymphoma kinase (ALK) gene product *(39)*. This is most often a result of a characteristic translocation of chromosomes

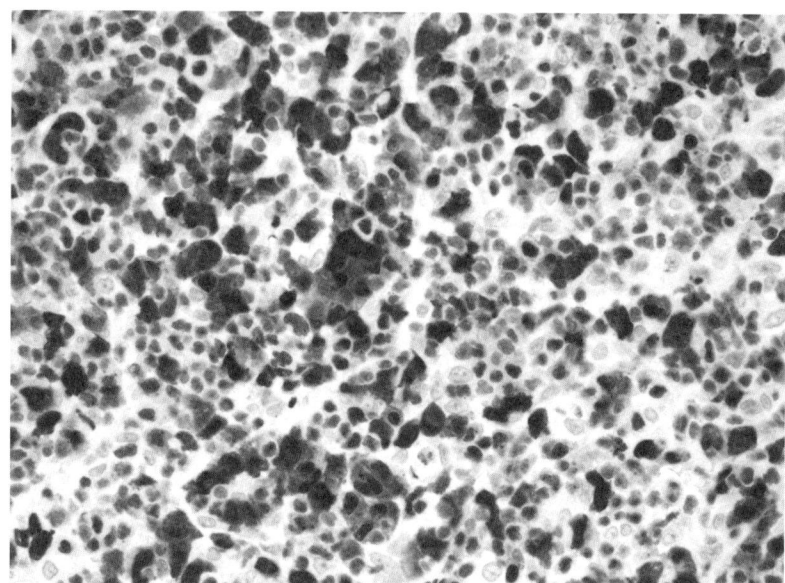

Fig. 18. Anaplastic lymphoma kinase expression in a case of anaplastic large cell lymphoma. The presence of both nuclear and cytoplasmic staining is associated with the presence of the translocation between chromosome 2 and chromosome 5.

2 and 5. The t(2;5) causes a fusion of the *ALK-1* gene on the short arm of chromosome 2 with the promoter region of the *nucleophosmin* (*NPM*) gene on the long arm of chromosome 5. When these genes are combined, they lead to over-expression of the ALK protein in both the nucleus and cytoplasm of the cell (**Fig. 18**). As in this case, overexpression of ALK in the cytoplasm, without nuclear expression, may be the result of variant cytogenetic translocation. Expression of the "ALK" tyrosine kinase protein product of the t(2;5) translocation or limitation of disease to the skin each predict excellent prognosis. Noncutaneous cases of ALK negative ALCL have a worse prognosis *(40)*.

These lymphomas variably express cytotoxic molecules with the majority expressing TIA-1 and a subset expressing granzyme B or perforin. As is typical of T-cell lymphomas in general, pan-T markers are present (CD2, CD3, CD5, CD7) but loss of individual pan-T antigens is common. There is often loss of surface CD3 with only cytoplasmic CD3 expression.

3.3.5. Bcl-2

Bcl-2 staining is common in many lymphomas *(26)*. It is present in about 75% of all B-cell lymphomas, including: most FL, a subset of DLBCL, most MCL, most MZL, and most CLL/SLL. It is also positive in many T-cell lymphomas.

Table 2
Immunohistochemical Differentiation of Follicular Hyperplasia and Follicular Lymphoma

Stain	Follicular hyperplasia	Follicular lymphoma
Bcl-2	Negative	Positive
Bcl-6	Positive	Positive
CD10	Positive	Positive
Ki-67	High	Low
CD23 (in FDC)	Positive	Positive

The presence of bcl-2 staining is not equivalent to the presence of the 14;18 translocation of the *bcl-2* gene with IgH heavy chain gene seen in FL and some DLBCL. Bcl-2 is expressed in cells that have a long life, such as normal mantle cells and T-cells.

A common consideration in practice is the differential diagnosis of follicular lymphoma vs follicular hyperplasia. Although there are several morphologic criteria that are valuable, immunohistochemical confirmation is always reassuring (**Table 2**). Bcl-2 is an antiapoptosis protein that is expressed in a variety of cells. In normal cells of the follicle center, it is not expressed, as benign germinal center cells need the capacity to undergo apoptosis as a function of clonal selection. In benign follicles, Bcl-2 protein is positive in the mantle zone cells but negative in follicle centers. Conversely, in follicular lymphoma, the B-cells of the follicle are positive for Bcl-2 in about 80% of cases (**Fig. 19**). It should be noted that 20% lack bcl-2 positivity.

3.3.6. Cyclin D1

Cyclin D1 is of particular importance in diagnosing MCL. Cyclin D1 overexpression correlates with a translocation of chromosomes 11 and 14 resulting in fusion of the *cyclin D1* gene with the immunoglobulin heavy chain locus. Cyclin D1 is a very specific stain in the context of lymphoma; its variable nuclear staining being almost pathognomonic of MCL (**Fig. 20**). It should be noted that both plasma cell neoplasms and hairy cell leukemias and, rarely, CLL *(40)* can also express cyclin D1. Its expression is also fairly common in non-hematopoietic neoplasms, and one of its earlier names, PRAD-1 derives from its overexpression in parathyroid adenomas.

3.3.7. CD10/bcl-6 in FL

CD10 and bcl-6 are both stains that (almost always) indicate that the cells are of follicular origin *(27,28)*. In cases where the architecture does not allow for

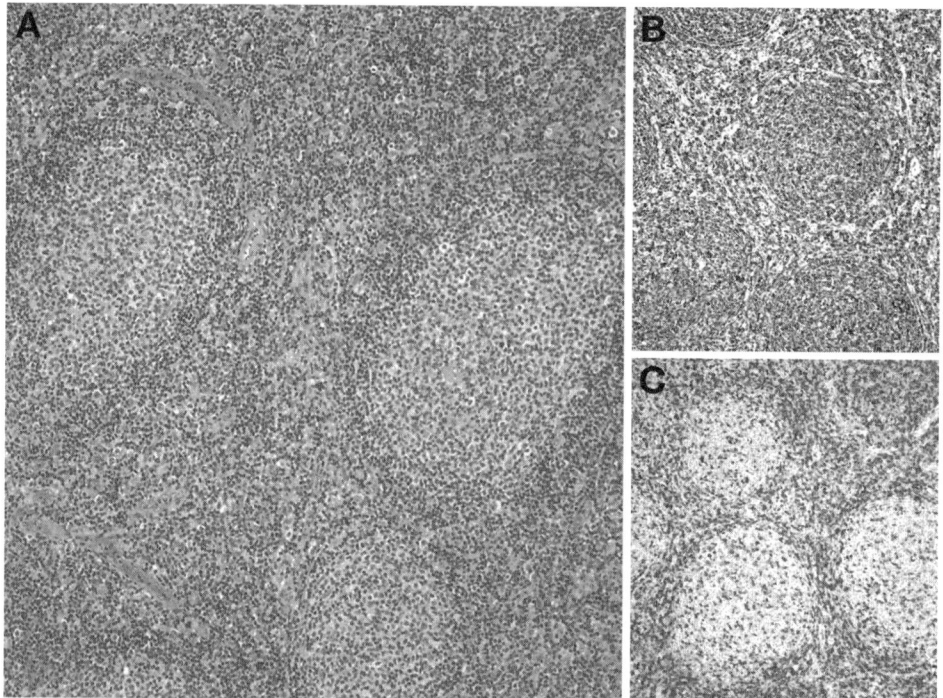

Fig. 19. Low-grade follicular lymphoma expressing bcl-2. **(A)** H&E section, **(B)** Bcl-2, and **(C)** CD3 expression. When interpreting a Bcl-2 stain it is important to compare results of a CD3 stain, as normal T cells are positive for Bcl-2.

interpretation of a follicular pattern, then either or both can be used to establish the follicular origin of cells.

3.3.8. CD10/bcl-2/bcl-6/MUM-1 in DLBCL

The literature has several reports concerning prognostication in DLBCL using IHC *(42,43)*. There have been several conflicting studies using CD10/bcl-2/bcl-6/MUM-1 on DLBCL and trying to correlate findings with the aggressiveness or treatability of DLBCL. Gene array studies have shown that there are three general types of DLBCL: (1) the germinal center type, (2) the activated B-cell type, and (3) a heterogeneous group provisionally called "type 3." In general, the germinal center type has a good prognosis and is highly curable, whereas the activated B-cell type tends to have a poor prognosis. Immunohistochemical studies have tried to replicate the gene array results by using a few, well-known markers. Although it is likely that specific markers will eventually be validated for good vs poor prognosis in DLBCL, it has not yet become clear what markers are best for this determination.

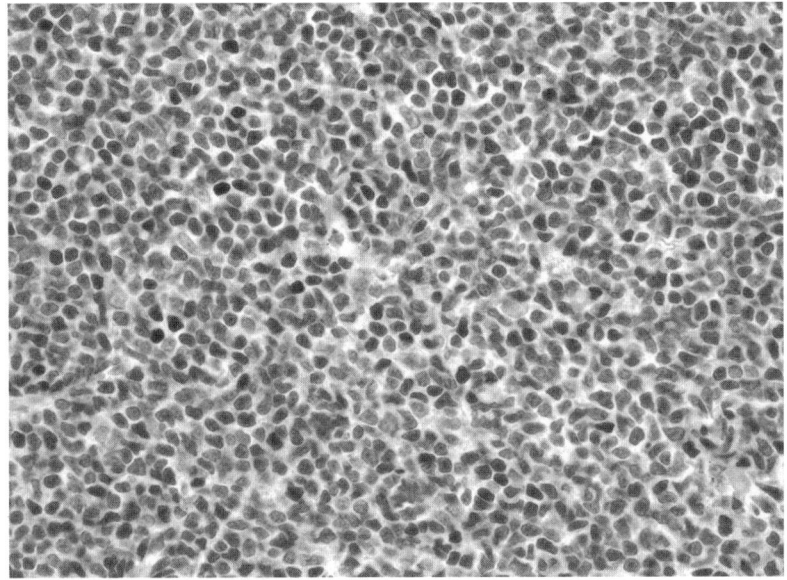

Fig. 20. Cyclin D1 expression in a case of mantle cell lymphoma. Varying intensity of nuclear staining is the expected result for the cyclin D1 stain.

3.3.9. CD5/CD20/CD10/CD23

Besides expression in T-cells, CD5 is positive in CLL/SLL and MCL and only rarely on other small B-cell lymphomas. In conjunction with CD23 and CD10, CD5 can be helpful to differentiate among the various small B-cell lymphomas. MCL would be CD5+/CD23−, CLL/SLL would be CD5+/CD23+, and virtually all cases of FL or MZL are negative for CD5 and negative for CD23 (**Table 3**).

3.3.10. CD3/CD4/CD8 and Other T-Cell Markers

Besides CD3, other pan T-cell markers such as CD2, CD5, and CD7 are expressed early in T-cell differentiation and throughout the life of T-cells. Selective loss of T-cell markers is common in the neoplastic cells of T-cell lymphomas, and can support the diagnosis. CD4 and CD8 are markers of T-cell differentiation. Most T-cell lymphomas express CD4, although, there are occasional CD8-positive lymphomas. Some lymphomas, including precursor T-cell neoplasms, can be either "double-positive" (CD4+CD8+) or "double negative" (CD4−CD8−). CD1a, most commonly utilized to identify Langerhans cell histiocytosis, will also identify immature T-cells. To evaluate cytotoxic differentiation in T- and natural killer cell proliferations, CD56, TIA-1, perforin, granzyme-B, as well as CD4 and CD8 are helpful.

Table 3
Comparison of Immunohistochemical Results in Several B-Cell Lymphomas

	CD20	CD3	Bcl-2	CD5	CD23	CD43	CyclinD1	Other
FL	+	−	+	−	+	−	−	CD10+
SLL	+	−	+	+	+	+	−	
MCL	+	−	+	+	−	+	+	
MZL	+	−	+/−	−	−	+/−	−	

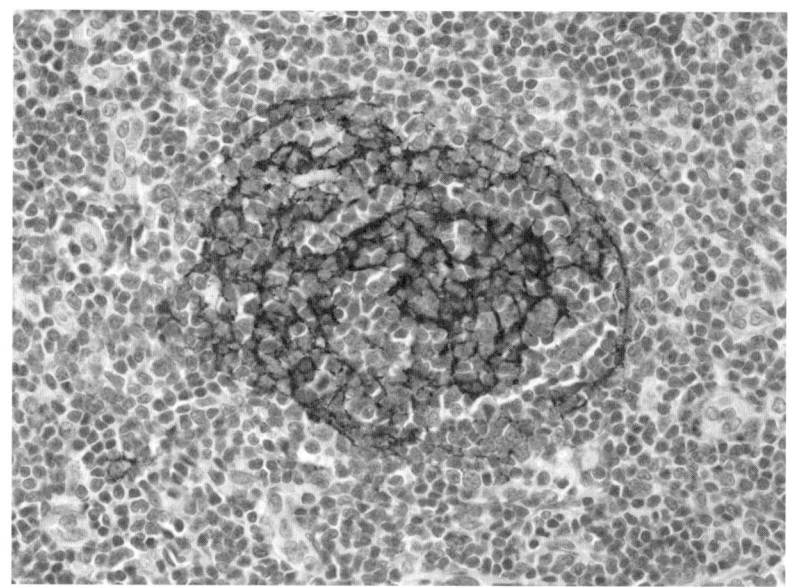

Fig. 21. Follicular dendritic cells are highlighted by a CD21 stain in the case of low-grade follicular lymphoma.

3.3.11. CD21/CD35/CD23/S-100 as Dendritic Cell Stains

Follicular dendritic cells (FDC) are accessory cells that help make up the skeleton of normal follicles. Because of their antigen presenting capability, they play an important role in the ongoing immune response and B-cells maturation. CD21 stain is a useful stain for staining FDC, although CD35 works as well (some use a cocktail of both) (**Fig. 21**). CD23 staining has a slightly different staining pattern than the other two markers.

Neoplastic proliferation of FDC may occur in lymph nodes or elsewhere (these are termed FDC sarcomas); they can be identified by CD21 immunostaining. In addition, assessing the distribution of FDC can be occasionally useful in differentiating subtypes of lymphomas. In follicular lymphoma, FDC are typically retained in the nodular portions of the lymphoid proliferation, where they form tight networks within the neoplastic follicles. In contrast, other lymphomas may have reduced or diminished numbers of FDC. Irregularly expanded FDC networks are typically seen in cases of angioimmunoblastic T-cell lymphoma.

Interdigitating reticulum cell (IDC) sarcoma may simulate FDC. However, they can be reliably distinguished by immunostaining with CD21 (and/or CD35) and S-100 (the latter being only positive in IDC). Additionally, ultrastructural examination of the FDC reveals the presence of desmosomes, distinguishing the process from IDC, which lack this type of cell junction.

3.4. Spleen

IHC is a valuable tool in the evaluation of splenic disorders. It provides unique challenges, however, because of the functional complexity of the spleen and the variety of its histological components. The purpose of this section is to provide general guidelines on evaluating the complex splenic microanatomy, stressing in particular the morphologic and the immunohistological characteristics of the white pulp and red pulp compartments *(44)*. The lymphoid components will not be specifically discussed.

As a functional compartment, the stroma of the spleen is often overlooked. It does, however, give rise to both neoplastic and nonneoplastic proliferations, which may be complex and difficult to evaluate. In addition, the stroma of the spleen may in itself, provide insight into the development of splenic disorders (e.g., myeloid metaplasia).

In terms of architecture, the splenic stroma can be divided into three main components: the vascular component, the reticuloendothelial or monocyte/macrophage component, and the remainder *(45)*. This remaining portion consists of various mesenchymal cells and extracellular matrix (ECM), which forms the structural framework of the spleen.

The large arteries, arterioles, and veins are similar to other sites in the body, and can be evaluated with the battery of immunostains used to stain endothelial cells as well as vascular tumors at other sites, i.e., CD34, CD31, factor VIII (von Willebrand factor), and, more recently, FLI-1 (**Figs. 22** and **23**). A specialized endothelial cell unique to the spleen is the littoral cell, which lines the vascular sinuses of the spleen. The littoral cells share features of both endothelial cells and monocyte/macrophages. They are usually flat, inconspicuous cells along the edges of sinuses. When activated, they become plump and appear larger. Some of the interesting features of the cells are that they are strongly and uniformly positive for CD8, a marker that is more commonly associated with cytotoxic or suppressor T-cells (**Fig. 24**). Therefore, CD8 is a useful stain in delineating the sinusoidal architecture in the spleen; however, the strong vascular reactivity with CD8 can make evaluation of CD8-positive T-cells somewhat

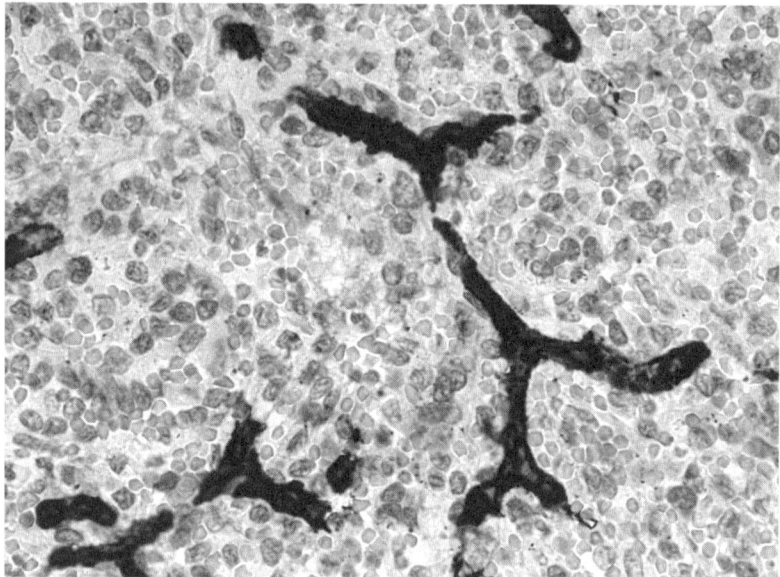

Fig. 22. CD34 expression in small vessels of the spleen. Note that the sinus-lining cells (e.g., littoral cells) are CD34 negative.

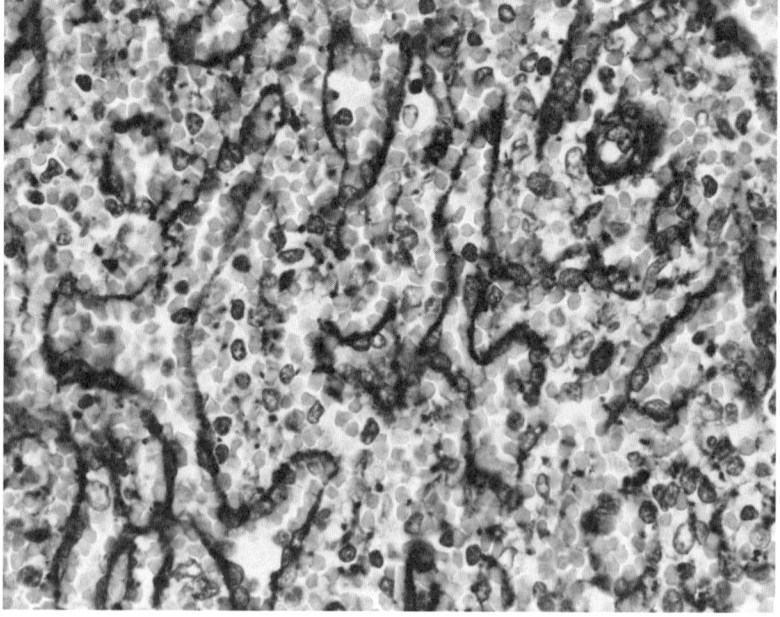

Fig. 23. Factor VIII antigen staining in a normal spleen. All vascular elements stain with factor VIII antigen.

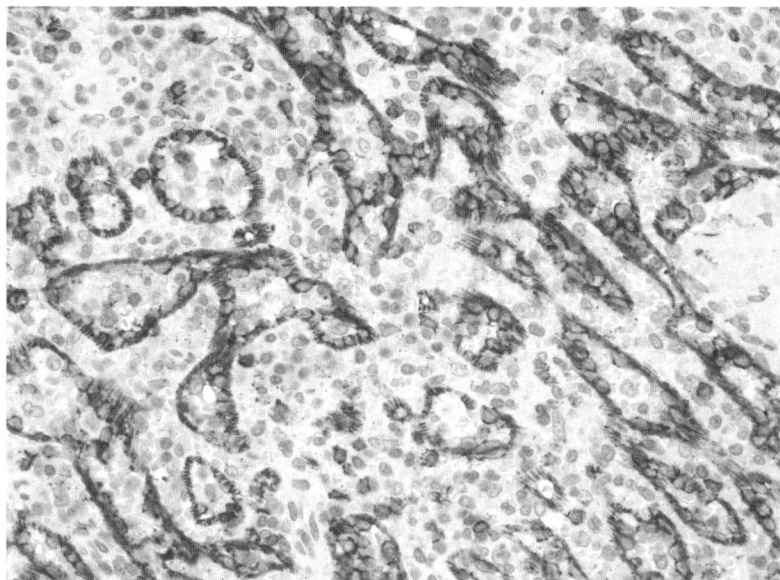

Fig. 24. CD8 staining of littoral cells in spleen. In addition, numerous circulating T-cells of the suppressor type (e.g., CD8 positive) are seen.

more difficult. CD8 is only inconsistently positive in the neoplastic counterpart of the sinusoidal endothelium, the littoral cell angioma.

The monocyte/macrophage system (MMS) is one of the more important anatomic and functional components of the spleen; it forms the bulk of the red pulp (cordal macrophages), but often receives little specific attention. Only when there is a significant derangement of the MMS, is it even noticed. Normally, the MMS serves as a functional filter for effete red blood cells and other less than desirable components of the circulating blood. In states in which there is an increase in destruction of circulating blood components, as in an autoimmune hemolytic anemia or immune thrombocytopenic purpura, the cordal macrophages will become engorged and hyperplastic within the spleen producing a picture of red pulp congestion. The cordal macrophages can also become engorged with metabolic products in storage diseases, infectious agents, or even abnormally produced immunoglobulins.

Evaluation of the MMS using IHC can be accomplished by a number of antibodies, which include CD68, lysozyme, antichymotrypsin, and others. When there is accumulation of intracellular material in macrophages, histological stains may be of considerable value, depending on the accumulated product. Most abnormal storage proteins are PAS positive. Infectious organisms can be evaluated by the judicious use of AFB, GMS, tissue Gram, and PAS stains. In

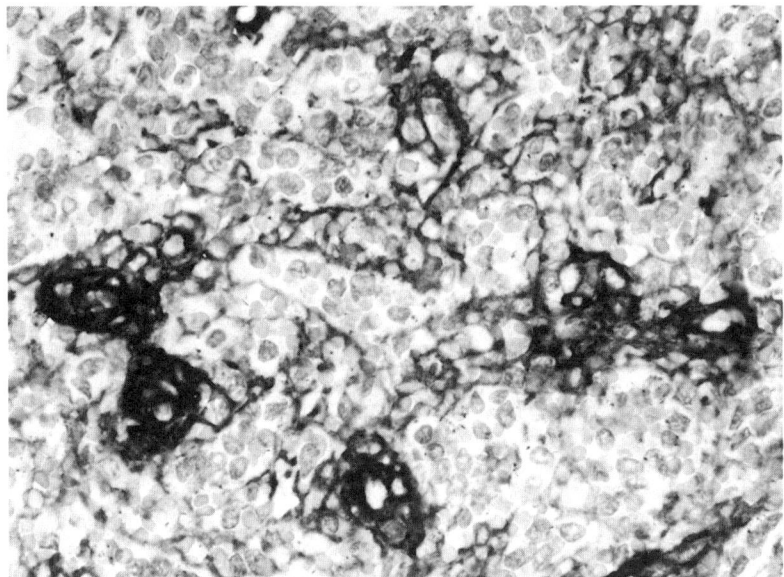

Fig. 25. Nerve growth factor receptor (NGFR) staining of red pulp of spleen. NGFR stains stromal elements of the spleen.

the case of immunoglobulin accumulation, IHC for κ and λ light chains may be of benefit.

A considerable portion of the spleen (white pulp) is devoted to its function as a lymphoid organ. Components that are notable parts of this are dendritic cells (FDC and IDC). Distinction of dendritic cells is usually accomplished by IHC. Dendritic cells are varyingly positive for monocyte/macrophage-associated markers such as CD68, S100, CD1a, lysozyme and, α-1-antitrypsin (as previously described).

Evaluation of structural mesenchymal cells and ECM by IHC can be performed using various antibodies. Low-affinity nerve growth factor receptor (ME20-4) identifies reticulum cells in the splenic cords, periarteriolar and pericapillary adventitial cells as well as FDCs (**Figs. 25** and **26**). The low-affinity nerve growth factor receptor positive cell subsets all share fibroblastic or spindle cell morphology and perform mainly structural functions. Smooth muscle actin (SMA; 1A4) can be used to identify pericytes and cells with myofibroblastic differentiation (myoid cells). SMA staining highlights a concentric reticular meshwork of SMA-positive cells present at the interface between red pulp and marginal zones (**Fig. 27**). SMA staining of perivascular cells within the red pulp can also be observed. The ECM can be evaluated by IHC for collagen IV (CIV22; basement membrane type collagen) and by reticulin staining. Collagen IV highlights the "ring fibers," which incompletely surround the littoral cells of

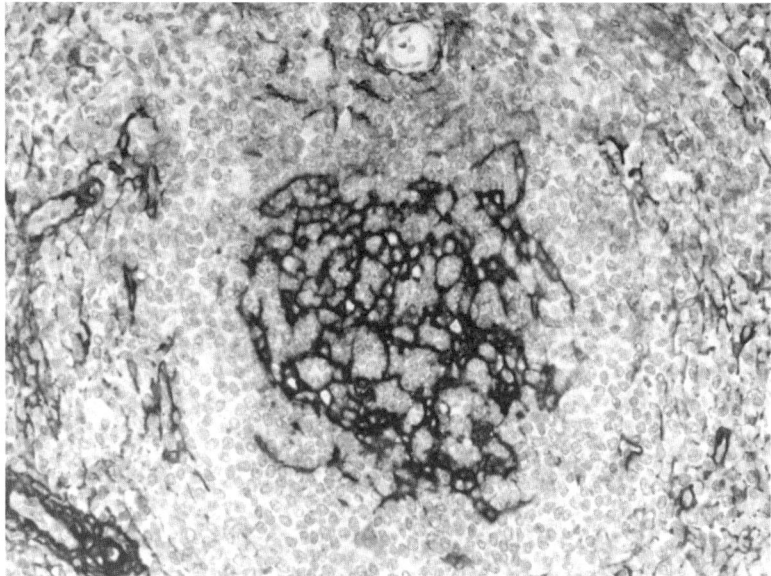

Fig. 26. Nerve growth factor receptor (NGFR) staining of white pulp of spleen. NGFR stains dendritic cells of white pulp.

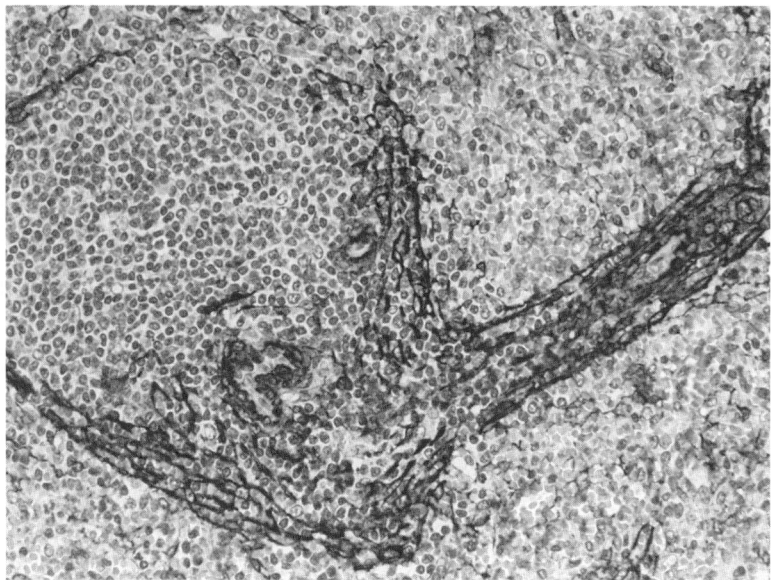

Fig. 27. Smooth muscle actin (SMA) staining in normal spleen. SMA highlights cells with myoid differentiation that define the boundaries between red and white pulp.

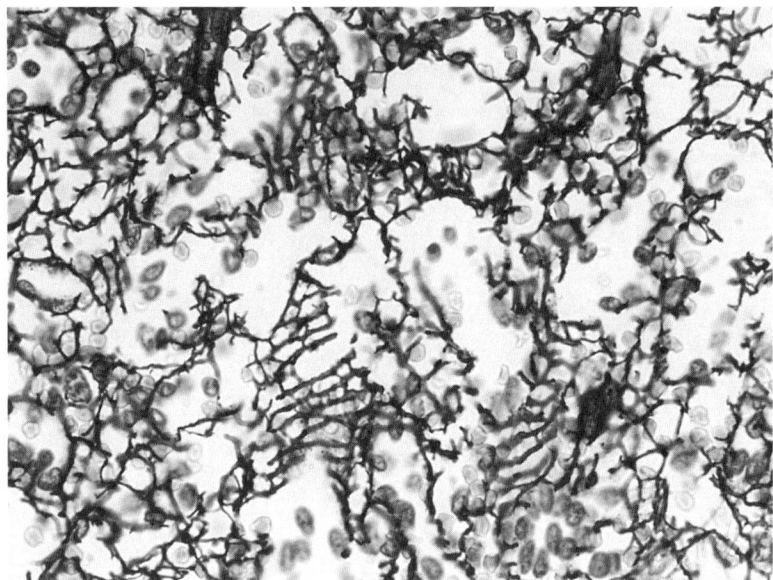

Fig. 28. Collagen type IV staining in normal spleen. This stain highlights the ring fibers of the splenic sinusoids.

the splenic sinusoids (**Fig. 28**). Other types of collagen are collectively stained by Gomori silver impregnation technique also known as reticulin stain. Various patterns of stromal cell hyperplasia or alterations in the architectural distribution of ECM proteins can be observed in a variety of splenic disorders.

References

1. Rudiger, T., Hofler, H., Kreipe, H. H., et al. (2002) Quality assurance in immunohistochemistry: results of an interlaboratory trial involving 172 pathologists. *Am. J. Surg. Pathol.* **26,** 873–882.
2. His, E. D. and Yegappan, S. (2001) Lymphoma immunophenotyping: a new era in paraffin-section immunohistochemistry. *Adv. Anat. Pathol.* **8,** 218–239.
3. Warnke, R. A. and Isaacson, P. G. (2001) Immunohistochemical analysis of lymphoid tissue. In: *Neoplastic Hematopathology,* (Knowles, D. M., ed.), Lippincott Williams and Wilkins, Philadelphia, PA, 227–253.
4. Gown, A.M. (2004) Unmasking the mysteries of antigen or epitope retrieval and formalin fixation. *Am. J. Clin. Pathol.* **121,** 172–174.
5. Jaffe, E. S., Banks, P. M., Nathwani, B., Said, J., and Swerdlow, S. H. (2004) Recommendations for the reporting of lymphoid neoplasms: a report from the Association of Directors of Anatomic and Surgical Pathology. *Mod. Pathol.* **17,** 131–135.
6. Orazi, A., Cattoretti, G., Schiro, R., et al. (1992) Recombinant human interleukin-3 and recombinant human granulocyte-macrophage colony-stimulating factor administered

in vivo after high-dose cyclophosphamide cancer chemotherapy: effect on hemato-poiesis and microenvironment in human bone marrow. *Blood* **79**, 2610–2619.

7. Pinkus, G. S. and Pinkus, J. L. (1991) Myeloperoxidase: a specific marker for myeloid cells in paraffin sections. *Mod. Pathol.* **4**, 733–741.

8. Manaloor, E. J., Neiman, R. S., Heilman, D. K., et al. (2000) Immunohistochemistry of routinely processed bone marrow biopsies can be used to subtype acute myeloid leukemia: comparison with flow cytometry. *Am. J. Clin. Pathol.* **113**, 814–822.

9. Orazi, A., O'Malley, D. P., Jiang, J., et al. (2004) Acute panmyelosis with myelofibrosis: an entity distinct from acute megakaryoblastic leukemia. *Mod. Pathol.* **10**, 1–12.

10. Rimsza, L. M., Larson, R. S., Winter, S. S., et al. (2000) Benign hematogone-rich lymphoid proliferations can be distinguished from B-lineage acute lymphoblastic leukemia by integration of morphology, immunophenotype, adhesion molecule expression, and architectural features. *Am. J. Clin. Pathol.* **114**, 66–75.

11. Orazi, A., Cotton, J., Cattoretti, G., et al. (1994) Terminal Deoxynucleotidyl Transferase staining in acute leukemia and normal bone marrow using routinely processed paraffin sections. *Am. J. Clin. Pathol.* **102**, 640–645.

12. Soligo, D., Delia, D., Oriani, A., et al. (1991) Identification of CD34+ cells in normal and pathological bone marrow biopsies by QBEND10 monoclonal anti-body. *Leukemia.* **5**, 1026–1030.

13. Kotylo, P., Seo, I. S., Heerema, N. A., et al. (2000) Flow cytometric immunophe-notypic analysis of pediatric and adult minimally differentiated acute myeloid leukemia (AML-M0). *Am. J. Clin. Pathol.* **113**, 193–200.

14. Nguyen, T. T., Schwartz, E. J., West, R. B., et al. (2005) Expression of CD163 (hemoglobin scavenger receptor) in normal tissues, lymphomas, carcinomas, and sarcomas is largely restricted to the monocyte/macrophage lineage. *Am. J. Surg. Pathol.* **29**, 617–624.

15. Robertson, P. B., Neiman, R. S., Worapongpaiboon, S., John, K., and Orazi, A. (1997) 013 (CD99) positivity in hematologic proliferations correlates with TdT positivity. *Mod. Pathol.* **10**, 277–282.

16. Orazi, A., Cattoretti, G., Soligo, D., Luksch, R., and Lambertenghi-Deliliers G. (1993) Therapy-related myelodysplastic syndromes: FAB classification, bone marrow histo-logy, and immunohistology in the prognostic assessment. *Leukemia* **7**, 838–847.

17. Baur, A. S., Meuge-Moraw, C., Schmidt, P. M., Parlier, V., Jotterand, M., and Delacretaz, F. (2000) CD34/QBEND10 immunostaining in bone marrow biopsies: an additional parameter for the diagnosis and classification of myelodysplastic syn-dromes. *Eur. J. Haematol.* **64**, 71–79.

18. Orazi, A., Neiman, R. S., Cualing, H., Heerema, N. A., and John, K. (1994) CD34 immunostaining of bone marrow biopsies is a reliable way to classify the phases of chronic myeloid leukemia. *Am. J. Clin. Pathol.* **101**, 426–428.

19. Orazi, A., Albitar, M., Heerema, N. A., Haskins, S., and Neiman, R. S. (1997) Hypoplastic myelodysplastic syndromes can be distinguished from acquired aplas-tic anemia by CD34 and PCNA immunostaining of bone marrow biopsy speci-mens. *Am. J. Clin. Pathol.* **107**, 268–274.

20. Contos, M. J., Kornstein, M. J., Innes, D. J., and Ben-Ezra, J. (1992) The utility of CD20 and CD43 in subclassification of low-grade B-cell lymphoma on paraffin sections. *Mod. Pathol.* **5,** 631–633.
21. Chen, C. C., Raikow, R. B., Sonmez-Alpan, E., and Swerdlow, S. H. (2000) Classification of small B-cell lymphoid neoplasms using a paraffin section immunohistochemical panel. *Appl. Immunohistochem. Mol. Morphol.* **8,** 1–11.
22. Saez, A. I., Artiga, M. J., Sanchez-Beato, M., et al. (2002) Analysis of octamer-binding transcription factors Oct2 and Oct1 and their coactivator BOB.1/OBF.1 in lymphomas. *Mod. Pathol.* **15,** 211–220.
23. Torlakovic, E., Torlakovic, G., Nguyen, P. L., Brunning, R. D., and Delabie, J. (2002) The value of anti-pax-5 immunostaining in routinely fixed and paraffin-embedded sections: a novel pan pre-B and B-cell marker. *Am. J. Surg. Pathol.* **26,** 1343–1350.
24. Loddenkemper, C., Anagnostopoulos, I., Hummel, M., et al. (2004) Differential Emu enhancer activity and expression of BOB.1/OBF.1, Oct2, PU.1, and immuno-globulin in reactive B-cell populations, B-cell non-Hodgkin lymphomas, and Hodgkin lymphomas. *J. Pathol.* **202,** 60–69.
25. O'Connell, F. P., Pinkus, J. L., and Pinkus, G. S. (2004) CD138 (syndecan-1), a plasma cell marker immunohistochemical profile in hematopoietic and non-hematopoietic neoplasms. *Am. J. Clin. Pathol.* **121,** 254–263.
26. Lai, R., Arber, D. A., Chang, K. L., Wilson, C. S., and Weiss, L. M. (1998) Frequency of bcl-2 expression in non-Hodgkin's lymphoma: a study of 778 cases with comparison of marginal zone lymphoma and monocytoid B-cell hyperplasia. *Mod. Pathol.* **11,** 864–869.
27. Dogan, A., Bagdi, E., Munson, P., and Isaacson, P. G. (2000) CD10 and BCL-6 expression in paraffin sections of normal lymphoid tissue and B-cell lymphomas. *Am. J. Surg. Pathol.* **24,** 846–852.
28. King, B. E., Chen, C., Locker, J., et al. (2000) Immunophenotypic and genotypic markers of follicular center cell neoplasia in diffuse large B-cell lymphomas. *Mod. Pathol.* **13,** 1219–1231.
29. Ohshima, K., Kawasaki, C., Muta, H., et al. (2001) CD10 and Bcl10 expression in diffuse large B-cell lymphoma: CD10 is a marker of improved prognosis. *Histo-pathology* **39,** 156–162.
30. Orazi, A., Cattoretti, G., John, K., and Neiman, R. S. (1994) Terminal deoxy-nucleotidyl transferase staining of malignant lymphomas in paraffin sections. *Mod. Pathol.* **7,** 528–586.
31. Stein, H., Foss, H. D., Durkop, H., et al. (2000) CD30(+) anaplastic large cell lym-phoma: a review of its histopathologic, genetic, and clinical features. *Blood* **96,** 3681–3695.
32. Miller, T. P., Grogan, T. M., Dahlberg, S., et al. (1994) Prognostic significance of the Ki-67-associated proliferative antigen in aggressive non-Hodgkin's lym-phomas: a prospective Southwest Oncology Group trial. *Blood* **83,** 1460–1466.
33. Budke, H., Orazi, A., Neiman, R. S., Cattoretti, G., John, K., and Barberis, M. (1994) Assessment of cell proliferation in paraffin sections of normal bone marrow by the monoclonal antibodies Ki-67 and PCNA. *Mod. Pathol.* **7,** 860–866.

34. Brown, D.C. and Gatter, K. C. (2002) Ki67 protein: the immaculate deception? *Histopathology* **40**, 2–11.
35. Segal, G. H., Stoler, M. H., and Tubbs, R. R. (1992) The "CD43 only" phenotype. An aberrant, nonspecific immunophenotype requiring comprehensive analysis for lineage resolution. *Am. J. Clin. Pathol.* **97**, 861–865.
36. Lai, R., Weiss, L. M., Chang, K. L., and Arber, D. A. (1999) Frequency of CD43 expression in non-Hodgkin lymphoma. A survey of 742 cases and further characterization of rare CD43+ follicular lymphomas. *Am. J. Clin. Pathol.* **111**, 488–494.
37. Boudova, L., Torlakovic, E., Delabie, J., et al. (2003) Nodular lymphocyte-predominant Hodgkin lymphoma with nodules resembling T-cell/histiocyte-rich B-cell lymphoma: differential diagnosis between nodular lymphocyte-predominant Hodgkin lymphoma and T-cell/histiocyte-rich B-cell lymphoma. *Blood* **102**, 3753–3758.
38. von Wasielewski, R., Mengel, M., Fischer, R., et al. (1997) Classical Hodgkin's disease. Clinical impact of the immunophenotype. *Am. J. Pathol.* **151**, 1123–1130.
39. Pittaluga, S., Wlodarska, I., Pulford, K., et al. (1997) The monoclonal antibody ALK1 identifies a distinct morphological subtype of anaplastic large cell lymphoma associated with 2p23/ALK rearrangements. *Am. J. Pathol.* **151**, 343–351.
40. ten Berge, R. L., de Bruin, P. C., Oudejans, J. J., Ossenkoppele, G. J., van der Valk, P., and Meijer, C. J. (2003) ALK-negative anaplastic large-cell lymphoma demonstrates similar poor prognosis to peripheral T-cell lymphoma, unspecified. *Histopathology* **43**, 472–469.
41. O'Malley, D. P., Vance, G. H., and Orazi, A. (2005) Chronic lymphocytic leukemia/small lymphocytic lymphoma with trisomy 12 and focal cyclin d1 expression: a potential diagnostic pitfall. *Arch. Pathol. Lab. Med.* **129**, 92–95.
42. Sanchez-Beato, M., Sanchez-Aguilera, A., and Piris, M. A. (2003) Cell cycle deregulation in B-cell lymphomas. *Blood* **101**, 1220–1235.
43. Colomo, L., Lopez-Guillermo, A., Perales, M., et al. (2003) Clinical impact of the differentiation profile assessed by immunophenotyping in patients with diffuse large B-cell lymphoma. *Blood* **101**, 78–84.
44. Neiman, R. S. and Orazi, A. (2001) Histopathologic manifestation of lymphoproliferative and myeloproliferative disorders involving the spleen. In: *Neoplastic Hematopathology, 2nd ed.,* (Knowles, D. M., ed.), Williams and Wilkins, Baltimore, MD, 1881–1914.
45. van Krieken, J. M. and Orazi, A. (2006) Spleen. In: *Histology for Pathologists, 2nd ed.,* (Sternberg, S. S., ed.), Lippincott-Raven Publishers, Philadelphia, PA, in press.

9

Bead-Based Multianalyte Flow Immunoassays

The Cytometric Bead Array System

Rudolf Varro, Roy Chen, Homero Sepulveda, and John Apgar

Summary

Analytical cytometry has significant potential beyond cellular analysis. The inherent capability of flow cytometers to efficiently discriminate between uniformly sized particles based on their intrinsic properties provides the foundation for multiplex bead assays. The technology can be exploited in designing immunoassays, Western blot-like antibody assays, and nucleic acid hybridization assays. This chapter focuses on immunoassay applications. The multiplex bead assays have recently evolved as a new and increasingly popular area for flow cytometry, becoming a good alternative to enzyme-linked immunosorbent assay for efficient evaluation of panels of analytes. This chapter provides detailed information about two bead platforms, the BD™ Cytometric Bead Array kits and the BD Cytometric Bead Array Flex Set Assays.

Key Words: CBA; multiplex bead immunoassays; preconfigured kits; Flex-Set assays; soluble proteins; cell signaling proteins; cell lysates.

1. Introduction

Bead-based, flow cytometric immunoassays have the ability to simultaneously and quantitatively measure multiple antigens or antibodies in a small volume of biological fluids. The flow cytometers support a broad dynamic assay range for the multiplex assays. The technology may be utilized to analyze the networks of mediators expressed by cells during immune and inflammatory responses. Cytokines (1), chemokines (2), inflammatory mediators and their receptors, as well as immunoglobulins (3), are frequently described as target molecules for multiplex assays. In addition, the bead assays can be applied to the simultaneous analysis of cell signaling molecules (4) and follow various activation pathways.

From: *Methods in Molecular Biology, vol. 378: Monoclonal Antibodies: Methods and Protocols*
Edited by: M. Albitar © Humana Press Inc., Totowa, NJ

The use of microspheres of different size or color is at the basis of constructing multiplexed immunoassays. Several analytes can be assayed in one tube using very small sample volumes. Three basic concepts were developed to establish multianalyte assays. Fulwyler *(5)* and McHugh *(6)* pioneered the flow multiplex area using beads of different sizes as carriers for antigens or antibodies. The beads carrying different analytes are differentiated by their different scatter characteristics. Binding of fluorescent detectors to the beads generate the immunoassay signal.

Beads of the same size may be identified and differentiated by one type of fluorescence, whereas the signal is generated by conjugates carrying a second type of fluorescent signal *(7)*. This concept is useful to create low-complexity bead sets *(8)*.

Combining two or more fluorescent indexing colors in individual beads further extended the usefulness of multiplex flow assays. The individual bead populations contain unique ratios of the incorporated dyes, and their differing fluorescent signature is used to identify a series of beads carrying different specificities. Bead indexing is achieved in multidimensional fluorescent space with the capability to reach up to 100 individual bead addresses in two dimensions *(9)*. The immunoassay signal is generated by antibodies coupled to a fluorescent dye, which is not interfering with the bead indexing. New instruments were designed to exploit the capabilities of multiplex bead assays without requiring the complex expertise of flow cytometry. The LabMAP 100 by Luminex and the BD FACSArray Bioanalyzer (**Fig. 1**) by BD Biosciences both support the utilization of the familiar microplate format. Both of these instruments have two lasers, a red laser that excites the two dyes in the dual color beads, and a green laser that is used for exciting the bead-bound conjugates. The signal generator is most often phycoerythrin (PE), thus the green laser excitation maximizes signal-to-noise ratios.

Multiplex assays are well suited to demonstrate a pattern of antibody responses against infectious agents, thus providing a bead assay analog to the Western blot method. McHugh *(10)* presented a prototype Hepatitis C virus antibody assay for potential use in the blood bank. Faucher *(11)* has demonstrated the capability of the multiplex assays to detect HIV-1 antibodies from fresh plasma and from dried bloodspot specimens. Khan *(12)* utilized the multiplex format to construct a serological assay, which detected 10 highly prevalent mouse infectious pathogens in a single reaction.

Two types of cytometric bead array (CBA) assays were developed at BD BioSciences. The BD CBA kits contain all the necessary components to perform the assay. The BD CBA Flex Set assays, on the other hand, provide all the necessary components and protocols to create customized multiplex panels, allowing a mix-and-match strategy.

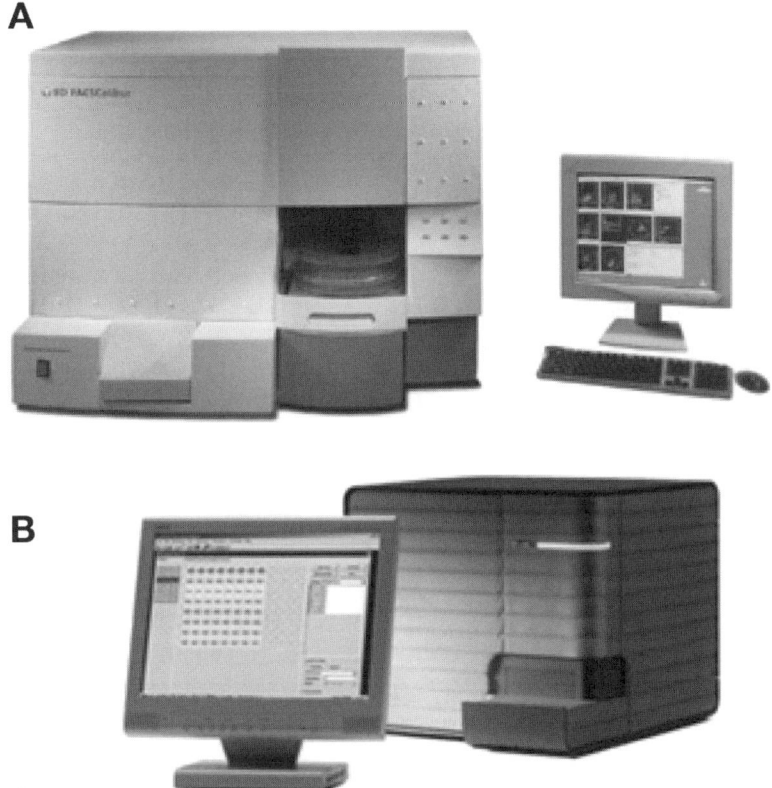

Fig. 1. BD Flow cytometers most often used with the cytometric bead array (CBA) assays. **(A)** BD FACSCalibur™ Flow Cytometer. The dual laser instrument is compatible with single color and dual color indexed CBA beads and assays constructed with these beads. **(B)** BD FACSArray™ bioanalyzer is a microplate-based instrument optimized for bead assays. The instrument utilizes a 635-nm red laser to index the dual color beads and a 532-nm green laser for exciting the signal generator phycoerythrin (PE) conjugate. Both single color and dual color indexed beads are compatible with the platform.

The CBA kits are utilizing beads, which are dyed with a single red fluorescent dye. Each different group of beads is labeled with a discrete level of fluorescent dye so that it can be distinguished by its mean fluorescence intensity (MFI) upon flow cytometric analysis. Beads within each group are covalently coupled with antibodies that can specifically capture a particular type of molecule present within biological fluids including serum, plasma, tissue culture supernatants, or cell lysates. The capture beads are mixed with PE-conjugated detection antibodies and standards, controls, or test samples to form sandwich complexes. Following acquisition of sample data using multicolor flow cytometry, the

Table 1
List of Available BD™ CBA Kits

Human CBA kits

Kit name	Specificities in kit
Allergy/asthma mediator kit – I	IL-3, IL-4, IL-5, IL-7, IL-10, GM-CSF
Allergy/asthma mediator kit – II	IL-3, IL-4, GM-CSF, G-CSF, eotaxin
Anaphylatoxin	C4a, C3a, C5a
Apoptosis kit	Cleaved PARP, Bcl-2, active caspase-3
Chemokine kit – I	IL-8, RANTES, MIG, MCP-1, IP-10
Inflammation kit	IL-8, IL-1β, IL-6, IL-10, TNF-α, IL-12p70
Th1/Th2 cytokine kit – I	IL-2, IL-4, IL-5, IL-10, TNF-α, IFN-γ
Th1/Th2 cytokine kit – II	IL-2, IL-4, IL-6, IL-10, TNF-α, IFN-γ

Nonhuman primate CBA kits

Nonhuman primate Th1/Th2 kit	IL-2, IL-4, IL-5, IL-6, TNF-α, IFN-γ

Mouse CBA kits

Immunoglobulin isotyping kit	IgG1, IgG2a, IgG2b ,IgG3 , IgA, IgM, IgE
Inflammation kit	IL-6, IL-10, MCP-1, IFN-γ, TNF-α, IL-12p70
Th1/Th2 cytokine kit	IL-2, IL-4, IL-5, TNF, IFN-γ

standard curves are compiled in graphic format and sample results are tabulated by the BD CBA software.

The assays are compatible with most of the BD flow cytometers, including FACScan, FACSCalibur, FACSVantage, FACSAria, FACSCanto, and FACSArray platforms. The performance characteristics of the multiplex assays, including sensitivity, spike recovery, dilution linearity, specificity, and intra- and interassay precision were determined for each kit.

The list of available CBA kits is summarized in **Table 1**. The immunoassay analysis is performed by a stand alone CBA software, which is compatible with both Apple Macintosh and PC computers. **Figure 2** shows six standard curves constructed with data using the Th1/Th2 CBA panel.

The CBA kits are often utilized to profile immunological processes. Tear samples from nonallergic and allergic donors were tested and reduced levels of interleukin (IL)-10 was found in allergic donors as compared to nonallergics *(13)*. This application was further developed by Sonoda *(14)*. Inflammatory cytokine CBA panel was used to monitor IL-6, IL-8, and IL-10 levels in pediatric patients who underwent cardiopulmonary bypass procedure *(15)*. A characteristic time-course of these cytokines was detected, with significant increase during the intraoperative phase and fast decrease in the postoperative phase.

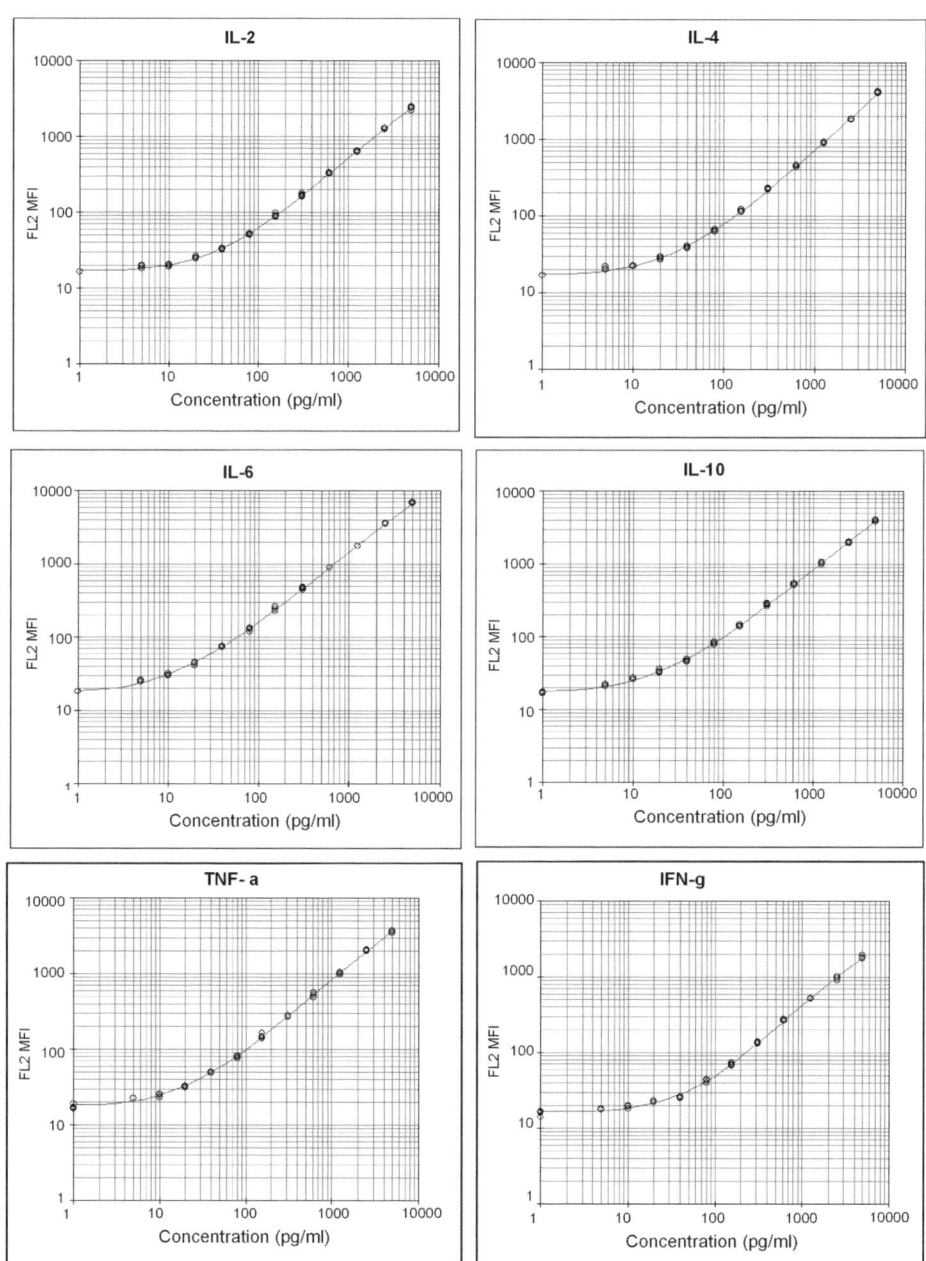

Fig. 2. Standard curves for the BD™ CBA Human Th1/Th2 panel (interleukin [IL]-2, IL-4, IL-6, IL-10, tumor necrosis factor-α, and interferon-γ), analyzed using BD CBA software.

Hodges evaluated plasma samples from neonates with confirmed bacterial infection using the inflammatory cytokine panel *(16)*. IL-6, IL-10, and IL-12 showed significant increase in *in utero* infected cases, whereas infection acquired after birth did not result in increased cytokine expression. Lipopolysaccharide induced cytokine and chemokine expression was evaluated in human carotid lesions using inflammatory cytokine, Th1/Th2 cytokine, and chemokine panels *(17)*. The chemokine panel was also useful in analyzing differences between uncomplicated influenza A and B cases and H5N1 influenza A infection *(18)*.

The kits were also evaluated in combination with cellular assays. Orfao reported simultaneous detection of secreted and cell-bound Th1/Th2 cytokines *(19)* using the CBA system.

Specificities and number of analytes are fixed in the CBA kits. Flexibility in combining analytes was achieved with BD CBA Flex Set assays, which are based on dual-color dyed beads (**Fig. 3B**).

The Flex Set system provides an open and configurable menu of bead-based reagents designed to create multiplex assays to specified requirements. Antibody conjugation chemistry, pair optimization strategies, and direct PE-detection reagents assure consistent assay performance in complex biological samples. Each antibody pair is evaluated for dynamic range, sensitivity, and parallel titration to native biological samples. The assay diluent and wash buffers are formulated to reduce potential interferences of serum and plasma samples. Direct PE conjugates are used as detection reagents, this minimizes the risk of increased background caused by endogenous biotin. The Flex Sets are compatible with serum, plasma, tissue culture supernatant, or cell lysate samples. A list of the available specificities and their bead location is summarized in **Table 2**. The standards are provided as unit-dose pellets, which can be easily combined with any number of additional pelletized standards. Common assay components, such as setup particles, buffers, and diluents are combined in a master buffer kit. The assays may be run either in tubes or in microplate format.

The Flex Set reagents require the use of dual-laser flow cytometers capable of detecting and distinguishing fluorescence emissions at 576, 670, and >680 nm. The Flex Set assays are compatible with the dual laser FACSCalibur, LSRII, FACSAria, FACSVantage, FACSCanto instruments, and the FACSArray Bioanalyzer.

Data analysis of the acquired FCS 2.0 data files is performed using FCAP Array software, which automatically clusters dual color CBA beads. It is a template-based system, which allows the design of customized Flex Set assay at the computer workstation. **Fig. 4** shows two standard curves, constructed for IL-6 and IL-8 by using the FCAP Array software. A 27-plex Flex Set assay, consisting of cytokines, chemokines, and other biological modifiers is demonstrated on **Fig. 5**.

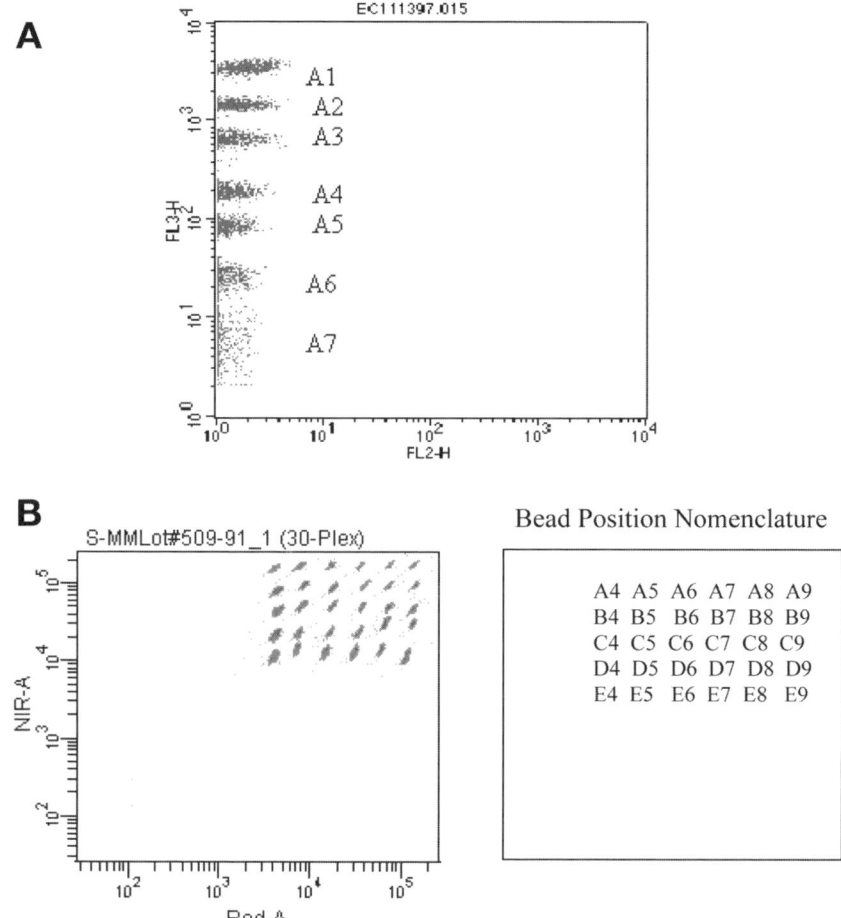

Fig. 3. Bead sets utilized in cytometric bead array (CBA) assays. (**A**) Single color fluorescent beads of graded red fluorescence. These uniform sized beads are discernable by their varying FL3 fluorescence. The single color beads are used in the BD™ CBA assay kits. (**B**) Dual color fluorescent beads. The 30 uniform sized beads are excited by the red laser and discernable in two dimensions by their individual red and near infrared fluorescence. The beads are utilized in the BD CBA Flex Set assays.

Fig. 6 shows the bead map of a 9-plex Flex Set assay which was configured to quantitatively measure T-cell activation in cell lysates. **Fig. 7** demonstrates the kinetics of Jurkat cell activation with CD3/CD28 treatment. Flex set assays were used to evaluate IgM signaling enhancement through ZAP 70 in chronic lymphoid leukemia (*20*).

In this chapter, we summarize the specifics of both the fixed panels and the Flex Set CBA assays. We are focusing on the assay methodology, for detailed

Table 2
List of Available BD™ CBA Flex Set Assays

Human soluble protein flex sets

Analyte	Bead position	Analyte	Bead position
Angiogenin	C4	IL-8	A9
Eotaxin	C7	IL-9	B6
Fas ligand	C6	IL-10	B7
Basic FGF	C5	IL-12p70	E5
G-CSF	C8	IP-10	B5
GM-CSF	C9	LT-a	D7
IFN-γ	E7	MCP-1	D8
IL-1β	B4	MIG	E8
IL-2	A4	MIP-1a	B9
IL-3	D5	MIP-1b	E4
IL-4	A5	RANTES	D4
IL-5	A6	TNFα	D9
IL-6	A7	VEGF	B8
IL-7	A8		

Mouse soluble protein flex sets

GM-CSF	B9	IL-9	B5
IFN-γ	A4	IL-10	C4
IL-2	A5	IL-12p70	D7
IL-3	A8	IL-13	B8
IL-4	A7	KC	A9
IL-5	A6	MCP-1	B7
IL-6	B4	TNF-α	C8

Rat soluble protein flex sets

IFN-γ	A6	IL10	A9
IL-4	B9	TNF-α	C8
IL-6	A9		

Phosphorylation site-specific flex sets

Btk (Y551)[a]	D5	PLCg (Y783)	B7
ERK1/2(T202/Y204)	C4	RSK (T573)	D7
Itk (Y511)	C6	Stat1 (Y701)	C5
JNK1/2 (T183/Y185)	B5	Syk (Y352)	B9
eNOS (S1177)	C7	ZAP-70 (Y319)	B8
p38/MAPKinase (T180/Y182)	B6		

(Continued)

Table 2 (*Continued*)

Total signaling protein flex sets			
Stat1	D4	ZAP-70	B8
Syk	B9		

[^a]The assays are specific for the phosphorylation sites displayed in brackets for each cell signaling molecule.

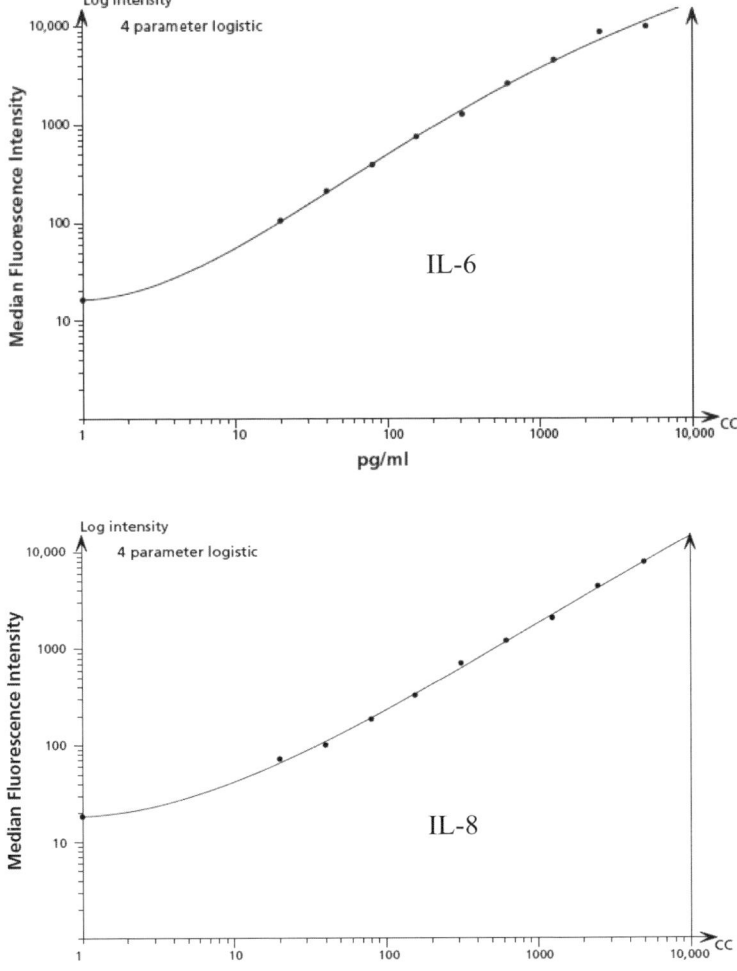

Fig. 4. CBA Flex Set standard curves for human interleukin (IL)-6 and IL-8. Data acquired on a BD FACSArray™ bioanalyzer and analyzed using the FCAP Array™ software.

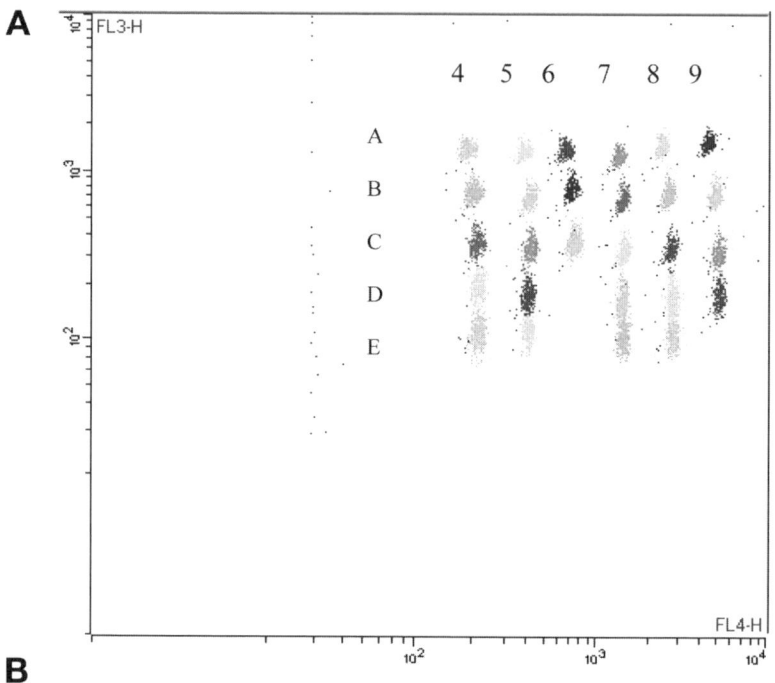

Analyte	Position	Analyte	Position	Analyte	Position	Analyte	Position
IL-2	A4	IL-9	B6	G-CSF	C8	IL-12p70	E5
IL-4	A5	IL-10	B7	GM-CSF	C9	IFNg	E7
IL-5	A6	VEGF	B8	RANTES	D4	MIG	E8
IL-6	A7	MIP-1a	B9	IL-3	D5		
IL-7	A8	Angiogenin	C4	LT-a	D7		
IL-8	A9	b-FGF	C5	MCP-1	D8		
IL_1b	B4	FasL	C6	TNF	D9		
IP-10	B5	Eotaxin	C7	MIP-1b	E4		

Fig. 5. A 27-plex Flex Set on a dual laser BD FACSCalibur™ instrument. (**A**) Dot plot representation of the 27-plex Flex Set. (**B**) List of the human specificities coupled to the different beads. Each unique bead position is defined as an alphanumeric address.

information on data handling using the BD CBA analysis software and FCAP Array software please refer to their respective user guides. Both of these documents are accessible at www.bdbiosciences.com. Additional technical information about FCAP Array software can be found at the Soft Flow website (www.softflow.com).

2. Materials

2.1. Th1/Th2 Human Cytokine Panel

This panel serves as an example of the ready-to-use CBA kits, which contain all the necessary assay components in a single package. Six bead populations

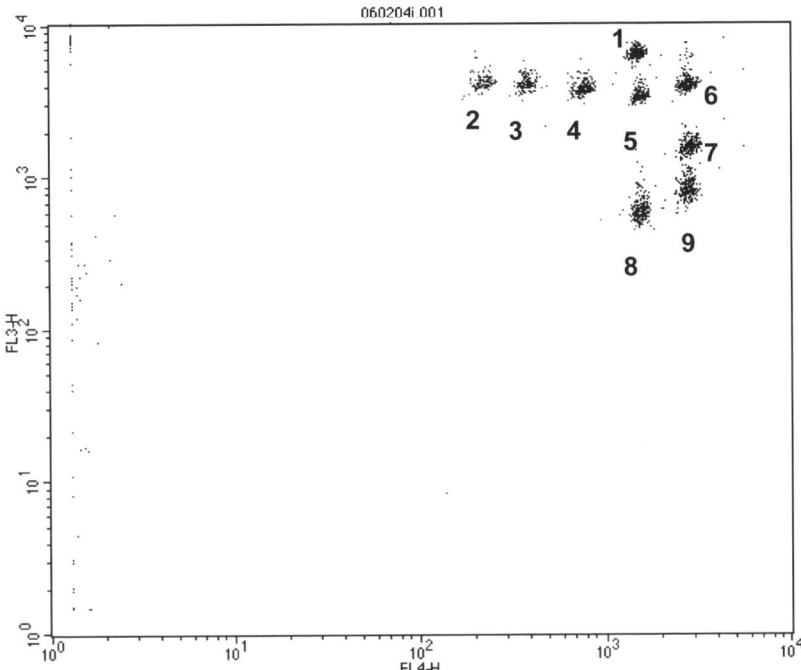

Fig. 6. A 9-plex Flex Set for testing T-cell activation. Key to the bead specificities: (1) Itk, (2) ERK, (3) JNK, (4) P38, (5) PLCγ, (6) ZAP70, (7) LAT, (8) c-Jun, (9) RSK.

with distinct fluorescence intensities have been coated with capture antibodies specific for IL-2, IL-4, IL-6, IL-10, tumor necrosis factor (TNF)-α, and interferon (IFN)-γ. The six individual bead populations are mixed together during the assay preparation. **Fig. 8** shows the FL3 histogram of the combined capture beads. The cytokine capture beads are combined with the PE-conjugated detection antibodies and then incubated with recombinant standards or test samples to form sandwich complexes. Following acquisition of sample data using the flow cytometer, the sample results are generated in graphical and tabular format using the BD CBA analysis software. The kit provides sufficient reagents for the quantitative analysis of 50 test samples and two standard curve sets.

2.1.1. Human Cytokine Capture Beads

There are 0.8 mL of each specific capture beads with discrete fluorescence intensity characteristics are supplied with the kit. The brightest bead in the kit is designated A1, the dimmest bead is A6. The beads are carrying the following specificities: A1= human IL-2, A2 = human IL-4, A3 = human IL-6, A4 = human IL-10, A5 = human TNF-α, A6 = human IFN-γ. The mixed capture bead

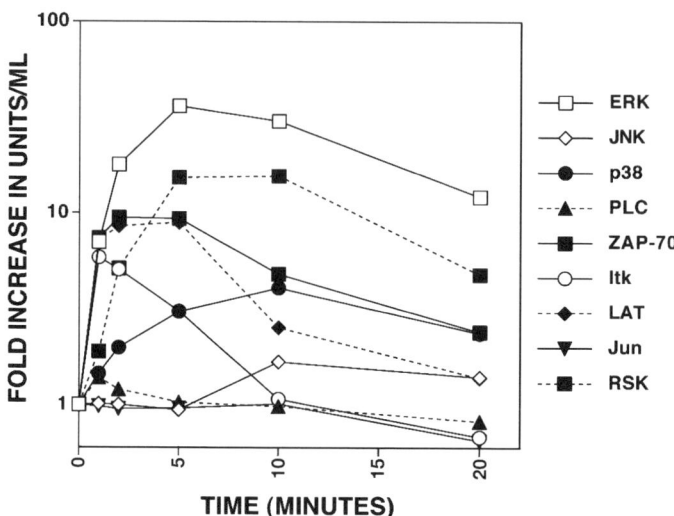

Fig. 7. Kinetics of T-cell activation using anti-CD3/CD28. Jurkat cells were activated with anti-CD3 and anti-CD28 for different lengths of time and the cells were lysed. A 9-plex BD CBA assay using 10 µg of lysate was run measuring phosphorylated ERK, JNK, p38, PLCγ, ZAP-70, Itk, LAT, c-Jun, and RSK. Using standard curves, concentration (U/mL) for each specificity was determined and the fold increase in activity was plotted.

reagent is formulated to support a 50-µL/test volume. The beads need to be stored at 4°C, and cannot be frozen.

2.1.2. PE-detection Reagent

Four milliliters of the mixed detector reagent is provided, containing PE-labeled monoclonal antibodies against human IL-2, IL-4, IL-6, IL-10, TNF-α, and IFN-γ. The combined detector reagent is formulated for use at 50 µL/test.

2.1.3. Cytokine Standards

Two vials of freeze-dried mixed standards are supplied with the kit, each vial containing a mixture of human recombinant IL-2, IL-4, IL-6, IL-10, TNF-α, and IFN-γ. Each vial should be reconstituted in 0.2 mL of assay diluent to prepare a 10X bulk standard. The reconstituted 10X bulk standard contains 50 ng/mL of each recombinant human IL-2, IL-4, IL-6, IL-10, TNF-α, and IFN-γ protein.

2.1.4. Instrument Setup Beads and Controls

One and a half-milliliter setup bead and 0.5 mL of each of a PE- and FITC-labeled controls are included in the kit. The PE control is a PE-conjugated antibody specific for the antigen coated on the setup bead, and formulated for

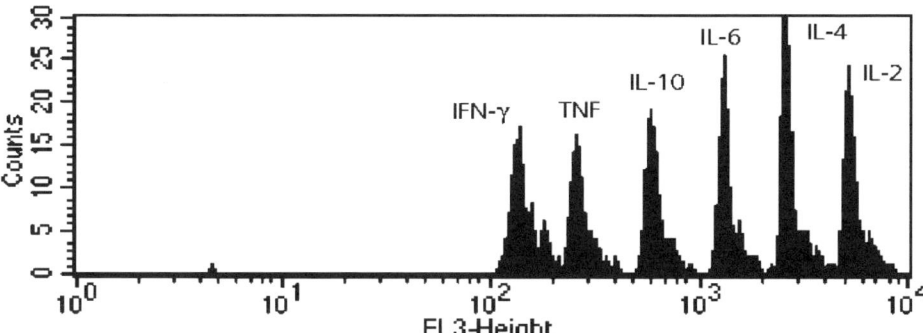

Fig. 8. FL3 histogram of the Th1/Th2 CBA kit beads. The individual bead peaks are labeled with the corresponding specificity.

use at 50 μL/test. The fluorescein (FITC) control is a FITC-conjugated antibody specific for the antigen coated on the setup bead, and formulated for use at 50 μL/test. The controls are used with the instrument setup bead to set the initial instrument compensation.

2.1.5. Buffers

One hundred-thirty milliliters wash buffer and 30 mL assay diluent is supplied in the kit. The wash buffer is phosphate-buffered saline (PBS) with protein and detergent additives. It is used for wash steps and to resuspend the washed beads for analysis. The assay diluent is a buffered protein solution used to reconstitute and dilute the human Th1/Th2 cytokine standards and to dilute test samples.

2.1.6. Instrumentation, Equipment, and Software Requirements

To run the CBA assay a flow cytometer equipped with a 488-nm laser capable of detecting and distinguishing fluorescence emissions at 576 and 670 nm (e.g., BD FACScan™ or BD FACSCalibur™ instruments) and BD CellQuest™ Software is required. Data analysis requires the BD CBA Software. Regular 12 × 75-mm sample acquisition tubes, such as BD Falcon™ tubes are used for the assay preparation and data acquisition.

2.2. Soluble Protein Flex Set Assays

The Soluble Protein Flex Set assay system allows combination of the available single bead assays (**Table 2**) to create multiplex panels, as required by the experimenter's needs. These assays are supporting human, mouse, and rat multiplex panels. Each individual capture bead population has a distinct and unique near-infra red and red fluorescence intensity signature. Each bead species are covalently coupled with a capture antibody specific for a given soluble protein. Each bead population is resolvable from the other bead species in the multiplex assay by their unique signature in the FL3 and FL4 channels of a FACSCalibur flow cytometer or in the near-infra red and red channels of a FACSArray Bioanalyzer. Each bead population is given an α-numeric position designation indicating its position relative to other beads in the BD CBA Flex Set system (**Table 2**, **Fig. 3B**). Beads with different positions can be combined in assays to create a multiplex assay. In a Flex Set assay the capture bead, PE-conjugated detection reagent, and standard or test samples are incubated together to form sandwich complexes. Following acquisition of sample data using the flow cytometer, the sample results are generated in a graphical and tabular format using the FCAP Array software.

2.2.1. Bead Reagents

1. Flex Set beads: each capture bead species supplied as bead suspensions in buffered saline solution containing fetal bovine serum and 0.09% sodium azide.
2. Instrument setup beads: setup beads defining the four corners of the Flex Set bead clusters (A1, A8, F1, F9 positions) are supplied as single-bead suspensions and are used to adjust the optimal instrument setup.
3. PE instrument setup bead: suspension of F1 beads, used for generating a PE positive bead population for instrument setup. The beads are covalently coupled with an anti-immunoglobulin antibody.

2.2.2. Antibody Reagents

1. Flex Set detectors: each analyte is defined by both the specific capture bead and the complementary PE-conjugated detector antibody reagent. The corresponding bead and detector specificities, together with lyophilized standards are supplied for each analyte in a single package. Each antibody conjugate is supplied in buffered saline solution containing bovine serum albumin (BSA) and 0.09% sodium azide. For the list of available soluble protein analytes to construct multiplex assays, *see* **Table 2**.
2. PE-positive control detector: a single vial of PE-conjugated antibody, formulated for use at 50 μL/test. This reagent is used with the PE instrument setup bead F1 to set instrument compensation settings. Store at 4°C. Do not freeze.

2.2.3. Flex Set Standards

For each assay, two vials of lyophilized standards are provided. The standards are lyophilized from an aqueous buffered protein solution containing BSA and Proclin™ 150. Each vial is reconstituted with 0.2 mL assay diluent.

2.2.4. Buffers and Diluents

1. Wash buffer: 1X PBS solution, containing protein and detergent, used for wash steps and to resuspend beads for analysis. Store at 4°C.

2. Assay diluent: 1X buffered solution used to dilute the BD™ CBA Human Soluble Protein Flex Set Standards and to dilute test samples. Store at 4°C.
3. Capture bead diluent for serum/plasma samples: 1X PBS solution containing protein used to resuspend capture beads prior to testing serum or plasma samples. Store at 4°C.
4. Capture bead diluent for cell culture supernatant samples: 1X PBS solution containing protein used to dilute capture beads prior to testing cell culture samples. Store at 4°C.
5. Detection reagent diluent: 1X PBS solution containing protein used to dilute the detection reagents. Store at 4°C.

2.2.5. Instrumentation, Equipment, and Software

A flow cytometer equipped with a 488- or 532-nm laser and a 635-nm laser capable of detecting and distinguishing fluorescence emission at 576 and 670 nm (off the 488-nm laser) and 660 nm (off the 635-nm laser) such as a FACSCalibur or 576 nm (off the 532-nm laser) and 660 and >680 nm (off the 635-nm laser) such as a FACSArray bioanalyzer is needed to perform CBA Flex Set bead assays. For assays run on the FACSCalibur 12 × 75-mm sample acquisition tubes are needed. FACSArray tests are run on microtiter plates, such as Millipore MultiScreen® BV 1.2-μm clear nonsterile filter plates. Plate washing is performed on a Millipore MultiScreen vacuum manifold, the plates are mixed on a digital microplate stirrer. Data acquisition and analysis requires availability of CellQuest, FACSComp, and FCAP Array software packages.

2.3. Cell Signaling Flex Set Assays

The cell signaling Flex Set assays are two-site sandwich multiplex immunoassays, which are available as total protein or phophorylated protein assays (**Table 2**). The assays are using cell lysates as samples and provide quantitative results based on standard curves constructed with recombinant protein standards. The sample data are analyzed using the FCAP Array software and the results are expressed as arbitrary U/mL for each analyte.

2.3.1. Bead Reagents

1. Flex Set beads: each capture bead species supplied as bead suspensions in buffered saline solution containing fetal bovine serum and 0.09% sodium azide.
2. Instrument setup beads: setup beads defining the four corners of the Flex Set bead clusters (A1, A8, F1, F9 positions) are supplied as single-bead suspensions and are used to adjust the optimal instrument setup.
3. PE instrument setup bead: suspension of F1 beads, used for generating a PE-positive bead population for instrument setup. The beads are covalently coupled with an anti-immunoglobulin antibody.

2.3.2. Antibody Reagents

1. Cell signaling Flex Set detectors: each analyte is defined by both the specific capture bead and the complementary PE-conjugated detector antibody reagent. The corresponding bead and detector specificities, together with lyophilized standards, are supplied for each analyte in a single package. The antibody conjugates are supplied in buffered saline solution containing BSA and 0.09% sodium azide.
2. PE-positive control detector: a single vial of PE-conjugated antibody that is formulated for use at 50 µL/test. This reagent is used with the PE instrument setup bead to set instrument compensation. Store at 4°C. Do not freeze.

2.3.3. Flex Set Standards

Each cell signaling flex set assay standard is formulated in aqueous solution containing 0.09% sodium azide. The standard is packaged together with the capture bead and the detector.

2.3.4. Buffers and Diluents

1. Wash buffer: 1X PBS solution containing protein and detergent used for wash steps and to resuspend beads for analysis. Store at 4°C.
2. Assay diluent: buffered solution used to dilute the cell signaling standards and to dilute test samples. Store at 4°C.
3. 5X Denaturation buffer: 5X sodium dodecyl sulfate solution used to denature test samples. Store at room temperature or 4°C.
4. Capture bead diluent: PBS solution containing protein. It is used to dilute capture beads prior to each experiment. Store at 4°C.
5. Detection reagent diluent: PBS solution containing protein. It is used to dilute the detection reagents prior to each experiment. Store at 4°C.

2.3.5. Instrumentation, Equipment, and Software

Same as described in **Subheading 2.2.5**.

3. Methods

3.1. Human Th1/Th2 Bead Assay

The human Th1/Th2 CBA Assay is used as a representative example of the ready-to-use CBA kits. **Table 1** summarizes the available kits and provides the list of analytes within each kit.

3.1.1. Preparation of Human Th1/Th2 Cytokine Standards

The human Th1/Th2 cytokine standards are lyophilized and should be reconstituted and serially diluted before mixing with the capture beads and the PE-detection reagent.

1. Reconstitute one vial of lyophilized human Th1/Th2 cytokine standards with 0.2 mL of assay diluent to prepare a 10X bulk standard. Allow the reconstituted standard to

equilibrate for at least 15 min before making dilutions. Agitate vial to mix thoroughly. Do not vortex.

2. Label 12 × 75-mm tubes (BD Falcon, cat. no. 352008) and arrange them in the following order: Top standard, 1:2, 1:4, 1:8, 1:16, 1:32, 1:64, 1:128, and 1:256.
3. Add 900 μL of assay diluent to the top standard tube.
4. Add 300 μL of assay diluent to each of the remaining tubes.
5. Transfer 100 μL of 10X bulk standard to the top standard tube and mix thoroughly.
6. Perform a serial dilution by transferring 300 μL from the top standard to the 1:2 dilution tube and mix thoroughly. Continue making serial dilutions by transferring 300 μL from the 1:2 tube to the 1:4 tube and so on to the 1:256 tube and mix thoroughly. The assay diluent serves as the negative control.

3.1.2. Preparation of Mixed Human Th1/Th2 Cytokine Capture Beads

The capture beads are bottled individually, and it is necessary to pool the six individual bead reagents immediately before mixing them together with the PE-detection reagent, standards, and samples.

1. Determine the number of assay tubes (including standards and controls) that are required for the experiment (e.g., 8 unknowns, 9 cytokine standard dilutions, and 1 negative control = 18 assay tubes).
2. Vigorously vortex each capture bead suspension for a few seconds before mixing.
3. Add a 10-μL aliquot of each capture bead, for each assay tube to be analyzed, into a single tube labeled "mixed capture beads" (e.g., 10 μL of IL-2 capture beads × 18 assay tubes = 180 μL of IL-2 capture beads required).
4. Vortex the bead mixture thoroughly. The mixed capture beads are now ready to be transferred to the assay tubes.

3.1.3. Preparation of Test Samples

The standard curve for each cytokine covers a defined set of concentrations from 20 to 5000 pg/mL. It may be necessary to dilute test samples to ensure that their mean fluorescence values fall within the limits or range of the generated cytokine standard curve. For best results, samples that are known or assumed to contain high levels of a given cytokine should be diluted as described next.

1. Dilute test sample by the desired dilution factor (i.e., 1:2, 1:10, or 1:100) using the appropriate volume of assay diluent.
2. Mix sample dilutions thoroughly before transferring samples to the appropriate assay tubes containing mixed capture beads and PE detection reagent.

3.1.4. Assay Procedure

Following the preparation and dilution of the standards and mixing of the capture beads, transfer these reagents and test samples to the appropriate assay tubes for incubation and analysis.

1. Add 50 μL of the mixed capture beads to the appropriate assay tubes. Vortex the mixed capture beads before adding to the assay tubes.

2. Add 50 µL of the human Th1/Th2 PE-detection reagent to the assay tubes.
3. Add 50 µL of the human Th1/Th2 cytokine standard dilutions to the control assay tubes.
4. Add 50 µL of each test sample to the test assay tubes.
5. Incubate the assay tubes for 3 h at room temperature and protect from direct exposure to light.
6. Add 1 mL of wash buffer to each assay tube and centrifuge at 200g for 5 min.
7. Carefully aspirate and discard the supernatant from each assay tube.
8. Add 300 µL of wash buffer to each assay tube to resuspend the bead pellet.
9. Begin analyzing samples on a flow cytometer. Vortex each sample for 3–5 s immediately before analyzing on the flow cytometer.

3.1.5. Data Acquisition and Data Analysis

Each assay tube is acquired on the flow cytometer using a CBA acquisition template. Acquisition template may be downloaded via the Internet from www.bdbiosciences.com/pharmingen/CBA//Dual-Laser.pdf. This template assures that each collected sample file contains approx 300 events for each capture bead species. To facilitate analysis of data files using the BD CBA software a numeric suffix is added to each file that corresponds to the assay tube number (i.e., tube no. 1 containing 0 pg/mL could be saved as RV032595.001). The acquired FACS files are saved and then analyzed using the BD CBA software. The outputs of the analysis are the calibration curves for the six analytes (**Fig. 2**) and tabulated concentrations of the six cytokines for each sample.

3.2. Soluble Human Protein Flex Set Bead Assay

3.2.1. Preparation of Human Soluble Protein Flex Set Standards

The two standards provided with each soluble protein Flex Set are provided as a 10X bulk recombinant protein (50,000 pg/mL) when reconstituted in 0.2 mL of assay diluent and should be serially diluted before mixing with the capture beads and the PE-detection reagent for a given assay. Each assay (single bead or multiplex) performed in a given experiment will need to have a standard curve prepared.

1. For multiplex experiments involving 10 or fewer soluble protein Flex Set assays, reconstitute each Flex Set standard vial with 0.2 mL of assay diluent to prepare a 10X bulk standard. Allow the reconstituted standard to equilibrate for at least 15 min before making dilutions. Mix reconstituted protein by pipet only. Do not vortex.
2. Label 12 × 75-mm tubes (BD Falcon, cat. no. 352008) and arrange them in the following order: top standard, 1:2, 1:4, 1:8, 1:16, 1:32, 1:64, 1:128, and 1:256.
3. Add 100 µL of each soluble protein standard to be run in the experiment to the top standard tube.

4. Add assay diluent to the top standard tube to bring the final volume to 1 mL.
   Example: if five soluble protein Flex Sets are being multiplexed for a given experiment, 100 μL of each soluble protein Flex Set standard needs to be added to the top standard tube (5 × 100 μL = 500 μL total volume) and then add 500 μL of assay diluent (1 mL assay diluent – 500 μL [volume of standards added] = 500 μL assay diluent). Adjust calculations accordingly for multiplexes of 10–20 soluble protein Flex Set assays.
5. Add 500 μL of assay diluent to each of the remaining tubes.
6. Perform a serial dilution by transferring 500 μL from the top standard to the 1:2 dilution tube and mix thoroughly. Continue making serial dilutions by transferring 500 μL from the 1:2 tube to the 1:4 tube and so on to the 1:256 tube and mix thoroughly. Mix by pipet only, do not vortex. Prepare one tube containing assay diluent to serve as negative control.

3.2.2. Preparation of Test Samples

The standard curve for each soluble protein Flex Set covers a defined set of concentrations from 20 to 5000 pg/mL. It may be necessary to dilute test samples to ensure that their mean fluorescence values fall within the limits or range of the generated standard curve. For best results, samples that are known or assumed to contain high levels of a given protein should be diluted as described next.

1. Dilute test sample by the desired dilution factor (i.e., 1:10 or 1:100) using the appropriate volume of assay diluent. Serum or plasma samples must be diluted at least 1:4 before transferring the samples to the assay tubes or wells.
2. Mix sample dilutions thoroughly before transferring samples to the appropriate assay tubes containing capture beads. Do not vortex. Mix by pipet only.

3.2.3. Preparation of Soluble Protein Flex Set Capture Beads

The capture beads provided with each soluble protein Flex Set are a 50X bulk (1 μL/test) and should be mixed with other soluble protein Flex Set capture beads and diluted to their optimal volume per test (50 μL/test) before adding the beads to a given tube or assay well.

1. Determine the number of soluble protein Flex Sets to be used in each tube or assay well in the experiment (size of the multiplex).
2. Determine the number of tubes or wells in the experiment.
3. Vortex each Soluble Protein Flex Set capture bead and then transfer 1 μL/test of each capture bead to a conical tube labeled "mixed capture beads."
   a. If testing cell culture supernatant samples, add capture bead diluent to the mixed capture beads tube to bring the final volume to 50 μL/test.
   b. If testing serum or plasma samples, add 0.5 mL of wash buffer to the mixed capture beads tube and centrifuge at 200*g* for 5 min to pellet the beads. Discard the supernatant by aspiration. Resuspend beads in capture bead diluent for serum/plasma to a final volume of 50 μL/test and incubate for 15 min at room temperature before proceeding to **step 5**.

Example: if five soluble protein Flex Sets are being multiplexed for a given 20 test experiment, you would add 1 μL/test of each capture bead to the mixed capture Bead tube (1 μL/test × 20 tests = 20 μL total volume of each soluble protein Flex Set capture bead) and then add capture bead diluent to bring the final volume to 50 μL/test by determining the remaining volume to add (the final volume of mixed capture beads is 20 tests × 50 μL/test = 1000 μL). A total of 100 μL of capture beads were added to the mixed capture beads tube previously listed when 20 μL total volume of each capture bead was added from the five soluble protein Flex Sets. The amount of capture bead diluent to add is 1000 μL total volume – 100 μL of capture beads = 900 μL).

5. Vortex the beads to mix thoroughly. Mixed capture beads are now ready to be used in the experiment.

3.2.4. Preparation of Flex Set PE-Detection Reagents

The PE-detection reagent provided with each soluble protein Flex Set is a 50X bulk (1 μL/test) and should be mixed with other soluble protein Flex Set PE-detection reagent and diluted to their optimal volume per test (50 μL/test) before adding the PE-detection reagents to a given tube or assay well.

1. Determine the number of soluble protein Flex Sets to be used in each tube or assay well in the experiment (size of the multiplex).
2. Determine the number of assay tubes or wells to be run in the experiment.
3. Transfer 1 μL/test of each soluble protein Flex Set PE-detection reagent to a conical tube labeled "mixed PE-detection reagent."
4. Add detection reagent diluent to the mixed PE-detection reagent tube to bring the final volume to 50 μL/test.
   Example: if five soluble protein Flex Sets are being multiplexed for a given 20 test experiment, you would add 1 μL/test of each soluble protein Flex Set PE-detection reagent to the mixed PE-detection reagent tube (1 μL/test × 20 tests = 20 μL total volume of each PE-detection reagent) and then add detection reagent diluent to bring the final volume to 50 μL/test by determining the remaining volume to add (the final volume of mixed PE-detection reagent is 20 tests × 50 μL/test = 1000 μL). A total of 100 μL of PE-detection reagent was added to the mixed PE-detection reagent tube previously listed when 20 μL total volume of each PE-detection reagent was added from the five soluble protein Flex Sets. The amount of detection reagent diluent to add is 1000 μL total volume – 100 μL of PE-detection reagents = 900 μL).
5. Vortex mixed PE-detection reagent briefly. Mixed PE-detection reagent is now ready to be used in the experiment.

3.2.5. Soluble Protein Flex Set Assay Procedure

Transfer the standards, capture beads, test samples, and PE-detection reagent to the appropriate assay tubes or wells for incubation and analysis.

1. For assays performed in filter plates, prewet the plate by adding 100 μL of wash buffer to each well. To remove excess volume, apply plate to vacuum manifold.

Do not exceed 10 inches of Mercury vacuum pressure 500*g*. Do not aspirate until wells are dry, leave a small amount of wash buffer in the wells.

2. Add 50 μL of the mixed capture beads to the appropriate assay tubes or wells. Vortex the mixed capture beads before adding them to the assay tubes or wells.

3. Add 50 μL of the soluble protein Flex Set standard dilutions to the control assay tubes or wells.

4. Add 50 μL of each test sample to the test assay tubes or wells.

5. For assays performed in tubes, mix assay tubes gently and incubate for 1 h at room temperature and protect from direct exposure to light. For assays performed in filter plate wells, mix the microwell plate for 5 min using a digital shaker at 500 and incubate plate for 1 h at room temperature, protecting from direct exposure to light.

6. Add 50 μL of the mixed PE-detection reagent to the assay tubes or wells.

7. For assay performed in tubes, mix assay tubes gently and incubate for 2 h at room temperature and protect from direct exposure to light. For assays performed in filter plate wells, mix the microwell plate for 5 min using a digital shaker at 50*g* and incubate plate for 2 h at room temperature, protecting from direct exposure to light.

8. For assays run in tubes, add 1.0 mL of wash buffer to each assay tube and centrifuge at 200*g* for 5 min. For assays run in filter plate wells, apply the plate to the vacuum manifold and vacuum aspirate (do not exceed 10" Hg of vacuum pressure) until wells are drained (2–10 s).

9. For assays run in tubes, carefully aspirate and discard the supernatant from each assay tube. For assays run in filter plate wells, proceed to **step 10**.

10. Add 300 μL of wash buffer to each assay tube or 150 μL of wash buffer to each assay well. Vortex assay tubes briefly or shake microwell plate on a digital shaker at 500*g* for 5 min to resuspend beads.

11. Begin analyzing samples on a flow cytometer. For assays run in tubes, it is recommended that each tube be vortexed briefly before analyzing on the flow cytometer.

3.2.6. Instrument Setup, Data Acquisition, and Analysis

FACSComp software is used for the daily setup the FACSCalibur flow cytometer. CellQuest software is required for analyzing samples and formatting data for subsequent analysis using the FCAP Array software. Setup for the FACSArray bioanalyzer is required only once a month. Sample acquisition is automated on the FACSCalibur, using the carousel loader, whereas the FACSArray instrument acquires the samples directly from the microplate wells. The data are analyzed using the FCAP Array software. The outputs of the Flex Set assays are the standard curves for each assay (**Fig. 5**) and the tabulated results for each analytes.

3.3. Cell Signaling Bead Assay

3.3.1. Preparation of Cell Signaling Flex Set Standards

The standard provided with each Cell Signaling Flex Set is provided as a 50X bulk recombinant protein (50,000 U/mL) and should be serially diluted before mixing with the capture beads and the PE-detection reagent for a given assay. The protocol listed next indicates how standards should be mixed and diluted for use in a cell signaling Flex Set assay. Each assay (single bead or multiplex) performed in a given experiment will need to have a standard curve prepared. Each cell signaling Flex Set standard was assigned an arbitrary unit value. In each case, the unit potency of the Flex Set standard will be kept consistent from lot to lot.

1. Warm standard vial to 37°C and vortex to mix thoroughly.
2. Label 12 × 75-mm tubes (BD Falcon, cat. no. 352008) and arrange them in the following order: top standard, 1:2, 1:4, 1:8, 1:16, 1:32, 1:64, 1:128, and 1:256.
3. Add 20 μL of each cell signaling Flex Set standard to be run in the experiment to the top standard tube.
4. Add assay diluent to the top standard tube to bring the final volume to 1 mL.
   Example: if five cell signaling Flex Sets are being multiplexed for a given experiment, 20 μL of each BD CBA cell signaling flex.
   Set standard needs to be added to the top standard tube (5 × 20 μL = 100 μL total volume) and will then add 900 μL of assay diluent (1 mL assay diluent – 100 μL [volume of standards added] = 900 μL assay diluent).
5. Add 500 μL of assay diluent to each of the remaining tubes.
6. Perform a serial dilution by transferring 500 μL from the top standard to the 1:2 dilution tube and mix thoroughly. Continue making serial dilutions by transferring 500 μL from the 1:2 tube to the 1:4 tube and so on to the 1:256 tube and mix thoroughly. The assay diluent serves as the negative control.

3.3.2. Preparation of Test Samples

The cell signaling Flex Sets are designed to measure total or phosphorylated proteins from denatured cell lysate samples. The tested cells need to be lysed and denatured using the 5X denaturation buffer (provided in the kit) before used in a Flex Set assay. The standard curve for each Flex Set covers a defined set of concentrations between 3.9 and 1000 U/mL. It may be necessary to dilute test samples to ensure that their mean fluorescence values fall within the limits or range of the generated standard curve. For best results, samples that are known or assumed to contain high levels of a given protein should be diluted. In cases where the samples are known or assumed to contain low levels of a given protein, the sample should be lysed in a lower volume of lysis buffer thereby concentrating the protein in the sample. It is important that the cell number or the total protein concentration of the cell lysate sample is known so that results determined using the Flex Sets can be normalized (e.g., U/mL/10^6 cells or U/mL/μg of cell lysate). It is necessary to heat the 5X denaturation buffer to 37°C before use (shake or vortex until all precipitates have gone back into solution). The final concentration of the denaturation buffer should reach 1X once mixed with cells to achieve denaturation of the cell lysate.

3.3.2.1. CELLS IN SUSPENSION

1. Count cells in sample. This is to give an approximate idea of protein concentration, which should be greater than 1 mg/mL (protein concentration is dependent on cell type, e.g., Jurkat = $100 - 200 \, \mu g/10^6$ cells whereas peripheral blood lymphocytes = $25 - 50 \, \mu g/10^6$ cells).
2. Treat cells to induce or inhibit protein phosphorylation as required for the experiment.
3. Add appropriate amount of 5X denaturation buffer so that the final concentration is 1X. Alternatively, ice-cold PBS can be added to the tube and the cells pelleted. Add an appropriate amount of 1X denaturation buffer (prepared by diluting the 5X denaturation buffer with water) to resuspend the cell pellet.
4. Immediately place in a boiling water bath for 5 min.
5. Determine protein concentration.
6. Dilute cell lysate sample by the desired dilution factor (i.e., 1:2, 1:10, or 1:20) using the appropriate volume of assay diluent. Sample must be diluted at least 1:2 to reduce the percentage of sodium dodecyl sulfate.
7. Mix sample dilutions thoroughly before transferring samples to the appropriate assay tubes containing capture beads.

3.3.2.2. ADHERENT CELLS

1. Count cells before plating. This is to give an approximate idea of protein concentration, which should be greater than 1 mg/mL.
2. Treat cells to induce or inhibit protein phosphorylation as required for the experiment.
3. Add the appropriate amount of 5X denaturation buffer so that the final concentration is 1X. Alternatively, aspirate off all liquid and add denaturation buffer diluted to 1X with water. Scrape or agitate cells to dislodge from plate.
4. Immediately place in a boiling water bath for 5 min.
5. Determine protein concentration.
6. Dilute cell lysate sample by the desired dilution factor (i.e., 1:2, 1:10, or 1:20) using the appropriate volume of assay diluent. Sample must be diluted at least 1:2.
7. Mix sample dilutions thoroughly before transferring samples to the appropriate assay tubes containing capture beads.

3.3.3. Preparation of Capture Beads

The capture beads provided with each cell signaling Flex Set are a 50X bulk (1 µL/test) and should be mixed with other cell signaling Flex Set capture beads and diluted to their optimal volume per test (50 µL/test) before adding the beads to a given tube or assay well.

1. Determine the number of BD CBA cell signaling Flex Sets to be used in each tube or assay well in the experiment (size of the multiplex).
2. Determine the number of assay of tubes or wells to be run in the experiment.

3. Vortex each cell signaling Flex Set capture bead and then transfer 1 µL/test of each cell signaling Flex Set capture bead to a conical tube labeled "mixed capture beads."

4. Add capture bead diluent to the mixed capture beads tube to bring the final volume to 50 µL/test.

   Example: if five cell signaling Flex Sets are being multiplexed for a given 20 test experiment, 1 µL/test of each cell signaling Flex Set capture bead needs to be added to the mixed capture bead tube (1 µL/test × 20 tests = 20 µL total volume of each cell signaling Flex Set capture bead) and then capture bead diluent is added to bring the final volume to 50 µL/test by determining the remaining volume to add (the final volume of mixed capture beads is 20 tests × 50 µL/test = 1000 µL). A total of 100 µL of capture beads were added to the mixed capture beads tube previously listed when 20 µL total volume of each cell signaling Flex Set capture bead was added from the five cell signaling Flex Sets. The amount of capture bead diluent to add is 1000 µL total volume – 100 µL of capture beads = 900 µL).

5. Vortex the beads to mix thoroughly. Mixed capture beads are now ready to be used in the experiment

3.3.4. Preparation of PE-Detection Reagents

The PE-detection reagent provided with each cell signaling Flex Set is a 50X bulk (1 µL/test) and should be mixed with other cell signaling Flex Set PE-detection reagent and diluted to their optimal volume per test (50 µL/test) before adding the PE-detection reagents to a given tube or assay well.

1. Determine the number of cell signaling Flex Sets to be used in each tube or assay well in the experiment (size of the multiplex).

2. Determine the number of assay tubes or wells to be run in the experiment.

3. Transfer 1 µL/test of each cell signaling Flex Set PE-detection reagent to a conical tube labeled "mixed PE-detection reagent."

4. Add detection reagent diluent to the mixed PE-detection reagent tube to bring the final volume to 50 µL/test.

   Example: if five cell signaling Flex sets are being multiplexed for a given 20 test experiment, 1 µL/test of each cell signaling Flex Set PE-detection reagent needs to be added to the mixed PE-detection reagent tube (1 µL/test × 20 tests = 20 µL total volume of each BD CBA cell signaling Flex Set PE-detection reagent) and then add detection reagent diluent to bring the final volume to 50 µL/test by determining the remaining volume to add (the final volume of mixed PE-detection reagent is 20 tests × 50 µL/test = 1000 µL). A total of 100 µL of PE-detection reagent was added to the mixed PE-detection reagent tube previously listed when 20 µL total volume of each cell signaling Flex Set PE-detection reagent was added from the five cell signaling Flex Sets. The amount of detection reagent diluent to add is 1000 µL total volume – 100 µL of PE-detection reagents = 900 µL.

5. Vortex mixed PE-detection reagent briefly. Mixed PE-detection reagent is now ready to be used in the experiment.

3.3.5. Assay Procedure

Transfer the standards, capture beads, test samples, and PE-detection reagent to the appropriate assay tubes or wells for incubation and analysis. Flex Set standards are run in each experiment to allow quantitation of test samples.

1. Add 50 µL of the mixed capture beads to the appropriate assay tubes or wells. Vortex the mixed capture beads before adding them to the assay tubes or wells.
2. Add 50 µL of the mixed PE-detection reagent to the assay tubes or wells.
3. Add 50 µL of the cell signaling Flex Set standard dilutions to the control assay tubes or wells.
4. Add 50 µL of each denatured cell lysate test sample to the test assay tubes or wells.
5. For assays performed in tubes, mix assay tubes gently and incubate for 4 h at room temperature and protect from direct exposure to light. For assays performed in filter plate wells, mix the microwell plate for 15 min using a digital shaker at 500g and incubate plate for 4 h at room temperature and protect from direct exposure to light.
6. For assays run in tubes, add 1.0 mL of wash buffer to each assay tube and centrifuge at 200g for 5 min. For assays run in filter plate wells, apply the plate to the vacuum manifold and vacuum aspirate (do not exceed 10" Hg of vacuum) until wells are drained (2–10 s).
7. For assays run in tubes, carefully aspirate and discard the supernatant from each assay tube. For assays run in filter plate wells, proceed to **step 8**.
8. Add 300 µL of wash buffer to each assay tube or 150 µL of wash buffer to each assay well. Vortex assay tubes briefly or shake microwell plate on a digital shaker at 50g for 5 min to resuspend beads.
9. Begin analyzing samples on a flow cytometer. For assays run in tubes, it is recommended that each tube be vortexed briefly before analyzing on the flow cytometer.

3.3.6. Instrument Setup, Data Acquisition, and Analysis

FACSComp software is used for setting up the FACSCalibur flow cytometer daily. BD CellQuest software is required for analyzing samples and formatting data for subsequent analysis using the FCAP Array software. Setup for the FACSArray Bioanalyzer required only once a month. Sample acquisition is automated on the FACSCalibur, using the carousel loader, whereas the FACSArray instrument acquires the samples directly from the microplate wells. The data are analyzed using the FCAP Array Software. The outputs of the Flex Set assays are the standard curves for each assay and the tabulated results for each analytes. **Fig. 6** shows the bead positions of a 9-plex cell signaling Flex Set combination. **Fig. 7** demonstrates the kinetics of T cell activation with CD3/CD28 treatment using Jurkat cells.

4. Notes

1. The BD CBA is not recommended for use on stream-in-air instruments where signal intensities may be reduced, adversely affecting assay sensitivity. Stream-in-air instruments include the FACStar Plus and FACS Vantage flow cytometers.
2. The antibody-conjugated beads will settle out of suspension over time. It is necessary to vortex the vial vigorously for 3–5 s before taking a bead suspension aliquot.
3. The human Th1/Th2 cytokine standards vials are stable until the kit expiration date. Following reconstitution, store the freshly reconstituted 10X bulk standard at 2–8°C and use within 12 h.
4. When running experiments with higher order multiplexes use the following instructions for reconstituting the soluble protein Flex Set standards. For multiplex experiments involving 10–20 soluble protein Flex Set assays, reconstitute each standard vial with 0.1 mL of assay diluent to prepare a 20X bulk standard. For multiplex experiments involving more than 20 soluble protein Flex Set assays, pour each standard protein sphere into a 15-mL conical tube and reconstitute all spheres together in 2 mL of assay diluent to prepare a top standard mixture.
5. To calibrate the flow cytometer and quantitate test samples, it is necessary to run the cytokine standards and the cytometer setup controls in each experiment.
6. For Flex Set assays that will be acquired on a FACSCalibur flow cytometer, it is recommended that additional dilutions of the standard be prepared (i.e., 1:512 and 1:1024) as it is possible that in multiplex experiments containing a large number of assays, the top standard and 1:2 standard dilution will not be analyzable by the FCAP Array software. In those cases, the top standard and 1:2 standard dilutions can be run on the experiment but will be excluded from the final analysis in the FCAP Array software.
7. Cell lysates may be stored at –70°C for up to 6 mo. Multiple freeze/thaw treatments of sample should be avoided.
8. It is necessary to analyze CBA samples on the day of the experiment. Prolonged storage of samples, once the assay is complete, can lead to increased background and reduced sensitivity.
9. The phospho-specific cell signaling Flex Set assays cannot be used in the same assay well with the total protein cell signaling Flex Set assays. An updated assay compatibility chart for the cell signaling Flex Sets is available at www.bdbiosciences.com/flexset.

References

1. Carson, R. T. and Vignali, D. A. (1999) Simultaneous quantitation of fifteen cytokines using a multiplexed flow cytometric assay. *J. Immunol. Meths.* **227,** 41–45.
2. Morgan, E., Varro, R., Sepulveda, H., et al. (2004) Cytometric bead array: a multiplexed assay platform with applications in various areas of biology. *Clin. Immunol.* **110,** 252–266.
3. Stall, A., Sun, Q., Varro, R., et al. (1998) A single tube flow cytometric multibead assay for isotyping mouse monoclonal antibodies. Abstract 1877, Experimental Biology Meeting.

4. Lund-Johansen, F., Davis, K., Bishop, J. E., and Malefyt, R. de W. (2000) Flow cytometric analysis of immunoprecipitates: high-throughput analysis of protein phosphorylation and protein-protein interactions. *Cytometry* **39,** 250–259.

5. Fulwyler, M. J., McHugh, T. M., Schwadron, R., et al. (1988) Immunoreactive bead (IRB) assay for the quantitative and simultaneous flow cytometric detection of multiple soluble analytes. *Cytometry* **2,** 19.

6. McHugh, T. M. (1994) Flow microsphere immunoassay for the quantitative and simultaneous detection of multiple soluble analytes. *Methods Cell Biol.* **42,** 575–595.

7. Camilla, C., Defoort, J. P., Delaage, M., et al. (1998) A new flow cytometry-based multi-assay system. 1. Application to cytokine immunoassays. *Cytometry* **8,** 132.

8. Chen, R., Lowe, L., Wilson, J. D., et al. (1999) Simultaneous quantification of six human cytokines in a single sample using microparticle-based flow cytometric technology. *Clin. Chem.* **9,** 1693–1694.

9. Fulton, R. J., McDade, R. L., Smith, P. L., Kienker, L. J., and Kettman, J. R. (1997) Advanced multiplexed analysis with the FlowMetrix system. *Clin. Chem.* **43,** 1749–1756.

10. McHugh, T. M., Viele, M. K., Chase, E. S., and Recktenwald, D. J. (1997) The sensitive detection and quantitation of antibody to HCV using a microsphere-based immunoassay and flow cytometry. *Cytometry* **29,** 106–112.

11. Faucher, S., Martel, A., Sherring, A., et al. (2004) Protein bead array for the detection of HIV-1 antibodies from fresh plasma and dried-blood-spot specimens. *Clin. Chem.* **50,** 1250–1253.

12. Khan, I. H., Kendall, L. V., Ziman, M., et al. (2005) Simultaneous serodetection of 10 highly prevalent mouse infectious pathogens in a single reaction by multiplex analysis. *Clin. Diagn. Lab. Immunol.* **12,** 513–519.

13. Cook, E. B., Stahl, J. L., Lowe, L., et al. (2001) Simultaneous measurement of six cytokines in a single sample of human tears using microparticle-based flow cytometry: allergics vs. non-allergics. *J. Immunol. Meths.* **254,** 109–118.

14. Sonoda, S., Uchino, E., Nakao, K., and Sakamoto, T. (2006) Inflammatory cytokine of basal and reflex tears analysed by multicytokine assay. *British J. Ophthalmology* **90,** 120–122.

15. Tárnok, A., Hambsch, J., Chen, R., and Varro, R. (2003) Cytometric bead array to measure six cytokines in twenty-five microliters of serum *Clin. Chem.* **49,** 1000–1002.

16. Hodge, G., Hodge, S., Haslam, R., et al. (2004) Rapid simultaneous measurement of multiple cytokines using 100 microliter sample volumes—association with neonatal sepsis. *Clin. Exp. Immunol.* **137,** 402–407.

17. Jatta, K., Wågsäter,D., Norgren, L., Stenberg, B., and Sirsjö, A. (2005) Lipopolysaccharide-induced cytokine and chemokine expression in human carotid lesions. *J. Vasc. Res.* **42,** 266–271.

18. Peiris, J. S., Yu, W. C., Leung, C. W., et al. (2004) Re-emergence of fatal human influenza A subtype H5N1 disease. *Lancet* **363,** 617–619.

19. Rodriguez-Caballero, A., Garcia-Montero, A. C., Bueno, C., et al. (2004) A new simple whole blood flow cytometry based method for simultaneous identification of activated cells and quantitative evaluation of cytokines released during activation. *Laboratory Investigation* **84,** 1387–1398.

20. Chen, L., Apgar, J., Huynh, L., et al. (2005) ZAP-70 directly enhances IgM signaling in chronic lymphocytic leukemia. *Blood* **105,** 2036–2041.

10

Cell-Free Bead-Based Detection of Total and Phosphorylated Proteins in Plasma and Cell Lysates

Detection of FLT3

Huai En Huang Chan, Iman Jilani, Richard Chang, and Maher Albitar

Summary

Frequently direct measurement of proteins or their phosphorylation in intact cells is not possible, for instance, when cells are too few, frozen, or subject to degradation. We have demonstrated that tumor cells pour their DNA, RNA, and protein content into circulation because of turnover and breakdown of cell structures. Proteins in solution most likely circulate as complexes, which protects them from degradation. We describe a cell-free, bead-based method that takes advantage of this phenomenon. Our approach is based on immunoprecipitation of the protein of interest on the surface of beads, followed by detection of the protein or its modification (phosphorylation) using a secondary antibody labeled with phycoerythrin at a 1:1 ratio. Fms-like tyrosine kinase-3, which is mutated in majority of cases of acute myeloid leukemia, is used as an example. This method could be applied to the quantitation of several other proteins without the need for intact cells.

Key Words: Proteins; phosphorylation; soluble; plasma; beads; FLT3; AML; MDS.

1. Introduction

The direct measurement of proteins and their phosphorylation in intact cells has been limited by the availability of viable cells. Proteins have been observed in plasma not as free or soluble moieties, but as circulating complexes *(1,2)*. In the following sections, we will describe the measurement of total and phosphorylated protein levels in plasma by flow cytometry, using Fms-like tyrosine kinase-3 (FLT3) as an example. FLT3 is a class III receptor tyrosine kinase that plays a pivotal role in survival, proliferation, and differentiation of hematopoietic progenitor cells. Somatic mutation of the *FLT3* gene in the form of an internal tandem duplication or point mutation (D835) in the coding sequence of

From: *Methods in Molecular Biology, vol. 378: Monoclonal Antibodies: Methods and Protocols*
Edited by: M. Albitar © Humana Press Inc., Totowa, NJ

the juxtamembrane domain has been observed in acute myeloid leukemia and myelodysplastic syndrome (*3–6*). These mutations activate FLT3 in a ligand-independent manner, leading to constitutive phosphorylation of downstream signal transducers.

2. Materials
2.1. FLT3 Protein and its Phosphorylation

1. Flow phosphate-buffered saline (PBS): prepare with 5.6 g sodium dibasic, 35.48 g sodium chloride, 2.8 g bovine serum albumin (BSA), and 4.0 g sodium azide. Add deionized water to 4 L; adjust pH to 7.4.
2. Carboxylated polystyrene beads (Bangs Laboratories, Fishers, IN).
3. Carbodiimide (Sigma Aldrich, St. Louis, MO).
4. Anti-human FLT3 antibody (R&D Systems, Minneapolis, MN).
5. Phycoerythrin (PE)-labeled anti-FLT3 (CD135) (BD Biosciences, San Jose CA).
6. PE-labeled anti-phosphotyrosine antibody (BD Biosciences).
7. Sorvall cell-washer 2 (Thermo Electron Corporation, Ashville, NC).

2.2. Flow Cytometric Analysis

1. FACSCalibur™ flow cytometer (BD Biosciences).
2. QuantiBRITE™ PE beads (BD Biosciences).
3. Cell Quest Pro acquisition and analysis software (BD Biosciences).

3. Methods

Our approach uses polystyrene beads coated with anti-FLT3 to capture circulating FLT3 protein in plasma. The captured FLT3 protein on the surface of the beads is quantified using either a secondary PE-labeled anti-FLT3 antibody or a secondary PE-labeled anti-phosphotyrosine antibody. Fluorescence is detected using flow cytometry and compared against a PE standard established with QuantiBRITE PE beads (*see* **Note 1**). This converts mean fluorescence intensities (MFI) into antibodies bound/bead.

3.1. Instrument Setup

1. The cytometer is calibrated prior to use according to the manufacturer's protocol using CaliBRITE 3 beads (BD Biosciences) with addition of APC-beads (BD Biosciences).
2. The FACSCalibur flow cytometer is prepared for acquisition by launching Cell Quest Pro software (BD Bioscience). It is recommended to check sheath fluid and waste levels prior to acquisition. The appropriate acquisition template and instrument settings are selected.
3. Standardization is performed before acquisition of samples using QuantiBRITE PE beads, which are reconstituted with 1 mL of flow PBS. Five thousand events are acquired on the FACSCalibur. An example of the results is shown in **Fig. 1**.

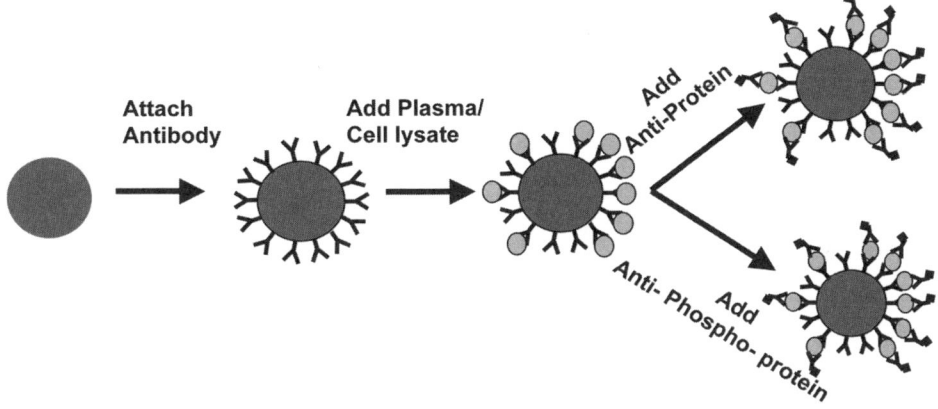

Fig. 1. Schematic representing bead conjugation, immunoprecipitation, and detection of protein to measure targeted protein in plasma by flow cytometry.

3.2. Bead Preconjugation With Anti-Human FLT3

1. Anti-human FLT3 antibody is conjugated onto beads with the following steps.
   a. 100 μL of 7.37 μ*M* polystyrene beads (Bangs Laboratories) are washed twice and diluted 1:10 with 0.05 *M* sodium bicarbonate.
   b. Beads are incubated in the presence of 0.01 g carbodiimide (Sigma Aldrich) for 30 min with mixing at room temperature.
   c. Beads are washed and resuspended in 1 mL 0.05 *M* sodium bicarbonate.
   d. 100 μL of beads are removed for beads check (*see* **Note 2**).
   e. The remaining 900 μL of beads are incubated with 100 μL anti-human FLT3 (R&D Systems) overnight at 4°C with mixing.

3.3. Bead and Sample Preparation for Quantitative Flow Cytometry

1. Beads are washed and resuspended in 1× PBS/5% BSA.
2. Lysate and plasma samples are diluted 1:20 and 1:10, respectively.
3. Samples are incubated with 5 μL 10% sodium dodecyl sulfate and denatured at 96°C for 5 min.
4. After cooling on ice, the samples are transferred to new tubes and incubated with 30 μL anti-FLT3-conjugated beads for 4 h at room temperature with mixing.
5. After being washed and resuspended in 1× PBS/5% BSA, beads are aliquoted into four tubes and incubated separately with 5 μL rabbit anti-phosphotyrosine (Zymed/Invitrogen, Carlsbad CA), IgG1 PE, or anti-human CD135 PE (BD Biosciences) (*see* **Note 3**).
6. After incubation for 1 h with mixing at room temperature, beads are washed and resuspended in 1× PBS/5% BSA.
7. Beads with rabbit anti-phosphotyrosine are then incubated with the appropriate secondary antibody (bovine anti-rabbit PE) for 1 h at room temperature, in the dark with mixing.

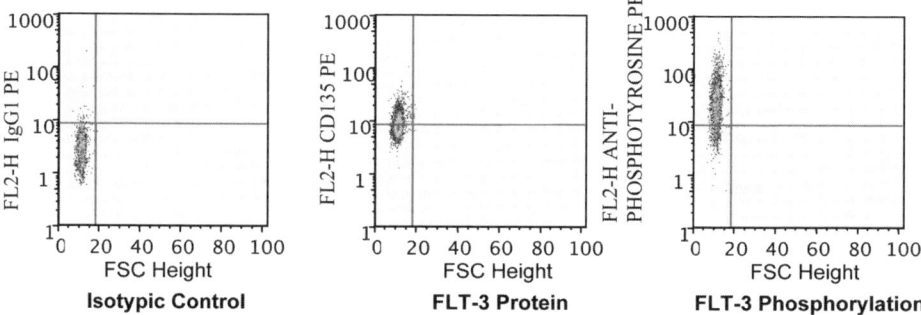

Fig. 2. Dot plots representing cells stained with FLT3 antibody and phosphorylated FLT3 antibody. An upward shift in FL2 (*x*-axis) represents detection of the antibody of interest.

8. Beads are washed and resuspended in 500 µL flow PBS for analysis on the FACSCalibur. An example of the result is shown in **Fig. 2**.

4. Discussion

This flow cytometry approach is based on immunoprecipitation of the protein of interest onto the surface of beads, followed by detection of the protein or its modification (phosphorylation) using a secondary antibody labeled with PE at a 1:1 ratio. This method could be applied to the quantitation of several other proteins without the need for intact cells. Measuring levels of total and phosphorylated FLT3 protein provides important information that may not be gleaned by analyzing only internal tandem duplication and D835 mutations. The use of plasma, rather than cells, provides the advantages of more sensitive detection, as plasma is highly enriched with the DNA, RNA, and protein content of leukemic cells. The specificity of antibodies should be validated using cell lines and ex vivo studies to manipulate the protein. This approach generates quantitative data on proteins and their modification without the need for intact cells (*see* **Note 4**).

5. Notes

1. QuantiBRITE PE beads are four different beads labeled with known amounts of PE antibody. These beads are acquired during every experiment and used as a fluorescence standard to covert MFI to antibody binding capacity (ABC).
2. It is preferable that the conjugation be confirmed by performing a detection step with anti-mouse PE. The conjugation is detected by incubation of diluted conjugated beads (1:10 with blocking buffer) with 5 µL anti-mouse PE for 15 min at room temperature in the dark. The beads are washed and resuspended in 500 µL flow PBS for flow analysis.

3. Though anti-phosphotyrosine detects all tyrosine kinases, only FLT3 kinase is present after immuno-precipitation with anti-human FLT3 conjugated beads. The IgG1 PE is used as the isotype control.
4. As flow cytometry output can be in terms of percentage positivity and MFI, it is recommended to analyze data in terms of a derived "index value," which combines both factors. Index = (percentage positivity) × ABC.

References

1. Albitar, M., Do, K. A., Johnson, M. M., et al. (2004) Free circulating soluble CD52 as a tumor marker in chronic lymphocytic leukemia and its implication in therapy with anti-CD52 antibodies. *Cancer* **101,** 999–1008.
2. Rogers, A., Joe, Y., Manshouri, T., et al. (2004) Relative increase in leukemia-specific DNA in peripheral blood plasma from patients with acute myeloid leukemia and myelodysplasia. *Blood* **103,** 2799–2801.
3. Kioyi, H., Towatari, M., Yokota, S., et al. (1998) Internal tandem duplication of the *FLT3* gene is a novel modality of elongation mutation which causes constitutive activation of the product. *Leukemia* **12,** 1333–1337.
4. Fenski, R., Flesch, K., Serve, S., et al. (2000) Constitutive activation of FLT3 in acute myeloid leukaemia and its consequences for growth in 32D cells. *Br. J. Haematol.* **108,** 322–330.
5. Nakao, M., Yokota, S., Iwai, T., et al. (1996) Internal tandem duplication of the *FLT3* gene found in acute myeloid leukemia. *Leukemia* **10,** 1911–1918.
6. Rombouts, W., Blokland, I., Lowenberg, B., and Plemacher, R. (2000) Biological characteristics and prognosis of adult acute myeloid leukemia with internal tandem duplications in the *FLT3* gene. *Leukemia* **14,** 675–683.

11

Measuring Humanized Antibodies in Plasma of Patients Treated With Antibody-Based Therapy Using Bead-Based Flow Cytometry

The Story of Alemtuzumab

Huai En Huang Chan, Iman Jilani, Richard Chang, and Maher Albitar

Summary

Alemtuzumab (Campath), the humanized rat monoclonal antibody that targets the CD52 surface antigen, is currently used for treatment of patients with resistant chronic lymphocytic leukemia. Monitoring levels of the antibody in plasma/serum could provide insight into the optimal dosing and scheduling of therapy. Current methods of detecting alemtuzumab in serum or plasma are complicated and difficult to adapt to high-throughput testing. We describe a novel bead-based assay that measures circulating alemtuzumab by taking advantage of remnant rat sequence in the antibody. Levels of total alemtuzumab complexed with CD52, and free alemtuzumab are quantitated in the serum or plasma by flow cytometry. This approach is applicable to the measurement of other humanized antibodies that contain an appropriate remnant animal sequence.

Key Words: Alemtuzumab; CAMPATH-1H; CD52; chronic lymphocytic leukemia; plasma.

1. Introduction

Alemtuzumab (Campath®; Berlex, Montville, NJ) is a humanized rat immunoglobulin (IgG1) monoclonal antibody directed against CD52, which is expressed on the surface of mature T- and B-cells, monocytes, and myeloid cells *(1,2)* but not in hematopoietic cells *(3)*. Alemtuzumab causes cell lysis through complement fixation in the host and antibody-dependent cellular cytotoxicity *(4)*. It has been clinically successful in previously treated patients with chronic lymphocytic leukemia, with response rates of up to 33% *(5)*.

From: *Methods in Molecular Biology, vol. 378: Monoclonal Antibodies: Methods and Protocols*
Edited by: M. Albitar © Humana Press Inc., Totowa, NJ

Alemtuzumab has also been studied for treatment of various T-cell malignancies such as graft-vs-host disease and autoimmune disease (6–9).

The original method of detecting and quantifying alemtuzumab in serum or plasma is based on capturing the alemtuzumab using cell line-expressing CD52 and quantifying the binding antibodies (10). This procedure is complicated and difficult to adapt for high-throughput analysis in clinical laboratories. More importantly, we have reported that free circulating CD52 can be detected in circulation, especially in patients with chronic lymphocytic leukemia and this free CD52 binds to the alemtuzumab in circulation forming immune complexes (11,12). It is important to measure total alemtuzumab, complexed alemtuzumab/CD52, and free alemtuzumab. Alemtuzumab is a fully humanized rat antibody in which most of the Ig framework is of human origin. However, sufficient rat sequence remains and we have reported the development of enzyme-linked immunosorbent assay based on capturing the rat portion of the alemtuzumab and detecting the human portion (13). Here, we report a simple bead-based assay that uses the same approach as that of the enzyme-linked immunosorbent assay with anti-rat Ig antibodies capturing the remnant rat sequence of alemtuzumab on beads instead of the surface of the plate then detecting the humanized portion using anti-human Ig antibodies. Furthermore, we report a method for the detection of the alemtuzumab/CD52 complexes as well as the free alemtuzumab. To detect the alemtuzumab/CD52 complexes, we first capture total alemtuzumab on the surface of beads using the anti-rat Ig antibodies, then we use anti-CD52 antibodies for detecting the complexes. As for detecting the free and not complexed alemtuzumab, we first immunoprecipitate the alemtuzumab/CD52 complexes from the plasma/serum sample using beads coated with anti-CD52, then we use this plasma/serum for detecting the alemtuzumab as previously described. These quantitative assays can be adapted for use in clinical laboratories.

2. Materials

2.1. Reagents and Equipment

1. 6.9 µM Carboxylated polystyrene beads (Bangs Laboratories, Fishers, IN).
2. Sodium bicarbonate (Sigma Aldrich, St. Louis, MO).
3. Carbodiimide (Sigma Aldrich).
4. Rabbit anti-rat IgG antibody (Sigma Aldrich).
5. Rat anti-human CD52 (Serotec, Raleigh, NC).
6. Phosphate-buffered saline (PBS) (Ca+/Mg+-free) (Sigma Aldrich).
7. Phycoerythrin (PE)-labeled rabbit anti-human IgG (BD Bioscience, San Jose, CA).
8. PE-labeled anti-CD52 (BD Biosciences).
9. Seven-color setup beads (BD Bioscience).
10. Sorvall Cellwasher 2 (Thermo Electron Corporation, Asheville, NC).

2.2. Buffer Preparation

1. Flow PBS: 5.6 g sodium phosphate dibasic, 35.48 g sodium chloride, 2.8 g bovine serum albumin (BSA), and 4.0 g sodium azide. Add deionized water to 4 L with and adjust pH to 7.4.
2. Blocking/dilution buffer (1× PBS/5% BSA): 10× PBS (Ca+/Mg+-free), 0.5 g BSA. Add deionized water to 1 L with and adjust pH to 7.4.
3. Activation buffer (0.05 M sodium bicarbonate): 4.2 g sodium bicarbonate. Add deionized water to 1 L with and adjust pH to 8.0.
4. Quenching solution (40 mM glycine): 3.02 g glycine. Add deionized water to 1 L and adjust pH to 7.4.

2.3. Flow Cytometric Analysis

1. FACSCanto™ flow cytometer (BD Biosciences).
2. FACSDiva™ software (BD Biosciences).
3. QuantiBRITE™ PE beads (BD Bioscience).
4. FlowJO analysis software (Treestar, Ashland, OR).

3. Methods

The methodology described here is based on immunoprecipation and detection on beads. Beads are either coated with antibodies directed against rabbit anti-rat IgG or anti-CD52. Upon exposure to plasma, the rat IgG-coated beads immunoprecipitate both total alemtuzumab and alemtuzumab–CD52 complexes; both of which can be separately quantitated with PE-labeled antibodies directed against the human component of the IgG or CD52, respectively. The CD52-coated beads immunoprecipitate alemtuzumab–CD52 complexes leaving free alemtuzumab in the supernatant. Free alemtuzumab is detected by immunoprecipitation with the IgG-coated beads and then detected with a PE-labeled human antibody.

3.1. Instrument Setup

1. Calibration should be performed prior to every acquisition using seven-color setup beads (BD Biosciences). Beads are prepackaged to be reconstituted with the provided buffer.
2. The FACSCanto is prepared by running "Fluidics Startup" and selecting the appropriate acquisition template and instrument settings on FACSDiva software.
3. Standardization is performed before acquisition of samples using QuatiBRITE PE beads, which are reconstituted with 1 mL flow PBS. Five thousand events are acquired on the FACSCanto.

3.2. Bead Conjugation and Preparation

1. All washes are performed with centrifugation at 17,949g or 2 min at room temperature unless otherwise stated. Beads are coated with antibodies directed against

rabbit anti-rat IgG or rat anti-human CD52 according to the manufacturer's protocol. The following is a brief description.

2. On day 1, 100 µL of 6.9 µ*M* carboxylated polystyrene beads are resuspended in
   1 mL of activation buffer (sodium bicarbonate) and washed twice.
3. After washing and resuspending in 1 mL of activation buffer, the beads are incubated
   in the presence of 10 mg carbodiimide for 25 min at room temperature with mixing.
4. The beads are then washed and resuspended in 1 mL activation buffer.
5. 100 µL of the beads are then incubated with either 100 µL rabbit anti-rat IgG or
   50 µL rat anti-human CD52 overnight at 4°C with mixing.
6. On day 2, the beads are washed and blocked with 1 mL blocking buffer for 90 min
   at 37°C with mixing.
7. The beads are washed with 1× PBS/5% BSA and incubated with quenching buffer
   for 30 min at room temperature with mixing.
8. The beads are then washed and resuspended with 1× PBS/5% BSA (*see* **Note 1**).

3.3. Sample Preparation

1. Plasmas are collected from the peripheral blood of a chronic myeloid lukemia
   (CML) patient and normal individuals. PBS is also used as a negative control.
2. The plasmas are diluted 1:10,000 in PBS/2% BSA and denatured in the presence
   of 2% SDS at 96°C for 5 min, followed by cooling to room temperature and
   centrifugation at 17,949*g* for 2 min (*see* **Note 2**).
3. 500 µL of denatured plasma is then aliquoted into two separate 1.5-mL microcentrifuge tubes.
4. Plasma is incubated with 30 µL of either IgG-conjugated beads or anti-CD52 conjugated beads for 3 h at room temperature with mixing.

3.4. Detection of Total and Complexed Alemtuzumab

1. The IgG-conjugated beads are centrifuged at 13,000*g* for 2 min.
2. After removal of supernatant, beads are washed three times with 1× PBS/5%
   BSA.
3. The beads are then split into two tubes and incubated with either 3 µL of anti-
   human PE (to detect total alemtuzumab) or 5 µL of CD52-PE (to detect complex
   alemtuzumab/CD52) for 1 h at room temperature with mixing.
4. Beads are washed in the cell washer and resuspended in 500 µL flow PBS for
   analysis. An example of the results is shown in **Fig. 1A,B**.

3.5. Detection of Free Alemtuzumab

1. The CD52-conjugated beads are centrifuged at 17,949*g* for 2 min.
2. The supernatant (which contains free CD52) is transferred to a fresh 1.5-mL
   microcentrifuge tube and incubated with 30 µL IgG-conjugated beads for 3 h at
   room temperature with mixing.
3. After centrifugation at 13,000*g* for 2 min, the beads are washed and resuspended
   in 1× PBS/5% BSA and then incubated with 3 µL anti-human PE for 1 h at room
   temperature in the dark with mixing.

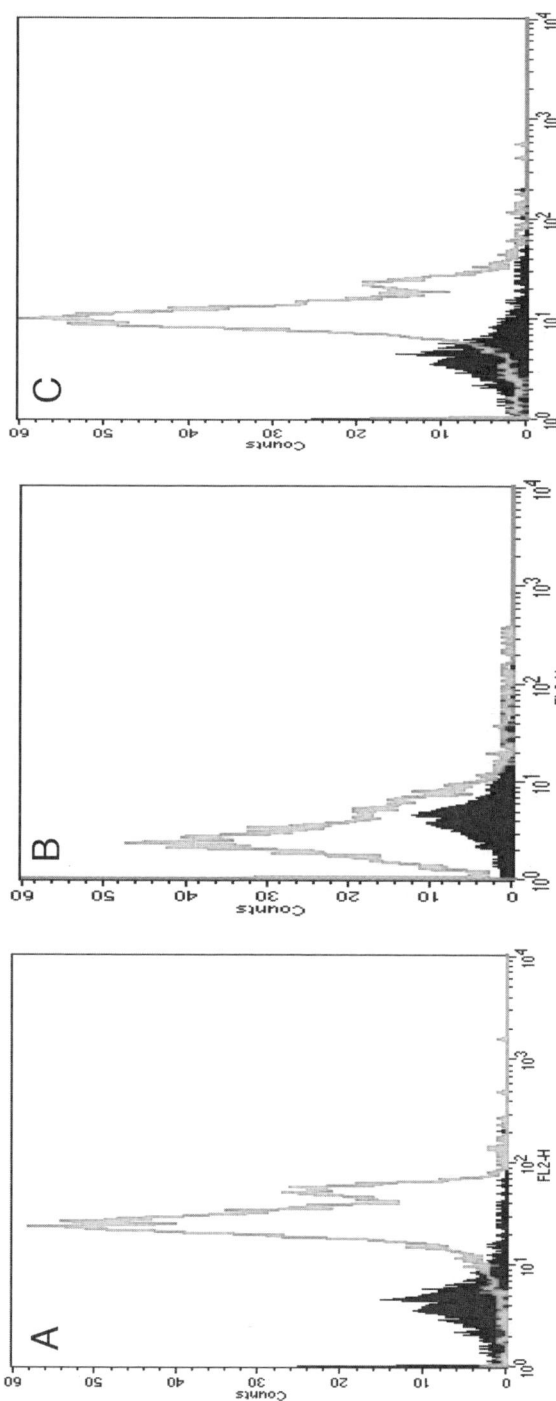

Fig. 1. Histogram overlays representing either unstained control beads (black) or stained beads (grey line). Beads are stained with either rabbit anti-human PE (to detect total Alemtuzumab) (**A**), anti-CD52 PE (to detect Alemtuzumab-CD52 complex) (**B**), or rabbit anti-human PE (to detect free Alemtuzumab) (C).

4. The beads are then washed in the cell washer and resuspended in 500 μL flow PBS for analysis. An example of the results is shown in **Fig. 1C**.

3.6. Acquisition and Analysis

1. The samples are acquired on the FACSCanto using FACsDiva software. Flow cytometry output is in the form of FCS files.
2. Quantitation is based on a fluorescence standard given by QuantiBRITE PE beads.
3. Data are analyzed using FlowJo software. Normal samples are used as the baseline for setting regional markers. Samples are analyzed based on gating according to the normal plasma samples.

3.7. Calculations

1. Index = % positive protein × antibody binding capacity (ABC) (*see* **Note 3**).
2. Ratio phosphorylated: total protein = index phosphorylated protein/index total protein.

4. Discussion

Proper dosing of therapeutic agents such as alemtuzumab may vary according to the tumor load and immune system in each patient. Thus, accurate measurement of alemtuzumab in the serum or plasma could provide the information necessary for tailoring therapy for individual patients. The assays described here take advantage of the minimal residual rat sequence in the alemtuzumab antibody, using antibodies against the rat Ig sequence. This approach can be used to monitor levels of alemtuzumab in patients during treatment and to correlate the results with clinical responses and adverse effects. Similar approach can be used for other humanized antibodies.

5. Notes

1. It is preferable that the conjugation be confirmed by performing a detection step with anti-mouse PE. The conjugation is detected by incubation of diluted conjugated beads (1:10 with blocking buffer) with 5 μL anti-mouse PE for 15 min at room temperature in the dark. The beads are washed and resuspended in 500 μL flow PBS for flow analysis.
2. The dilution factor of plasma should be determined empirically.
3. Fluctuations of intracellular proteins manifests as changes in percent of cellular positivity and fluorescence intensity. The index is a derived value that accounts for both. Index = (% positivity) × (ABC).

References

1. Hale, G., Swirsky, D. M., Hayhoe, F. G., et al. (1983) Effects of monoclonal anti-lymphocyte antibodies in vivo in monkeys and humans. *Mol. Biol. Med.* **1**, 321–334.
2. Hale, G. and Waldmann, H. (1994) Campath-1 monoclonal antibodies in bone marrow transplantation. *J. Hematother* **3**, 15–31.

3. Gilleece, M. H. and Dexter, T. M. (1993) Effects of Campath-1H antibody on human hematopoietic progenitors in vitro. *Blood* **82,** 807–812.
4. Schulz, H., Winkler, U., Staak, J. O., and Engert, A. (2000) The monoclonal antibodies Campath-1H and rituximab in the therapy of chronic lymphocytic leukemia. *Onkologie* **23,** 526–532.
5. Keating, M. J., Flinn, I., Jain, V., et al. (2002) Therapeutic role of alemtuzumab (Campath-1H) in patients who have failed fludarabine: results of a large international study. *Blood* **99,** 3554–3561.
6. Pawson, R., Matutes, E., Brito-Babpulle, V., et al. (1997) Treatment of T-cell prolymphocytic leukemia with human CD52 antibody. *J. Clin. Oncol.* **15,** 2667–2672.
7. Ferrajoli, A., O'Brien, S., Kurzock, R., et al. (2000) Phase II clinical trial of Campath-1H in refractory hematological malignancies expressing the surface antigen CD52. *Proc. Am. Soc. Clin. Oncol.* **19,** 8–22.
8. Hale, G., Jacobs, P., Wood, L., et al. (2000) CD52 antibodies for prevention of graft-versus-host disease and graft rejection following transplantation of allogeneic peripheral blood stem cells. *Bone Marrow Transplant* **26,** 69–76.
9. Lim, S. H., Hale, G., Marcus, R. E., Wadlmann, H., and Baglin, T. P. (1993) CAMPATH-1 monoclonal antibody therapy in severe refractory autoimmune thrombocytopenic purpura. *Br. J. Haematol.* **84,** 542–544.
10. Rebello, P. and Hale, G. (2002) Pharmacokinetics of CAMPATH-1H: assay development and validation. *J. Immunol. Methods* **260,** 285–302.
11. Albitar, M., Do, K. A., Johnson, M. M., et al. (2004) Free circulating soluble CD52 as a tumor marker in chronic lymphocytic leukemia and its implication in therapy with anti-CD52 antibodies. *Cancer* **101,** 999–1008.
12. Giles, F. J., Vose, J. M., Do, K. A., et al. (2003) Circulating CD20 and CD52 in patients with non-Hodgkin's lymphoma or Hodgkin's disease. *Br. J. Haematol.* **123,** 850–857.
13. Jilani, I., Keating, M., Giles, F. J., O'Brien, S., Kantarjian, H. M., and Albitar, M. (2004) Alemtuzumab: validation of a sensitive and simple enzyme-linked immunosorbent assay. *Leuk. Res.* **28,** 1255–1262.

12

Detection of Chromosome Translocations by Bead-Based Flow Cytometry

Huai En Huang Chan, Iman Jilani, Richard Chang, and Maher Albitar

Summary

Chromosome translocations resulting in fusion genes have been implicated in leukemogenesis. The paradigm involves the fusion of the genes encoding *BCR* and *ABL*, leading to a constitutively active tyrosine kinase. The detection of BCR-ABL has been limited to fluorescence *in situ* hybridization analysis, reverse transcription-polymerase chain reaction, of mRNA, and Western blot of analysis downstream effectors in the *BCR-ABL* activated pathway. Here, we describe a novel immunoassay that directly measures levels of *BCR-ABL* fusion protein and its phosphorylation in peripheral blood plasma and cell lysates. This approach has the potential for widespread application in the detection and quantitation of other fusion genes involved in hematological malignancies.

Key Words: CML; *BCR-ABL*; targeted therapy; quantitative flow cytometry; leukemia; imatinib mesylate.

1. Introduction

The molecular analysis of recurring chromosome rearrangements such as translocations and inversions has provided valuable insight into the pathogenesis of hematologic malignancies. Many translocations result in the fusion of genes located at the translocation breakpoints. The paradigm is the t(9;22)(q34;q11) translocation resulting in the *BCR-ABL* fusion gene, which encodes a cytoplasmic protein with constitutive tyrosine kinase activity. BCR-ABL is present in patients with chronic myeloid leukemia (CML) and in a subset of patients with acute lymphoblastic leukemia. The BCR-ABL fusion protein has been successfully targeted for therapy by a tyrosine kinase inhibitor, imatinib mesylate (Gleevec®; Novartis Pharmaceuticals Corporation, East Hanover, NJ) *(1–3)*. As resistance to this drug has been observed in patients

From: *Methods in Molecular Biology, vol. 378: Monoclonal Antibodies: Methods and Protocols*
Edited by: M. Albitar © Humana Press Inc., Totowa, NJ

with mutations affecting the *ABL* kinase domain *(4)*, several new, more specific, kinase inhibitors are in development.

Conventional approaches to the detection of BCR-ABL are limited. Fluorescence *in situ* hybridization analysis largely depends on the availability of intact and informative interphase nuclei. Reverse transcription-polymerase chain reaction is hindered by inherent variability in amplification and standardization of quantitation *(1,5)*. Monitoring the activity of the BCR-ABL protein itself is also difficult. In clinical material, the unstable fusion protein is subject to rapid degradation and dephosphorylation. Western blot analysis of downstream effectors of BCR-ABL, such as AKT and CRKL, has been used to monitor BCR-ABL activity *(6)*. However, these strategies are complicated by the presence of kinases other than BCR-ABL that may contribute to the activation of downstream effectors. Diagnostic tests adaptable to clinical laboratories are needed for direct and quantitative measurement of total and phosphorylated BCR-ABL protein.

We describe a simple and reliable immunoassay for measuring levels of BCR-ABL protein and its phosphorylation state in plasma. Monitoring the activity of BCR-ABL protein in CML patients would provide information on patient response and efficacy of therapy. This approach could be applied to other fusion genes in the monitoring of residual disease.

2. Materials

2.1. Reagents and Equipment

1. 6.9-μM Carboxylated polystyrene beads (Bangs Laboratories, Fishers, IN).
2. Carbodimide (Sigma Aldrich, St. Louis, MO).
3. Sodium dodecyl salt (10% [w/v]) (Bio-Rad Laboratories, Hercules, CA).
4. BCR antibody (Santa Cruz Biotechnology, Santa Cruz, CA).
5. c-ABL antibody (Santa Cruz Biotechnology).
6. Phospho-ABL (Thr) and Phospho-ABL (Tyr) rabbit monoclonal antibody (Cell Signaling Technology, Beverly, MA).
7. Phycoerythrin (PE)-labeled goat anti-rabbit IgG (Santa Cruz Biotechnology).
8. PE-labeled rabbit anti-mouse IgG (Jackson ImmunoResearch, West Grove, PA).
9. Seven-color setup beads (BD Bioscience, San Jose, CA).
10. QuantiBRITE™ PE beads (BD Bioscience).
11. Sorvall cell-washer 2 (Thermo Electron Corporation, Asheville, NC).
12. Microcentrifuge.
13. 37°C Incubator.
14. Tube rotator.

2.2. Buffer Preparation

1. Flow phosphate-buffered saline (PBS): 5.6 g sodium phosphate dibasic, 35.48 g sodium chloride, 2.8 g bovine serum albumin (BSA), and 4.0 g sodium azide. Add deionized water to 4 L; adjust pH to 7.4.

2. Blocking buffer (1X PBS + 5% BSA): 10X PBS (Ca+/Mg + free) and 0.5 g BSA. Add deionized water to 1 L; adjust pH to 7.4.
3. Activation buffer (0.05 *M* sodium bicarbonate): 4.2 g sodium bicarbonate. Add deionized water to 1 L; adjust pH to 8.0.
4. Quenching solution (40 m*M* glycine): 3.02 g glycine. Add deionized water to 1 L; adjust pH to 7.4.

2.3. Flow Cytometric Analysis

1. FACSCanto™ (BD Bioscience).
2. FACSDiva™ (BD Bioscience).
3. FlowJO™ analysis software (Treestar, Ashland, OR).
4. QuantiBRITE PE beads (BD Bioscience).

3. Methods

The number of total and phosphorylated BCR-ABL protein molecules bound per bead (ABC) is measured by quantitative flow cytometry. Polystyrene beads are used for immunoprecipitation of BCR-ABL protein from patient plasma. BCR-ABL protein is quantitated with antibodies that have PE conjugated at a 1:1 ratio. Fluorescence values obtained from beads are compared against a fluorescence standard established with QuantiBRITE PE beads, a set of four-bead populations each with a known number of bound PE molecules/bead. The use of 1:1 labeling allows the staining intensity on the bead surface to be converted to number of molecules bound per bead.

3.1. Instrument Setup

1. Calibration should be performed prior to every acquisition using seven-color setup beads (BD). Beads are prepackaged to be reconstituted with provided buffer.
2. The FACSCanto is prepared by running "Fluidics Startup" and selecting the appropriate acquisition template and instruments settings on FACSDiva software (BD Bioscience).
3. Standardization is performed before acquisition of samples using QuatiBRITE PE beads, which are reconstituted with 1 mL of flow PBS. Five thousand events are acquired on the FACSCanto. An example of the result is shown in **Fig. 1**.

3.2. Bead Conjugation/Preparation

1. All washes are performed with centrifugation at 17,949*g* for 2 min at room temperature unless otherwise stated.
2. Carboxylated polystyrene beads are coated with antibodies directed against BCR protein according to the manufacturer's protocol.
3. After washing and dilution (1:10) in activation buffer, the beads are activated with carbodimide (0.01 g/100 µL of original bead volume) for 20 min at room temperature with mixing.

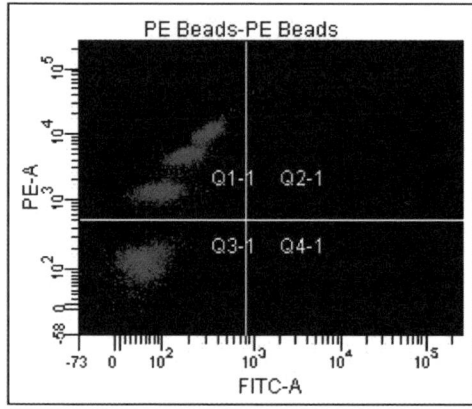

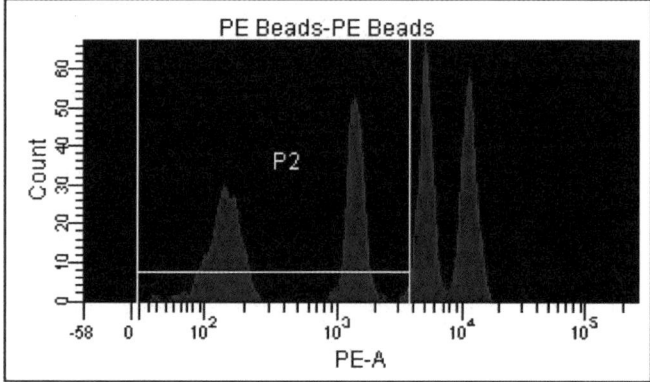

Fig. 1. Histogram and dot plot representing QuantiBRITE phycoerythrin (PE) beads, a set of four beads conjugated with known levels of PE fluorochrome. These beads are acquired in every experiment and used as a fluorescence standard to convert main fluorescent intensity (MFI) to antibody-binding capacity (ABC).

4. The beads are then incubated with 100 μL anti-BCR mouse monoclonal antibody per 100 μL original bead volume overnight at 4°C with mixing.
5. The beads are centrifuged and washed three times in *activation buffer* (1 mL/100 μL of original bead volume), then resuspended in *blocking buffer* (1 mL/100 μL of original bead volume) for 1.5 h at 37°C with mixing. Finally, the beads are centrifuged and resuspended in *quenching buffer* (1 mL/100 μL of original bead volume) for 30 min at room temperature with mixing.
6. The beads are then centrifuged and washed three times and resuspended in blocking buffer (1 mL/100 μL of original bead volume) (*see* **Note 1**; **Fig. 2**).

3.3. Sample Preparation

1. Plasmas are collected from the peripheral blood of a CML patient and normal individuals. PBS is also used as a negative control.

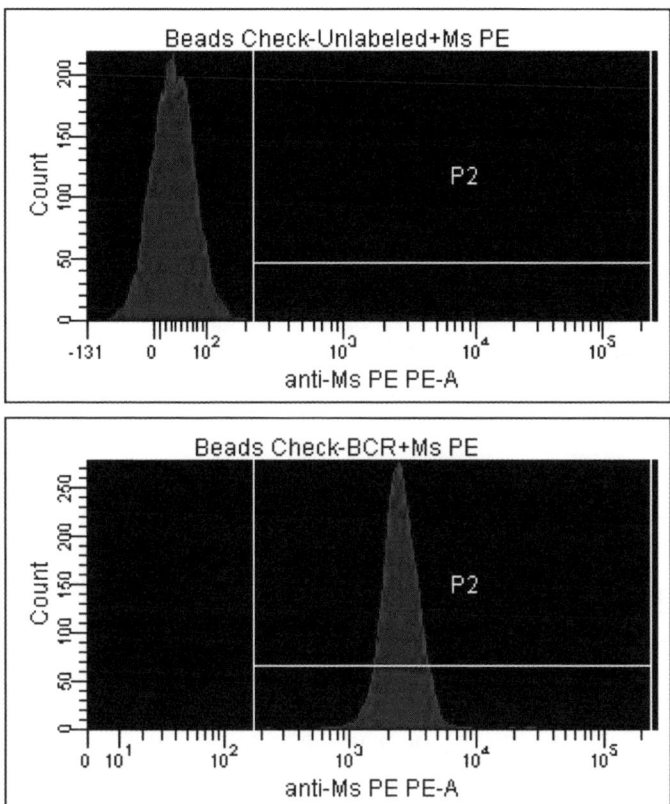

Fig. 2. Histrograms representing anti-BCR-coated beads before and after incubation with anti-mouse phycoerythrin. This "beads-check" is performed to ensure conjugation has occurred.

2. The plasmas are diluted 1:50 in PBS/2% BSA and denatured in the presence of 2% sodium dodecyl salt at 96°C for 4 min, followed by centrifugation at 17,949g for 2 min at room temperature.
3. The supernatant is incubated with 30 μL anti-BCR conjugated beads at room temperature for 2 h with mixing, followed by washes and resuspension in PBS/2% BSA.
4. Each sample is divided into three equal aliquots and incubated in the presence of 5 μL total ABL, phospho-ABL (Thr735), and phospho ABL Tyr 245 for 1 h at room temperature, respectively.
5. The beads are washed in the cell washer and resuspended in PBS/2% BSA, followed by incubation with 10 μL PE-labeled goat-anti-rabbit antibody for 30 min at room temperature with mixing.
6. The beads are washed and resuspended in 500 μL flow PBS for analysis.

3.4. Acquisition and Analysis

1. The samples are acquired on the FACSCanto using FACsDiva software. Flow cytometry output is in the form of FCS files.
2. Quantitation is based on a fluorescence standard given by QuantiBRITE PE beads (BD).
3. Data is analyzed using Flow-Jo software (TreeStar). An example of the result is shown in **Fig. 3**.
4. Normal samples are used as baseline for setting of regional markers. Samples are analyzed based on gating according to the normal plasma samples. Positive shifts less than 5% above normal control are considered to be negative for the presence of BCR-ABL protein (*see* **Note 2**).

3.5. Calculations

$$\text{Index} = \% \text{ positive protein} \times \text{ABC}$$

Ratio phosphorylated: total protein = index phosphorylated protein/index total protein

3.6. Discussion

The methodology described here offers several advantages over the conventional detection and quantitation of fusion genes formed by chromosome translocations. Fluoresence *in situ* hybridization analysis is largely limited by the availability of informative cells. PCR-based assays are hindered by amplification bias and difficulties of standardization. Furthermore, the reverse transcription-polymerase chain reaction assay for *BCR-ABL* mRNA measures the ratio of leukemic cells to normal cells. The ratio of hematopoietic cells to normal cells may fluctuate depending on the sample. Western blots assays of BCR-ABL downstream effectors are indirect and may be affected by other intracellular kinases. Western blots also do not discern different cellular populations.

Our approach quantitates the BCR-ABL protein itself and its kinase activity, providing the most direct measure of disease activity, progression, and response to treatment. The phosphorylation state of Thr-725 and Tyr-245 residues in the ABL domain indicate the level of BCR-ABL kinase activity. The use of plasma with this approach allows for the direct monitoring of BCR-ABL protein, thereby accounting for the effects of any posttranscriptional regulatory mechanisms on synthesis of BCR-ABL *(7,8)*. This method is adaptable for routine analysis in clinical laboratories and could be applied to the detection of several other oncogenic fusion genes that are caused by chromosome rearrangements.

4. Notes

1. Preferably, the conjugation should be confirmed by performing a detection step with anti-mouse PE. The conjugation is detected by incubation of diluted conjugated

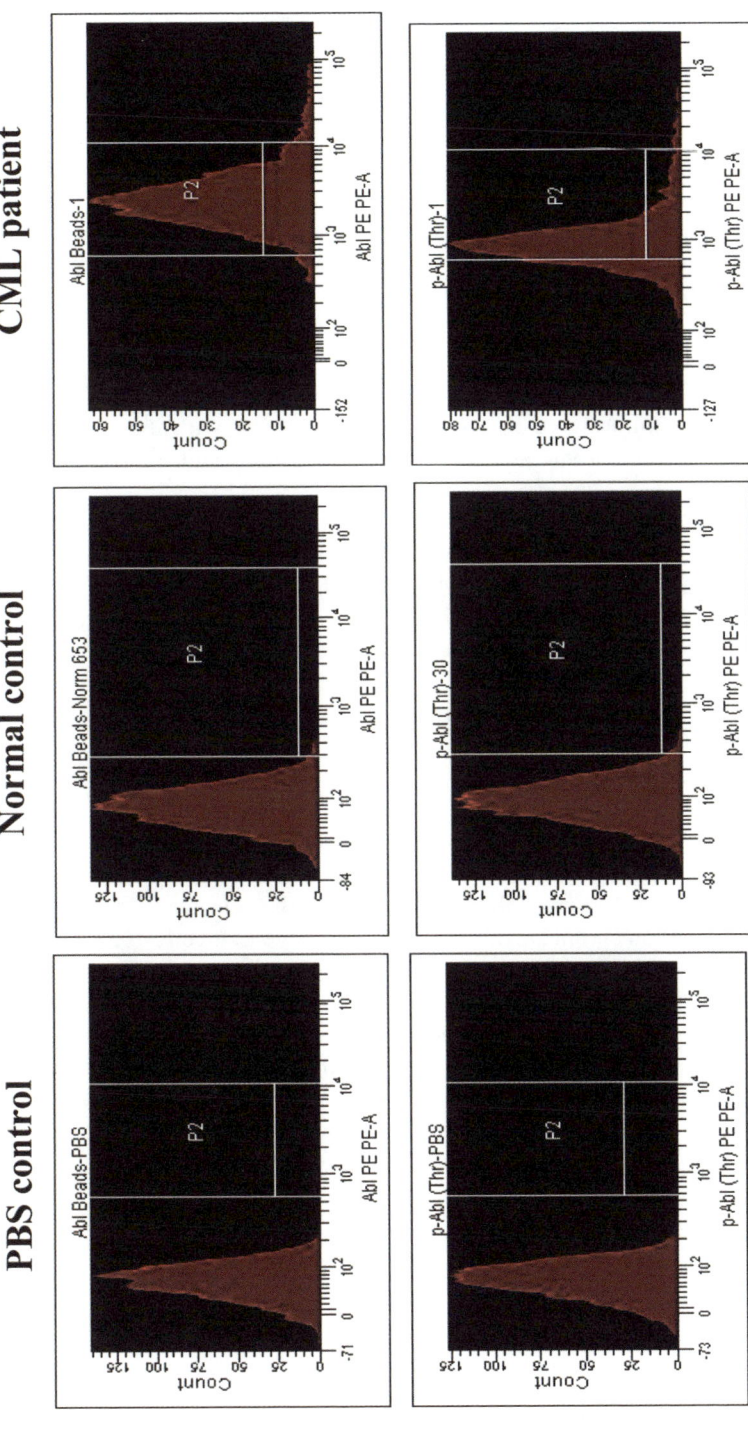

Fig. 3. Detection of BCR-ABL protein and its phosphorylation. Plasma samples prepared from peripheral blood plasma of a normal subject and an untreated chronic myeloid leukemia patient were incubated with anti-BCR coated beads, followed by incubation with antibody directed against ABL (upper row) or phosphorylated Tyr245 of ABL (lower row). PBS served as a negative control.

173

beads (1:10 with blocking buffer) with 5 μL anti-mouse PE for 15 min at room temperature in the dark. The beads are washed and resuspended in 500 μL flow PBS for flow analysis. An example of the result is shown in **Fig. 2**.

2. If normal samples exceed 5% shift more than PBS controls, newly conjugated beads are recommended. If all samples display a 100% shift more than normal, reblock and quench beads before use. If the scatter profile of beads is dispersed and excessive noise is present in the forward vs side scatter plot, there may be contamination in the blocking/dilution buffer.

References

1. Kantarjian, H. M., Talpaz, M., Cortes, J., et al. (2003) Quantitative polymerase chain reaction monitoring of BCR-ABL during therapy with imatinib mesylate (STI571; gleevec) in chronic-phase chronic myelogenous leukemia. *Clin. Cancer Res.* **9**, 160–166.
2. O'Brien, S. G., Guilhot, F., Larson, R. A., et al. (2003) Imatinib compared with interferon and low-dose cytarabine for newly diagnosed chronic-phase chronic myeloid leukemia. *N. Engl. J. Med.* **348**, 994–1004.
3. Deininger, M., Buchdunger, E., and Drucker, B. J. (2005) The development of imatinib as a therapeutic agent for chronic myeloid leukemia. *Blood* **105**, 2640–2653.
4. Gorre, M., Mohammed, M., Ellwood, K., et al. (2001) Clinical resistance to STI-571 cancer therapy caused by BCR-ABL gene mutation or amplification. *Science* **293**, 876–880.
5. Muller, M. C., Gattermann, N., Lahaye, T., et al. (2003) Dynamics of BCR-ABL mRNA expression in first line therapy of chronic myelogenous leukemia patients with imatinib or interferon alpha/ara-C. *Leukemia* **17**, 2392–2400.
6. Marley, S. B., Lewis, J. L., Schneider, H., Rudd, C. E., and Gordon, M. Y. (2004) Phosphatidylinositol-3 kinase inhibitors reproduce the selective anti-proliferative effects of imatinib on chronic myeloid leukaemia progenitor cells. *Br. J. Haematol.* **125**, 500–511.
7. Albitar, M., Do, K. A., Johnson, M. M., et al. (2004) Free circulating soluble CD52 as a tumor marker in chronic lymphocytic leukemia and its implication in therapy with anti-CD52 antibodies. *Cancer* **101**, 999–1008.
8. Rogers, A., Joe, Y., Manshouri, T., et al. (2004) Relative increase in leukemia-specific DNA in peripheral blood plasma from patients with acute myeloid leukemia and myelodysplasia. *Blood* **103**, 2799–2801.

13

Detection of the MDR1 P-Glycoprotein Expression and Function

Eugene Mechetner

Summary

Acquired and intrinsic multidrug resistance is the major reason for the failure of anticancer chemotherapy. The most important component of clinical multidrug resistance is mediated by P-glycoprotein (Pgp), an ABC transporter encoded by the *MDR1* gene and expressed on the membrane of tumor and normal cells. Sensitive and reproducible detection of Pgp expression and function are critical for the development of new MDR1 drugs and clinical protocols aimed at modulating Pgp-mediated multidrug resistance. The most commonly used methods for detecting Pgp distribution and functional activity have major flaws when used in routine clinical diagnostics. In this chapter, we describe and compare these techniques and introduce a new method for simultaneous detection of Pgp expression and function—the UIC2 Shift assay.

Key Words: MDR1; P-glycoprotein; drug resistance; flow cytometry.

1. Introduction
1.1. MDR1 P-glycoprotein and the Multifactorial Nature of Tumor Drug Resistance

Selection of mammalian cells in vitro and in vivo for resistance to cytotoxic agents frequently results in the development of cross-resistance to many other drugs that share little structural similarity with the primary selective agent and act at different intracellular targets. This phenomenon was termed multidrug resistance *(1,2)*.

Multidrug resistance in tumor cells involves several distinct molecular mechanisms. These mechanisms include ATP-dependent efflux of cytotoxic agents by membrane protein pumps encoded by the *MDR* or *MRP* genes,

From: *Methods in Molecular Biology, vol. 378: Monoclonal Antibodies: Methods and Protocols*
Edited by: M. Albitar © Humana Press Inc., Totowa, NJ

Lung Resistance Protein (LRP)-related drug sequestration in intracellular vesicles, DNA alterations caused by overexpression of topoisomerase II α, enhanced detoxification of alkylating agents by glutathione-linked enzyme systems, and other yet poorly understood multidrug resistance phenomena. In contrast, individual drug resistance to cancer chemotherapy drugs is caused by elevated levels of enzymes involved in intracellular drug metabolism. This group of drug resistance-associated enzymes includes such enzymes as thymidylate synthase conferring resistance to 5-fluorouracil, and O^6-methylguanine DNA methyltransferase contributing to clinical resistance to alkylating agents *(3)*.

The best characterized and understood molecular mechanism of multidrug resistance is membrane efflux mediated by P-glycoprotein (Pgp) encoded by the *MDR1* gene. Pgp expression permits tumor cells to evade the cytotoxic effects of several chemotherapy agents, thus contributing to clinical resistance to natural product-based chemotherapeutics, including taxanes, anthracyclines, vInca alkaloids, podophyllotoxins, and camptothecins *(1–3)*. Pgp functions as an ATP-dependent transporter of a structurally diverse group of substances from the cytosol and/or plasma membrane to the extracellular space *(4)*. The *MDR1* gene is a member of a large superfamily of integral membrane proteins known as the ATP-binding cassette (ABC) *(5)*. ABC also includes several other multi-drug resistance membrane proteins, such as the MRP superfamily, *BCRP* and *SPGP* gene products, the product of the cystic fibrosis gene, the TAP peptide transporters encoded by the major histocompatibility complex genes, etc. Overall, more than 100 ABC transporters have been identified in humans, other vertebrates, yeast, insects, plants, and bacteria *(6)*. However, in addition to *MDR1*, only two ABC genes, *MRP* and *BCRP*, contribute to the multidrug hesitance phenotype in clinical situations *(6,7)*. The clinical significance of *MDR1* over-expression has been substantiated by studies showing (1) significant increase in Pgp expression at relapse, and (2) presence of functional Pgp on normal cells that constitutively express this efflux pump and give rise to the malignant clones. Thus, both acquired and intrinsic MDR1 expression mechanisms contribute to clinical drug resistance *(3,8)*.

Pgp is constitutively expressed in a variety of human organs and tissues, such as the brush border of renal proximal tubules, the biliary surface of hepatocytes, the apical surface of mucosal intestinal cells, the adrenal cortex, and capillary endothelial cells of the blood–brain and blood–testis barriers *(9,10)*. Pgp expression has also been reported on the membrane of human hematopoietic stem cells and peripheral blood lymphocytes *(11,12)*. Based on the tissue distri-bution, it has long been proposed that Pgp plays a role in protecting cells and tissues against toxic xenobiotics and metabolites by active extrusion of these compounds into bile, urine, or intestinal lumen, and by preventing accumula-tion in critical organs, such as the brain *(13)*. The function of Pgp may also include the transmembrane transport of cellular products, such as steroid hormones and growth factors *(14–16)*. Pgp expression in epithelial cells has been shown to be associated with the transmembrane trafficking of ATP, regulation of membrane potentials and cell volume regulation via ATP-dependent, chloride-selective anion channels. Because Pgp is able to transport some natural steroid hormones, a physiological role of this protein in steroid secretion has been suggested *(17,18)*.

Although Pgp-mediated drug efflux appears to be the major component of clinical resistance to chemotherapy, there is accumulating evidence that any of the multidrug resistance mechanisms, or their combinations, can be associated with poor clinical outcomes in different cancer types. It has been also shown that substrate specificities of different multidrug resistance mechanisms may overlap *(19,20)*. Therefore, a sensitive tumor may become resistant to a certain drug via two or more molecular pathways (e.g., doxorubicin in the case of MDR1- and MRP-positive cells). It is because of the multifactorial nature of clinical drug resistance that it is essential to differentially detect individual components of the overall tumor drug response *(19–21)*.

Furthermore, the pharmacokinetics of drugs—MDR1 transport substrates can be significantly altered by the ubiquitous expression of MDR1 and other membrane pumps in normal tissues. For example, because high Pgp expression levels in the blood–brain barrier prevent MDR1 substrates from entering the brain, current chemotherapy protocols for brain tumors do not include several powerful anticancer drugs (such as doxorubicin, taxanes, vinblastine) *(22)*. Additionally, the ubiquitous expression of MDR1 and other ABC transporters results in significant side effects due to drug interference with normal physiological functions of multidrug resistance pumps in normal tissues, such as kidney, liver, gastrointestinal tract, adrenal, brain, hematopoietic stem cells. Although various adverse side effects of several small molecule MDR1 modulators were observed in several Phase I and I/II clinical trials *(23)*, their maximum-tolerated doses yielded serum levels considerably less than the levels needed to effectively inhibit MDR1 function *(24)*. It has been suggested that significant adverse side effects of Cyclosporine A, a transplantation drug and a known Pgp substrate, are associated with its interference with Pgp physiological functions *(3,24)*.

Thus, functional Pgp expressed in tumor cells, as well as normal organs and tissues, can seriously reduce anticancer effects of chemotherapy and alter pharmacokinetics, thereby negatively affecting the therapeutic window of many commonly used drugs—Pgp efflux substrates. Thus, efficient and selective detection of Pgp expression and function is essential for developing new drugs, conducting clinical trials, and designing new meaningful treatment protocols in cancer patients.

1.2. Existing Methods for Detecting Pgp Expression and Function

It has been shown in several solid tumor and leukemia/lymphoma systems that MDR1 expression levels determined on the protein or mRNA level correlated with in vitro and in vivo drug response and clinical outcomes in cancer patients *(19–22)*. However, a direct evidence of the causative relationship between clinical resistance and any of the known multidrug resistance mechanisms has not been provided. The major reason for this failure is that despite apparent clinical value of Pgp assays for assessing tumor multidrug resistance and extensive efforts to increase their sensitivity and specificity, of existing Pgp tests exhibit significant deficiencies, particularly when used on human-derived specimens in clinical laboratory routine (**Table 1**).

Although MDR1 testing based on highly sensitive and quantitative molecular biology techniques (reverse transcription-polymerase chain reaction [RT-PCR], Northern blotting) has been widely used in research laboratories, its use for clinical testing was hindered by several essential flaws. First, because every tumor sample contains both tumor and normal (e.g., connective tissue, blood vessels, and infiltrating hematopoietic cells) cells and because total specimen lysates are utilized for RNA isolation, it is impossible to discern specific Pgp expression in tumor vs normal cells. It has been shown that Pgp expression levels in nonmalignant stromal cells and peripheral blood lymphocytes (PBLs) infiltrating the tumor may be comparable to that in the tumor itself *(12)*. Therefore, the assay may generate falsely positive data because of the presence of nontumor Pgp-expressing cells in tissue specimens. Second, molecular biology based techniques are limited by the necessity of using total tumor lysates as the primary source of mRNA, and therefore no morphological analysis of individual Pgp-positive vs Pgp-negative cells can be performed. Finally, the use of this approach leads to ignoring posttranslational modifications of Pgp and does not determine Pgp expression and functional status levels on the protein level. It has been demonstrated that MDR1 mRNA data obtained using RT-PCR-based techniques does not necessarily correlate with the expression levels and functional activity of Pgp on the cell membrane *(25)*.

Pgp detection on the protein level can be carried out by Western blotting, immunohistochemistry (IHC), and flow cytometry using monoclonal antibodies (MAbs) against Pgp. These immunological techniques are potentially more accurate than molecular biology-based testing. For example, IHC allows a pathologist to discern tumor cells from infiltrating PBLs and stromal elements and assess tumor cell heterogeneity in tissue sections. However, Western blotting and conventional immunostaining methods share two common problems: low sensitivity and inability to detect Pgp functional activity.

Table 1
Pgp Detection Methods

Method	End-point	Disadvantages	Advantages
RNA-based (RT-PCR, Northern blotting)	*MDR1* RNA expression	Highly sensitive	No specific Pgp detection in tumor vs normal cells No cell morphology and biomarker detection No detection of Pgp function
Western blotting	Pgp expression	Pgp molecular weight verification	Low sensitivity No specific Pgp detection in tumor vs normal cells No cell morphology and biomarker detection No detection of Pgp function
Immunostaining (flow cytometry, immunohisto-chemistry (IHC))	Pgp expression	Specific detection of Pgp and biomarkers (flow cytometry) or morphology (IHC) in tumor cells	Relatively low sensitivity; no information on Pgp functional activity
Efflux assays (fluorescent dyes in flow cytometry, radioactive Pgp substrates in vitro)	Pgp function	High sensitivity detection of Pgp functional activity	No specific detection of Pgp vs other efflux mechanisms; relatively low reproducibility
In vitro cytoxicity assays	Pgp function	Detection of Pgp functional activity Clinically relevant drug testing	Low sensitivity and reproducibility No specific detection of Pgp vs other efflux mechnisms No cell morphology and biomarker detection
UIC2 shift assay (flow cytometry)	Pgp expression, Pgp function	Higher sensitivity vs conventional flow cytometry Highly specific detection of Pgp expression and function can be combined with efflux and immunostaining assays	Not applicable in IHC

Furthermore, MAbs reactive with internal Pgp epitopes (such as JSB-1 and, particularly, C219) are cross-reactive with other intracellular proteins and, therefore, their specificity to Pgp is limited *(26–28)*. On the other hand, MAbs against Pgp conformational extracellular epitopes are highly specific but sensitive to IHC fixatives and, therefore, can be used almost exclusively on living tumor cells in flow cytometry. Because of relatively low *MDR1* gene expression levels in tumor cells *(1,21,22)*, the sensitivity of highly specific monoclonal antibodies against extracellular epitopes of Pgp (such as MRK16, UIC2, 4E3, and MM12.10) has sometimes been too poor to provide accurate assessment of Pgp expression *(25)*. Thus, the sensitivity of both groups of anti-Pgp MAbs is limited, and many cases of low Pgp expressing tumors remain un- or under detected. The problem of low sensitivity is further compounded by cases of membrane expression of nonfunctional Pgp and the inability of MAB-based immunostaining techniques to detect Pgp-mediated transport activity *(29,30)*.

Two groups of tests are currently used to determine Pgp functional activity in tumor cells. While flow cytometry based assays measure direct efflux of fluorescent dyes (e.g., Rh 123, $DiOC_2$, Calcein AM) or drugs (e.g., daunorubicin) from MDR1-positive tumor cells under physiological conditions, cytotoxicity-based tests analyze tumor cells exposed in vitro to toxic drugs that are MDR1 efflux substrates. The percentage of cell death or cell growth inhibition is usually used as the end-point in this latter group. The first major deficiency of dye efflux and in vitro cytotoxicity based assays is that they are not suitable for the analysis of cell morphology. Another major limitation is a result of the multifactorial nature of drug resistance, i.e., the expression of other membrane efflux pumps and other mechanisms of drug resistance *(25,31)*. For example, it has been shown that Rho 123, a Pgp-transported fluorescent dye that is commonly used for the detection of Pgp-mediated efflux, is also a substrate for the MRP1 membrane pump *(32)*, thereby preventing accurate discrimination between functional activities of these multidrug resistance pumps. The overlap in substrate specificities exhibited by various members of the ABC transport system and other extrusion mechanisms (e.g., LRP) is the major reason why it has been so difficult to identify natural compounds that are truly Pgp specific. In addition, these tests are time/cost consuming and highly operator-dependent, making it difficult to standardize functional MDR1 testing between different labs.

Thus, new assays are needed to accurately and specifically detect MDR1 expression and function. In this chapter, we will describe a new method for Pgp detection, the UIC2 Shift assay, which can be utilized to quantitatively assess Pgp expression and function in a range of experimental configurations.

1.3. The UIC2 MAb and the UIC2 Shift Assay

It had been proven difficult to generate MAbs against external epitopes of Pgp because only 7% of the protein is exposed on the cell surface *(1)*. Despite multiple efforts, only a few MAbs reactive with extracellular epitopes have been developed. In 1992, we described a mouse IgG2a MAb, UIC2, that recognized human Pgp on the cell surface of normal and malignant cells *(33)*. We also found that UIC2 inhibited the efflux of Rh123, $DiOC_2$, and other fluorescent dyes and drugs transported by Pgp from MDR cells and reversed the in vitro resistance of MDR1 cells to Pgp-transported drugs in a dose-dependent fashion. Schinkel et al. *(12)* demonstrated that observed variation in binding specificity between UIC2 vs other anti-Pgp MAbs paralleled the reported functional differences in the ability of these antibodies to inhibit Pgp-mediated drug efflux.

Our epitope mapping studies revealed the conformational nature of the UIC2 epitope and suggested that it consists of (1) several paratopes that belong to the predicted Pgp extracellular domains, and (2) one Pgp domain located inside the cell membrane. Some of the identified UIC2 paratopes completely or partially overlapped with MRK16 paratopes, end these two MAbs strongly competed for Pgp binding in flow cytometry experiments (Mechetner and Roninson, unpublished). However, only UIC2 was capable of efficient inhibition of Pgp-mediated efflux function. Therefore, we hypothesized that conformational transitions that are associated with Pgp efflux activity result in "opening up" the Pgp epitope and permit UIC2 binding to the otherwise unavailable intramembrane stretch of amino acids. This hypothesis lead to the prediction that coincubation of MDR1 cells with Pgp transport drugs under physiological conditions should result in altered (increased or decreased) binding of UIC2. In our subsequent flow cytometry experiments, we indeed observed enhanced (up to 10- to 15-fold) binding of UIC2 (but not MRK16) to the cell surface when Pgp-positive cells were incubated at 37°C with multiple Pgp substrates. Both UIC2 affinity and the number of UIC2-binding sites on the cell surface were drastically increased in drug-treated MDR1 cells. This phenomenon, defined as an increase in UIC2 immunoreactivity under physiological conditions with functional vs nonfunctional Pgp, was termed "UIC2 shift" *(34,35)*.

Our subsequent studies on MDR1 cell lines expressing wild-type and mutant forms of Pgp confirmed that UIC2 shift was associated with conformational changes of functioning Pgp and showed that it was related to its ATPase status. This data suggested the existence of at least two possible functional conformations. One of these conformations ("closed") is characterized by lower UIC2 reactivity (revealed by conventional UIC2 staining, i.e., without exposure to a Pgp substrate), binding of two ATP molecules to Pgp, and complete absence of the efflux function. The second ("open") conformation is detectable by UIC2 staining in the presence of a Pgp substrate under physiological conditions, generates UIC2 shift, is linked to the dissociation of ATP from the ATP-binding domains, and involves active Pgp-mediated drug efflux. This model was further supported by data generated in different experimental systems using UIC2 as a probe for Pgp conformation and efflux activities (*see* **ref. 35** for review).

Based on the UIC2 shift phenomenon, we developed and validated a new flow cytometry test, the UIC2 Shift assay, which allows for simultaneous quantitative detection of Pgp expression and function in human MDR1 cells *(35)*. This test is based on the increased reactivity of an anti-Pgp MAb, UIC2, in the presence of Pgp-transported compounds at physiologic conditions (**Fig. 1**).

1.4. Applications of the UIC2 Shift Assay

1.4.1. Testing of Cell Lines and Clinical Tumor Specimens

The UIC2 shift phenomenon was more pronounced in MDR1 cell lines with low levels of Pgp expression, reflecting lower molar Pgp/drug ratio in these cells, as compared with high Pgp expressors *(34)*. This feature makes the UIC2 shift assay particularly attractive for Pgp detection in human tumors, the vast majority of which are characterized by low MDR1 expression levels *(19–22)* (**Table 2**).

We used a series of MCF7 breast carcinoma-derived cell lines as a model of clinical breast cancer for standardization and comparison of different Pgp detection methods (**Table 2**). Three microbead calibrated cell lines, MCF7-P4 (low level of MDR1 resistance), MCF7-P10 (low-medium), and MCF7-P19 (high) were derived from parental MCF7-WT cells through in vitro selection for doxorubicin resistance. Results of the UIC2 Shift Assay with 25 μM vinblastine strongly correlated with the number of Pgp molecules per cell by flow ($r = 0.98$), IHC scores on formalin-fixed, paraffin-embedded samples ($r = 0.98$), image analysis on cytospins ($r = 0.97$), and IC_{50} values derived in a 4-d cytotoxicity assay ($r = 0.78$). UIC2 shift values were higher by a factor of four in low and low-medium Pgp expressing MCF7-P4 and MCF7-P10 cell lines (compared with the high expressor, MCF70-P19). This data, as well as other results generated on KB calibrator cell lines (**Fig. 1**), *MDR1* retrovirus infected K562 cells, and MDR1-transfected NIH 3T3 cells *(21)*, proved the usefulness of the UIC2 shift assay for detecting Pgp expression and function in transformed cells with low levels of Pgp expression.

To validate the UIC2 shift assay on clinical samples, we analyzed in flow cytometry 163 fresh tumor specimens (117 solid tumor and 46 hematological specimens) positive for Pgp in conventional UIC2/MRK16/4E3 MAb staining. UIC2 shift was observed in 81% of solid tumors and 91% of hematological

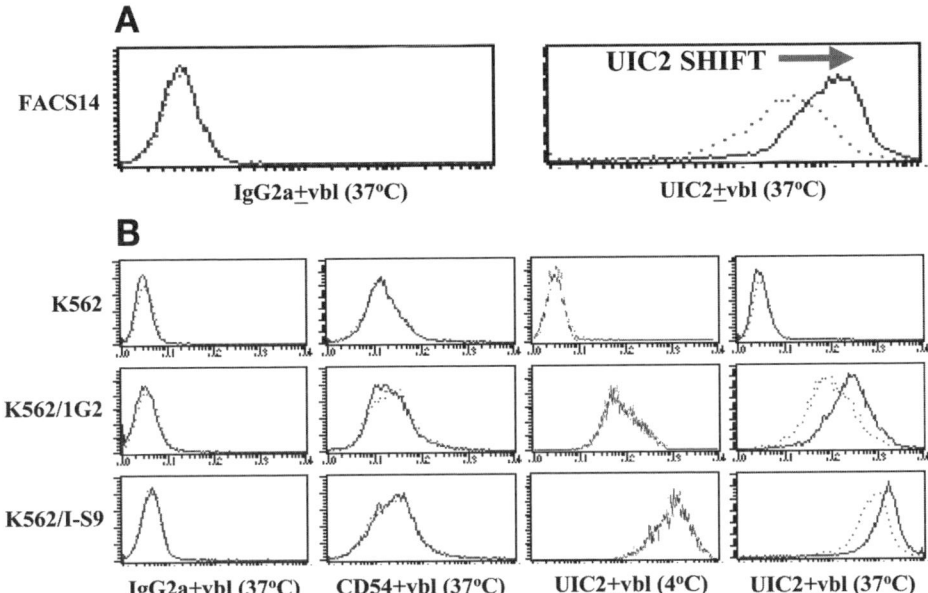

Fig. 1. The UIC2 shift assay on MDR1 cell lines. (**A**) Flow cytometric analysis of Pgp–positive FACS14 cell line stained with IgG2a labeled with phycoerythrin (PE; left) or UIC2-PE (right) in the presence of 25 μ*M* of vinblastine (solid line) or diluent (DMSO; dotted line) at 37°C. UIC2 staining is increased in the presence of vinblastine, whereas IgG2a binding is not affected by vinblastine treatment. The UIC2 shift (arrow) is defined as the difference between UIC2 binding in conventional UIC2 staining and UIC2 staining in the presence of MDR1-transported substrates under physiologic conditions. (**B**) UIC2 shift in the parental K562 cell line and its subclones with intermediate (K562/1G2) and high (K562/i-S9) levels of Pgp expression. As compared with diluent controls (dotted line), exposure to 25 μ*M* of vinblastine (solid line) does not affect nonspecific binding of IgG2a (isotype control) or specific binding of an anti-ICAM (CD54) monoclonal antibody at 37°C. Because functional Pgp is required for altered UIC2 reactivity, UIC2 binding to the K562/1G2 and K562/i-S9 cell lines is increased in the presence of vinblastine at 37°C but not at 4°C. There are no UIC2 staining and UIC2 shift in the parental K562 cell line.

samples and strongly correlated with conventional UIC2 staining (test for Pgp expression) and DiOC$_2$ dye efflux (test for Pgp functional activity). A 2- to 10-fold increase in Pgp detection sensitivity was achieved using the UIC2 shift assay *(36)*. At this point in time, it is not clear why the remaining Pgp-positive specimens did not produce UIC2 shift. The discordance between Pgp expression detected by MAbs and Pgp-mediated efflux in clinical samples was first documented by Leith et al. in a series of 60 AML patients *(30)*. This phenomenon can be explained by Pgp mutations that do not affect UIC2/MRK16/4E3

Table 2

	IC50[a]	Flow cytometry			Immunohistochemistry	
		Immunobead calibration	U1C2 shift assay		IHC score	Image analysis
			No drug	+ vinblastine		
MCF7-WT	0.15[b]	0[c]	2.5[d]	2.5[d]	0[e]	0[f]
MCF7-P4	1.8	7491	6.3	29	15	20
MCF7-P10	6.0	14,692	14	58	135	38
MCF7-P19	7.4	60,037	1893	2147	360	81
r[g]	0.78		0.98	0.98	0.98	0.97

[a]Determined for doxorubicin in the EDR assay.
[b]Doxorubicin concentration (μM).
[c]Molecules/cell.
[d]Median immunofluorescence (FL2) channel.
[e]IHC scores were determined as described in **Subheading 2**.
[f]Absorbance product (*see* **Subheading 2.**).
[g]Correlation coefficient from Pearson regression analysis; the date was correlated vs number of Pgp molecules/cell as determined by immunobead calibration.

binding in the "low" (conventional) conformation but alter the intramembrane Pgp domain involved in the "high" UIC2-reactive conformation. Alternatively, this incongruity can be caused by inadequate sample handling: the half-time of Pgp on the cell surface is relatively high (>2 d; **ref. 1**), whereas the UIC2 shift assay requires healthy, non-ATP-depleted Pgp-positive cells. Some of our preliminary data indicate that overnight preincubation of tumor samples at 37°C in culture with 10% fetal calf serum or increasing the drug concentration to cell number ratio significantly improve the UIC2 shift ssay results *(37)*.

In vitro cytotoxicity based Oncotech's extreme drug resistance and differential staining cytotoxicity assays were used to correlate drug response to doxorubicin (a potent Pgp substrate) and 4-HC (a non-Pgp drug) with the UIC2 shift assay results in 124 clinical tumor samples. These assays have been extensively validated on more than 120,000 clinical tumor specimens to predict tumor drug resistance with high probability (>99.2%) *(21)*. In our study, as expected, no correlation was found between the results of the UIC2 Shift assay and in vitro drug response in 4-HC-treated samples by extreme drug resistance or differential staining cytotoxicity. In contrast, doxorubicin drug resistance significantly correlated with Pgp expression determined by conventional UIC2 staining ($p = 0.04$) and the UIC2 shift assay ($p = 0.02$). These data demonstrates the link between the UIC2 shift assay and clinical Pgp-mediated drug resistance and suggests that prognostic value of the UIC2 Shift assays is higher than that of conventional immunostaining *(36,37)*.

1.4.2. UIC2 Shift Assay in Drug Screening and Monitoring

Introduction of time- and cost-efficient tests for high-throughput MDR1 analysis is greatly needed to facilitate the development of new, safe, and clinically efficient Pgp modulators, as well as pharmaceuticals that do not interfere with patients' physiological MDR mechanisms. Information on drug resistance substrate specificity profiles for new drug candidates is critical for rational design of new drugs and for managing of clinical trials on drug resistance modulators, as well as other drug candidates whose pharmacokinetic parameters can be affected by Pgp activity in various normal tissues. MDR1 detection tests are currently being used in drug development programs for the following two reasons.

First, one of the major problems with newly synthesized chemotherapeutic compounds is the development of tumor drug resistance mediated by Pgp or other drug resistance mechanisms. When entering preclinical and clinical drug safety studies, it is possible to avoid unnecessary expenses and shorten the testing time by identifying and eliminating of drug candidates—substrates for different drug resistance mechanisms. Although such drug candidates demonstrate high efficacy in vivo, their therapeutic window in animal models and, further down the line, in clinical trials is inevitably altered by the failure of reaching their cellular targets. Furthermore, experimental drug candidates may act as MDR1 modulators, thereby causing multiple side effects and resulting in insurmountable safety problems. In the worst-case scenario, a drug candidate—MDR substrate could strongly interfere with Pgp expressed in normal tissues (e.g., GI tract, kidney, or blood–brain barrier) resulting in strong adverse effects and termination of the entire drug development program.

Second, MDR1 detection tests are widely utilized to identify new molecules that modulate drug resistance. It was shown that Pgp expression can be reversed by such modulators, resulting in enhanced therapeutic efficacy in cellular and animal models of drug resistance *(4,19,38)*. Furthermore, tumor selection for increased Pgp expression can be prevented in cellular models by coadministration of MDR1-related cytotoxic drugs and modulators. Currently, 65 clinical trials on 16 different MDR1 modulators are conducted on patients with more than 12 MDR1-resistant tumor types *(24)*, with more clinical trials using potential Pgp substrates in progress. All existing MDR1 screening systems are based exclusively on in vitro cytotoxicity assays and flow cytometry techniques. These expensive and sometimes irreproducible functional tests for Pgp inhibition are not MDR1-specific (**Table 1**).

To address these issues and validate the utility of the UIC2 shift assays in drug screening and evaluation, we first used this method to analyze MDR1 substrate specificity on Pgp-positive tumor cell lines. At that point in time (1996), it was unclear if SN-38, an active species of a new chemotherapeutic drug CPT-11, was a Pgp substrate. The UIC2 Shift assay was performed on MDR1-positive KB-8-5 cells in the presence of different concentrations of SN-38, cyclosporine A (Pgp substrate positive control), and BSO (non-Pgp substrate negative). SN-38 induced a weak but statistically significant UIC2 shift in KB-8-5 cells, thereby providing the first evidence of it being a Pgp substrate *(39)*. This finding was later (1998) confirmed by other researchers using in vitro cytotoxicity tests *(40,41)*. Because CPT-11 chemotherapy protocols are used primarily on colorectal cancers, 80–100% of which are characterized by high Pgp expression levels, and recently on brain tumors, this information is essential for the understanding of its pharmacokinetics and assessing its therapeutic window.

In the late 1990s, normal human cells became increasingly utilized in the functional analysis of MDR1-related pharmacokinetics. The Bates' group at the National Institutes of Health (NIH) was first to introduce a Rhodamine 123 efflux-based multicolor flow cytometry technique that used CD56-positive PBLs as a surrogate marker of Pgp antagonism in PSC 833 clinical studies *(42)*. To extend and simplify this approach, we validated the use of the UIC2 Shift assay on normal PBLs *(35)*. In three-color flow cytometry on human PBL subsets in the presence of 25 μM vinblastine, Pgp expression was detected using the UIC2 Shift assay on 44–81% of T, CD4, CD8, B, and natural killer cells vs only 23–35% in conventional immunostaining. In addition to increased sensitivity, the UIC2 Shift assay provided information on the functional status of human PBLs. In a series of experiments combining the UIC2 Shift assay with $DiOC_2$ efflux analysis, a highly significant correlation ($r = 0.99$; **Fig. 2**) was found between the results of the two tests, both at the single-cell level and in terms of the percentage of PBL populations expressing functional Pgp. We then used PBL subsets to confirm Pgp substrate specificities of known MDR1 agents and successfully identify a series of new Pgp substrates, including monensin and retinol *(35)*. These results further validated the utility of the UIC2 shift assay for screening for new MDR1 agents and monitoring drug pharmacokinetics parameters, particularly in cells with low Pgp expression levels.

These data also emphasize the notion that accurate assessment of MDR1 expression and function in tumor specimens is impossible without precise gating on malignant cells present in the sample. In flow cytometry, this could be achieved by using additional tumor type-specific MAb markers (e.g., HER2 to gate on breast cancer cells) and/or by excluding normal cells present in the tumor bed (e.g., CD45 to gate out infiltrating PBLs).

In summary, the UIC2 shift assay is a new, highly specific, and sensitive technique for detecting the activity of the MDR1 efflux pump, which complements other conventional immunostaining and functional Pgp assays. Based on the specific reactivity of UIC2 with the active conformational epitope unique to Pgp,

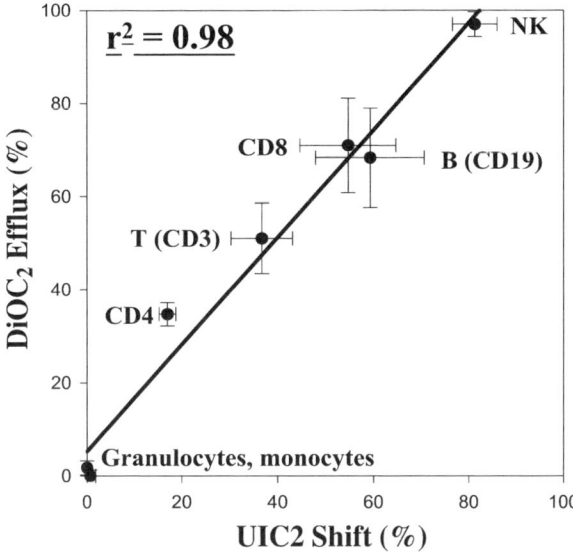

Fig. 2. Correlation between the UIC2 shift and the DiOC^2 efflux assays. The percentage of cells positive for P-glycoprotein in the UIC2 shift assay and DiOC^2-dim cells in the dye efflux assay were calculated as described in the figure. T-cells were defined as CD3+, CD4+ T-cells as CD3+CD4+, CD8+ T-cells as CD3+CD8+, B-cells as CD19+, natural killer (NK) cells as CD3+CD56+, monocytes as CD14+, and granulocytes as CD15+. Data (mean + standard deviation) from at least three independent combined experiments for each cell population are presented.

the UIC2 shift assay can selectively identify MDR1 functional activity on the background of other drug efflux mechanisms. The enhanced sensitivity of Pgp detection in the UIC2 shift assay allows for characterization of tumor and normal cells with low Pgp expression. The UIC2 shift assay simultaneously quantifies MDR1 expression and function in the same cell, making it possible to directly correlate cellular phenotypes with Pgp efflux activity. This technique can be utilized for direct analyses of Pgp-mediated membrane transport and provides a new method for screening and monitoring new pharmaceuticals.

2. Materials

2.1. Cell Culture

1. Complete medium: RPMI-1640 supplemented with 10% heat-inactivated fetal bovine serum (FBS) (both from Gibco/Invitrogen, Carlsbad, CA).
2. The K562/i-S9 cell line generated by retroviral transfer of the human *MDR1* gene into human CML-derived K562 cell line, followed by flow cytometry selection for Pgp-positive cells without exposure to cytotoxic drugs, is maintained in drug-free complete medium *(34,35)* (**Note 4.1**).

3. PBL are isolated by density gradient separation using Histopaque 1083 (Sigma, St. Louis, MO) from buffy coats obtained from healthy donors according to manufacturer's recommendations. Cells are washed twice in RPMI-1640 and adjusted to 10^6 cells/mL in RPMI-1640.

4. UIC2 and UIC2/A hybridoma cell lines secreting UIC2 in complete or protein-free medium, respectively, can be purchased from ATCC (accession nos. HB11207 and HB11287).

5. UIC2 shift assay buffers, AB: PBS supplemented with 2% FBS.

6. UIC2 shift assay stop buffer for flow cytometry, SSB: PBS supplemented with 2% FBS and 0.01% sodium azide.

2.2. Antibodies

1. Nonlabeled azide-free UIC2 MAb (mouse IgG2a) purified from serum-free hybridoma tissue culture supernatants can be purchased from Chemicon (MAB4334Z; Chemicon International, Temecula, CA) or purified using Protein A affinity chromatography from protein-free hybridoma supernatants as described in our previous reports *(34,35)*.

2. Phycoerythrin (PE) conjugated UIC2 is purchased from Chemicon (cat. no. MAB4334PE).

3. Control antibodies: IgG2a-PE (negative MAb control to UIC2-PE) (Sigma); IgG1-FITC and -PE, CD3-APC, CD4-FITC, CD8-FITC, CD14-FITC, CD15-FITC, CD19-FITC, CD45-FITC, CD14-PE, and CD54-PE (Becton Dickinson Immunocytometry Systems [BDIS], San Jose, CA); IgG1-APC, IgG2a-APC, and CD56-FITC (ExAlpha, Boston, MA).

4. Unconjugated purified IgG1, IgG2a, and IgG2b (negative controls to primary MAbs used at matching concentrations in indirect immunostaining) and PE-conjugated goat anti-mouse IgG2a (for secondary detection) were from Caltag (Burlingame, CA).

2.3. Fluorescent Dyes

1. 3,3-Diethyloxacarbocyanine iodide, $DiOC_2(3)$, is available from Molecular Probes (Eugene, OR). $DiOC_2$ solution is prepared in 96% ethanol and kept in 0.1-mL aliquots at 70°C for long-term storage or ambient temperature for weeks until analysis.

2. Solution of 1 µg/mL propidium iodide (PI; Molecular Probes/Invitrogen, Eugene, OR).

2.4. Chemotherapy Agents

1. Vinblastine (Sigma) solution is prepared in tissue-culture grade water at 25 µ*M*, sterilized using the 0.22 µ cellulose acetate filter unit (Corning, Corning, NY), and stored in 0.1-mL aliquots at –20°C.

2. Depending on solubility of other compounds tested in the UIC2 shift assay, their stock solutions can be prepared in water, DMSO, RPMI-1640, or complete medium.

3. Control diluents used to prepare drug stock solutions are added to achieve the same final concentrations in the UIC2 shift assay.

3. Methods

3.1. Pgp Expression and Function: UIC2 Shift Assay

1. A protocol for the UIC2 shift assay was described in detail in **refs. *34*** and ***35***.
2. Wash K562/i-S9 cells or PBL (from 10^5 to 10^6 cells per tube) two times in AB.
3. Resuspend cells in 1 mL of AB and equilibrate to 37°C in a water bath for 10 min (**Note 4.2**).
4. Add 5 µL of 25 µ*M* vinblastine, or drug stock solution, or control diluent; optimal concentrations for each stock solution have to be determined in preliminary titration experiments.
5. Incubate for another 10 min with periodic agitation at 37°C to load cells with the drug and engage the MDR1 pump.
6. Add 5 µL of UIC2-PE or IgG2a-PE isotype control to directly stain membrane Pgp experiments and incubated at 37°C for additional 15 min; 5 µL of unconjugated purified UIC2 or mouse IgG2a are added for 15 min in indirect staining experiments, followed by two ice-cold AB washes, and subsequent 15 min staining with a secondary detection reagents (e.g., PE-conjugated goat anti-mouse IgG2a).
7. Wash cells twice with ice-cold SSB (**Note 4.3**).
8. For additional immunostaining (e.g., subset analysis of PBL), stain on ice in SSB for additional 15 min with other directly conjugated primary antibodies (e.g., FITC- or APC-conjugated MAbs against CD antigens).
9. Wash twice in ice-cold SSB and resuspend in SSB containing 1 µg/mL PI to exclude dead cells; keep on ice in dark place or under metal foil to protect from light until analysis.
10. Typically, at least four samples are included in UIC2 shift experiments:
    a. Staining with IgG2a-PE or IgG2a in the presence of the diluent (isotype control for conventional UIC2 staining).
    b. Staining with IgG2a-PE or IgG2a in the presence of 25 µ*M* vinblastine or the tested compound (isotype control for UIC2 shift staining).
    c. Staining with UIC2-PE or UIC2 in the presence of the diluent (conventional UIC2 staining).
    d. Staining with UIC2-PE or UIC in the presence of 25 µ*M* vinblastine or the tested compound (UIC2 shift staining).
11. In quantitative terms, UIC2 shift is defined as the difference between UIC2 binding in the presence vs in the absence of a Pgp substrate (e.g., 25 µ*M* vinblastine) under physiologic conditions and expressed as the difference between the respective median FACS channels (**Fig. 1**) (**Notes 4.4** and **4.5**).

3.2. Pgp Expression: Conventional Pgp Immunostaining

1. After two washes in ice-cold SSB, resuspend target cells, 10^5 to 10^6 cells per tube, in 50 µL of staining buffer (SSB + 1 m*M* EDTA) containing 20 µg/mL of a 1:1 mixture of IgG$_1$ and IgG2b MAb (Sigma) to block Fc receptors.

2. After a 15-min preincubation and two subsequent washes with the staining buffer, add purified UIC2 (or control IgG2a), at 1 μg/sample, and incubate for 30 min.
3. Wash the cells twice, resuspend in 50 μL of staining buffer, and add goat anti-mouse IgG2a-PE at predetermined concentrations for 30 min.
4. After washing twice in SSB, resuspended the cells in 300 μL of SSB and 1 μg/mL propidium iodide for flow cytometry analysis.

3.3. Pgp Function: DiOC^2 Effux Assay

1. Load target cells with $DiOC_2$ at a final concentration of 1 μg/mL in RPMI-1640 on ice for 15 min in the dark.
2. Immediately after loading, wash the cells twice in ice cold RPMI-1640 with 2% FBS, resuspend at 37°C in RPMI-1640 with 2% FBS, transfer to tissue culture flasks (10^6 cells in 10 mL), and allowed to efflux at 37°C in 5% CO_2 for 3–5 h (typically, 15 min to 1 h for high Pgp expressors and 2–5 h for low Pgp expressors) on a rocker.
3. Incubations at 4°C or with known Pgp substrates (e.g., vinblastine, verapamil, and so on) are to be included as efflux background controls.
4. After efflux, wash the cells twice with ice-cold SSB and analyze by flow cytometry at 4°C in the presence of 1 μg/mL PI.
5. If necessary, target cells can be processed for further immunostaining performed at 4°C to prevent cells from further $DiOC_2$ efflux.

4. Notes

1. It is critical to characterize target cells for the levels of Pgp expression and functional activity using conventional immunostaining and the $DiOC_2$ efflux test. The UIC2 Shift assay produces the overall best results when using low and medium-low Pgp-expressing cells (e.g., human natural killer lymphocytes) and cell lines (e.g., KB-8-5 or MCF7-P10).
2. Maintaining target cells at 37°C is absolutely essential for Pgp function. Make sure that your sample volumes do not exceed 1 mL and plastic tubes are fully immersed in the water bath to ensure consistent results of the UIC2 Shift assay and the $DiOC_2$ efflux test.
3. Similarly, keeping cells at 4°C at all times is needed to prevent control Pgp-positive cells from "leaking" the dye during the $DiOC_2$ efflux test: residual levels of Pgp activity at higher temperatures may result in detectable $DiOC_2$ efflux.
4. Keep Pgp-positive cell lines free of MDR1 drugs for at least 1 wk before UIC2 Shift experiments to prevent their interference with the UIC2 Shift and $DiOC_2$ efflux assay results.
5. Pgp-positive cell lines may spontaneously lose some or all membrane Pgp as a result of long-term in vitro maintenance without continuous positive selection using MDR1 drugs or, preferably, cell sorting for Pgp-positive variants. To ensure consistent results, target cell have to be periodically checked for Pgp expressions levels using conventional immunostaining and, if needed, the $DiOC_2$ efflux test.

References

1. Roninson, I. B. (ed). (1990) *Molecular and Cellular Biology of Multidrug Resistance in Tumor Cells.* Plenum Press, New York.
2. Gottesman, M. M. and Pastan, I. (1993) Biochemistry of multidrug resistance mediated by the multidrug transporter. *Annu. Rev. Biochem.* **62,** 385–427.
3. Lehnert, M. (1996) Clinical multidrug resistance in cancer: a multifactorial problem. *Eur. J. Cancer* **32A,** 912–920.
4. Ambudkar, S. V., Dey, S., Hrycyna, C. A., Ramachandra, M., Pastan, I., and Gottesman, M. M. (1999) Biochemical, cellular, and pharmacological aspects of the multidrug transporter. *Annu. Rev. Pharmacol. Toxicol.* **39,** 361–398.
5. Higgins, C. F. (1992) ABC transporters: from microorganisms to man. *Annu. Rev. Cell Biol.* **8,** 67–113.
6. Klein, I., Sarkadi, B., and Varadi, A. (1999) An inventory of the human ABC proteins. *Biochim. Biophys. Acta.* **1461,** 237–262.
7. Borst, P., Zeker, N., and van Helvoort, A. (2000) ABC transporters in lipid transport. *Biochim. Biophys. Acta.* **1486,** 128–144.
8. Sikic, B. (1999) New approaches in cancer treatment. *Ann. Oncol.* **10,** 149–153.
9. Cordon-Cardo, C., O'Brien, J. P., Boccia, J., Bertino, J. R., and Melamed, M. R. (1990) Expression of a multidrug resistance gene product (P-glycoprotein) in human normal and human tissues. *J. Histochem. Cytochem.* **38,** 1277–1287.
10. Thiebaut, F., Tsuruo, T., Hamada, H., Gottesman, M. M., Pastan, I., and Willingham, M. (1987) Cellular localization of the multidrug resistance gene product in normal human tissues. *Proc. Natl. Acad. Sci. USA* **84,** 7735–7738.
11. Chaudhary, P. M., Mechetner, E. B., and Roninson, I. B. (1992) Expression and activity of the multidrug resistance p-glycoprotein in human preipheral blood lymphocytes. *Blood* **80,** 2735–2739.
12. Chaudhary, P. M. and Roninson, I. B. (1991) Expression and activity of P-glycoprotein, multidrug efflux pump, in human hematopoietic stem cells. *Cell* **66,** 85–94.
13. Schinkel, A. H., Smit, J. M., van Tellingen, O., et al. (1994) Disruption of the mouse mdr1a p-glycoprotein gene leads to a deficiency in the blood-brain barrier and to increased sensitivity to drugs. *Cell* **77,** 491–502.
14. Ueda, K., Okamura, N., Hirai, M., et al. (1992) Human P-glycoprotein transports cortisol, aldosterone, and dexamethasone, but no progesterone. *J. Biol. Chem.* **34,** 24,248–24,252.
15. Ernest, S. and Bello-Reuss, E. (1999) Secretion of platelet-activating factor is mediated by MDR1 P-glycorpotein in cultured human mesangial cells. *I. Am. Soc. Nephrol.* **10,** 2306–2313.
16. Ernest, S. and Bello-Reuss, E. (1998) P-glycorpotein functions and substrates: possible role of MDR1 gene in the kidney. *Kidney Int. Suppl.* **65,** 11–17.
17. Valverde, M. A., Diaz, M., Sepulveda, F. V., Gill, D. R., Hyde, S. C., and Higgins, C. F. (1992) Volume-regulated chloride channels associated with the human multidrug-resistance P-glycoprotein. *Nature* **355,** 830–833.
18. Roepe, P. D. (2000) What is the precise role of human MDR1 protein in chemotherapeutic drug resistance? *Curr. Pharm. Des.* **6,** 241–260.

19. Sonneveld, P. (2000) Multidrug resistance in haematological malignancies. *J. Intern. Med.* **247,** 521–534.

20. Robert, J. (1999) Multidrug resistance in oncology: diagnostic and therapeutic approaches. *Eur. J. Clin. Invest.* **29,** 536–545.

21. Mechetner, E., Kyshtoobayeva, A., Zonis, S., et al. (1998) Levels of multidrug resistance (MDR1) P-glycoprotein expression by human breast cancer correlate with in vitro resistance to taxol and doxorubicin. *Clin. Cancer Res.* **4,** 389–398.

22. Trock, B. J., Leonessa, F., and Clarke, R. (1997) Multidrug resistance in breast cancer: a meta-analysis of MDR1/gp170 expression and its possible functional significance. *J. Natl. Cancer Inst.* **89,** 917–931.

23. van den Heuvel-Eibrink, M. M., Wiemer, E. A., de Boevere, M. J., et al. (2001) MDR1 expression in poor-risk acute myeloid leukemia with partial or complete monosomy 7. *Leukemia* **15,** 398–405.

24. Bradshaw, D. M. and Arceci, R. J. (1998) Clinical relevance of transmembrane drug efflux as a mechanism of multidrug resistance. *J. Clin. Oncol.* **16,** 3674–3690.

25. Beck, W. T., Grogan, T. M., Willman, C. L., et al. (1996) Methods to detect P-glycoprotein-associated multidrug resistance in patients' tumors: consensus recommendations. *Cancer Res.* **56,** 3010–3020.

26. Liu, B., Sun, D., Xia, W., Hung, M. C., and Yu, D. (1997) Cross-reactivity of C219 anti-p170(mdr-1) antibody with p185(c-erbB2) in breast cancer cells: cautions on evaluating p170(mdr-1). *J. Natl. Cancer Inst.* **89,** 1524–1529.

27. Chan, H. S. and Ling, V. (1997) Anti-P-glycoprotein antibody C219 cross-reactivity with c-erbB2 protein: diagnostic and clinical implications. *J. Natl. Cancer Inst.* **89,** 1473–1476.

28. Rao, V. V., Anthony, D. C., and Piwnica-Worms, D. (1995) Multidrug resistance P-glycoprotein monoclonal antibody JSB-1 crossreacts with pyruvate carboxylase. *J. Histochem. Cytochem.* **43,** 1187–1192.

29. Bailly, J. D., Muller, C., Jaffrezou, J. P., et al. (1995) Lack of correlation between expression and function of P-glycoprotein in acute myeloid leukemia cell lines. *Leukemia* **9,** 799–807.

30. Leith, C. P., Chen, I. M., Kopecky, K. J., et al. (1995) Correlation of multidrug resistance (MDR1) protein expression with functional dye/drug efflux in acute myeloid leukemia by multiparameter flow cytometry: identification of discordant MDR-/efflux+ and MDR1+/efflux- cases. *Blood* **86,** 2329–2342.

31. Ferry, D. R. (1998) Testing the role of P-glycoprotein expression in clinical trials: applying pharmacological principles and best methods for detection together with good clinical trials methodology. *Int. J. Clin. Pharmacol. Ther.* **36,** 29–40.

32. Zaman, G. J., Flens, M. J., van Leusden, M. R., et al. (1994) The human multidrug resistance-associated protein MRP is a plasma membrane drug-efflux pump. *Proc. Natl. Acad. Sci. USA* **91,** 8822–8826.

33. Mechetner, E. B. and Roninson, I. B. (1992) Efficient inhibition of P-glycoprotein-mediated multidrug resistance with a monoclonal antibody. *Proc. Natl. Acad. Sci. USA* **89,** 5824–5828.

34. Mechetner, E. B., Schott, B., Morse, B. S., et al. (1997) P-glycoprotein function involves conformation transitions detectable by differential immunoreactivity. *Proc. Natl. Acad. Sci. USA* **94,** 12,908–12,913.
35. Park, S. W., Lomri, N., Simeoni, L. A., Fruchauf, J. P., and Mechetner, E. (2003) Analysis of P-glycoprotein-mediated membrane transport in human peripheral blood lymphocytes using the UIC2 shift assay. *Cytometry A.* **53,** 67–78.
36. Mechetner, E., Tee, L., Park, S., and Fruehauf, J. P. (1998) The UIC2 Shift Assay: improved detection of MDR1 in human tumors based on conformational transitions of functional P-glycoprotein. Proceedings of the American Association for Cancer Research Meeting, New Orleans, LA, 1998.
37. Mechetner, E., Tee, L., and Fruehauf, J. P. (1999) The UIC2 Shift Assay detects functional P-glycoprotein in tumors and correlates with in vitro drug response to doxorubicin. Proceedings of the American Association for Cancer Research Meeting, Philadelphia, PA, 1999.
38. Kobayashi, H., Takemura, Y., Miyachi, H. (2001) Novel approaches to reversing anticancer drug resistance using gene-specific therapeutics. *Hum. Cell.* **14,** 172–184.
39. Mechetner, E., Tee, L., Pavich, D., et al. (1998) High throughput screening for Mdr1 substrate specificity using the MDR1 Shift™ Assay. Proceedings of the American Association for Cancer Research Meeting, New Orleans, LA, 1998.
40. Jansen, W. J., Hulscher, T. M., van Ark-Otte, J., Giaccone, G., Pinedo, H. M., and Boven, E. (1998) CPT-11 sensitivity in relation to the expression of P170-glycoprotein and multidrug resistance-associated protein. *Br. J. Cancer* **77,** 359–365.
41. Hoki, Y., Fujimori, A., and Pommier, Y. (1997) Differential cytotoxicity of clinically important camptothecin derivatives in P-glycoprotein-overexpressing cell lines. *Cancer Chemother. Pharmacol.* **40,** 433–438.
42. Robey, R., Bakke, S., Stein, W., et al. (1999) Efflux of rhodamine from CD56+ cells as a surrogate marker for reversal of P-glycoprotein-mediated drug efflux by PSC 833. *Blood* **93,** 306–314.

14

Detection of Human Antibodies Generated Against Therapeutic Antibodies Used in Tumor Therapy

Jochen Reinsberg

Summary

Application of monoclonal antibodies (MAb) for therapeutic purpose may induce the formation of human antibodies directed against the immunogenic epitopes, which are presented on the therapeutic MAb. Formation of such human antibodies mostly is an undesired side effect, but in the case of newly developed immunotherapeutic tumor treatment strategies it represents the underlying therapeutic effect. Especially the formation of so-called "internal image" antibodies, which are directed against the antigen-combining site (paratope) of the therapeutic antibody, is supposed to evoke specific immune responses against tumor antigens mediated via idiotype–anti-idiotype interactions within the immunoregulatory network. For the monitoring of the immune response after antibody application, the newly formed human antibodies can be measured with immunoassay procedures involving the applied therapeutic antibody as test antibody. Because the original antigen is directed against the therapeutic antibody and inhibits the binding of "internal image" antibodies, a special assay design is needed to avoid interferences with samples containing the antigen. We describe an immunoassay procedure that allows the correct quantification of antiidiotypic antibodies including "internal image" antibodies that are not affected by the original antigen or other serum components that may interact with the therapeutic antibody.

Key Words: Antiidiotypic; antiiso/allotypic; immunotherapy; "internal image"; idiotypic network; immune response.

1. Introduction

Facilitated by their better availability monoclonal antibodies (MAbs) are increasingly used for therapeutic purposes. Especially for the therapy of neoplasm MAbs are applied either conjugated with cytotoxic agents or in native

From: *Methods in Molecular Biology, vol. 378: Monoclonal Antibodies: Methods and Protocols*
Edited by: M. Albitar © Humana Press Inc., Totowa, NJ

form *(1–7)*. In every case, antibody application may induce the formation of human antibodies directed against the immunogenic iso-, allo-, and idiotypic epitopes presented on the therapeutic MAb. For therapy with conjugated antibodies the formation of such human antibodies is an undesired side effect that negatively affects the pharmacokinetics and may diminish therapeutic activity *(8–10)*. However, in the last year different immunotherapeutic treatment strategies have been developed for cancer therapy intended to induce a tumor-specific humoral response of the host organism by triggering the idiotypic network, which leads to formation of a cascade of highly specific antiidiotypic antibodies *(11–14)*.

Antiidiotypic antibodies are directed against idiotypic epitopes (idiotopes), which are formed by the hypervariable region on the Fab portion of an antibody and, which are unique and representative for the specific antibody clone. Thus, antiidiotypic antibodies formed after antibody therapy react highly specific with the therapeutic antibody. A subset of antiidiotypic antibodies bind to the antigen-combining site (paratope) of the therapeutic antibody. These so-called "internal image" antibodies can functionally mimic a part of the three-dimensional structure of the original antigen *(15)* and their binding to the therapeutic antibody is inhibited by the antigen. For the immunotherapeutic treatment strategies the formation of "internal image" antibodies plays an essential role; it is supposed that vaccination with adequate antibodies may evoke specific immune responses against tumor antigens mediated via idiotype–anti-idiotype interactions of "internal image" antibodies within the immunoregulatory network *(11–16)*.

Formation of human antibodies against isotypic and allotypic epitopes that are located on the constant regions of the Fc and the Fab portions of the antibody only occurs when therapeutic antibodies with immunogenic nonself iso/allotypes are administered. Thus, the vast majority of MAbs clinically used for targeted cancer therapy are humanized to evade antiiso/allotypic immune responses and to minimize the immunogenicity of the antibodies, but in some cases antiidiotypic immune responses have been observed also with humanized antibodies *(17,18)*. On the other hand, for the immunotherapeutic concept an immune response with antibody formation represents the desired effect so that therapeutic antibodies with high immunogenicity are required. In every case, monitoring of the immune response to antibody application by measuring the newly formed human antibodies is a useful tool to assess the course of therapy. Especially for immunotherapy it is important to discriminate the newly formed antibodies according to their specificity. Thus, assay systems are needed that can specifically detect antiiso/allotypic antibodies, antiidiotypic antibodies, and internal image antibodies, respectively.

2. Materials

2.1. Absorption of Interfering Antiiso/Allotypic Human Anti-Mouse Antibodies

1. Mouse IgG-agarose suspension: polyclonal mouse IgG coupled to cyanogen bromide-activated agarose (Sigma-Aldrich, Deisenhofen, Germany). Resuspend settled gel by repeated shaking immediately before filling the pipet (*see* **Note 1**).
2. Phosphate-buffered saline with Tween (PBS-T): prepare 10X stock with 0.027 *M* KCl, 1.37 *M* NaCl, 0.1 *M* Na$_2$HPO$_4$, 0.018 *M* KH$_2$PO$_4$, and 1% Tween-20. Store at 4°C. Prepare working solution by dilution of one part with nine parts water.
3. Conical 4.5-mL polystyrene test tubes (Sarstett, Nümbrecht, Germany) (*see* **Note 2**).

2.2. Determination of Human Antiidiotypic Anti-OC125 Antibodies

1. Anti-human IgG-agarose suspension: Fc-specific anti-human IgG goat antibodies coupled to cyanogen bromide-activated agarose (Sigma-Aldrich). Resuspend settled gel by repeated shaking immediately before filling the pipet (*see* **Note 3**).
2. Conical 4.5-mL polystyrene test tubes (Sarstett) (*see* **Note 2**).
3. PBS-T: prepare 10X stock with 0.027 *M* KCl, 1.37 *M* NaCl, 0.1 *M* Na$_2$HPO$_4$, 0.018 *M* KH$_2$PO$_4$, and 1% Tween-20. Store at 4°C. Prepare working solution by dilution of one part with nine parts water.
4. Mouse IgG solution: polyclonal mouse IgG (reagent grade; Sigma-Aldrich) is dissolved at 12 mg/mL in PBS-T and stored in single use (0.4 mL) aliquots in 10 mL tubes at –20°C.
5. Detector antibody solution: the therapeutic antibody is used as detector antibody (*see* **Note 4**). These instructions assume the use of ^{125}I-labeled OC125 detector antibodies provided as tracer of the CA-125-II ^{125}I IRMA, DiaSorin, Stillwater, MN (*see* **Note 5**). The original tracer solution is diluted 10-fold with PBS-T and supplemented with 0.8 mg/mL polyclonal mouse IgG by addition 0.6 mL of the tracer solution to a 0.4-mL aliquot of mouse IgG solution together with 5 mL PBS-T (*see* **Note 6**).
6. Standard solutions: a serum pool with elevated levels of antiidiotypic antibodies can serve as arbitrary standard material. In the present protocol we use a serum pool made of samples drawn from two ovarian cancer patients treated repeatedly with OC125 antibodies. After absorption of antiiso/allotypic antibodies (*see* **Note 7**) the serum supernatant is stored as master standard stock solution in single use (60 µL) aliquots at –80°C. Working standard solutions are prepared by 1:2, 1:4, 1:8, 1:16, and 1:32 dilution of master standard with PBS-T. The concentration of the antiidiotypic antibodies is expressed as arbitrary units per milliliter (arb.units/mL). A nominal value of 1×10^3 arb.units/mL of antiidiotypic anti-OC125 antibodies is assigned to the master standard stock solution.
7. Diluent: a serum pool free of antiiso/allotypic human anti-mouse antibodies (HAMA) and antiidiotypic antibodies diluted 1:5 with PBS-T serves as diluent. The diluent is stored in single use (500 µL) aliquots at –80°C.

2.3. Inhibition Assay

1. Antigen solution: A high amount of the therapeutic antibody is directed against the antigen and is used to inhibit binding of the detector antibodies to "internal image" antibodies. Thus, these instructions assume the use of the cancer antigen 125 (CA-125) which is the corresponding antigen to the OC125 antibody (*see* **Note 8**). Two-hundred fifty microliters of CA-125 stock solution (1×10^6 arb.units/mL, Fitzgerald Industries International, Concord, MA) is diluted 10-fold with 2.25 mL PBS-T and stored in single use (0.4 mL) aliquots at –20°C.
2. Detector solution A (without antigen): the detector solution A corresponds to the detector antibody solution described in **Subheading 2.2**. The original OC125 tracer provided with the CA-125-II ^{125}I IRMA, DiaSorin is diluted 10-fold with PBS-T and supplemented with 0.8 mg/mL polyclonal mouse IgG by addition 0.6 mL of the tracer solution to a 0.4-mL aliquot of mouse IgG solution together with 5 mL PBS-T (*see* **Note 6**).
3. Detector solution B (with 2000 arb.units/mL CA-125): 0.3 mL of the original OC125 tracer is mixed with 0.2 mL of mouse IgG solution, 60 µL antigen solution, and 2.44 mL PBS-T (*see* **Note 6**).
4. Detector solution C (with 10,000 arb.units/mL CA-125): 0.3 mL of the original OC125 tracer is mixed with 0.2 mL of mouse IgG solution, 300 µL antigen solution, and 2.2 mL PBS-T (*see* **Note 6**).

3. Methods

The serum concentration of human antibodies newly formed in response to the application of a therapeutic antibody can be measured in serum samples prepared in the common way from blood collected by venipuncture into plain tubes. A serum volume of 1 mL is adequate for analysis. Serum samples can be stored at –20°C for several months without any effect on antibody concentration.

Antiiso/allotypic anti-murine antibodies (HAMAs) are found in a high percentage of patients treated with murine antibodies. For direct determination of the concentration of such HAMAs, specific assays are commercially available (*see* **Note 9**). HAMAs generally can falsify the results of immunometric assays that involve murine test antibodies by cross-linking capture and detector antibodies *(19,20)*. To avoid those interferences, HAMAs can be removed from serum samples by absorption onto mouse-IgG-agarose gel before measurement of antiidiotypic antibodies. Furthermore, HAMA activity can be blocked by addition of nonspecific murine antibodies to the assay buffer *(21)*.

Human antiidiotypic antibodies formed by patients after antibody therapy are measured by an immunometric assay procedure involving the applied therapeutic antibody as detector antibody. These instructions describe the determination of human antibodies developed after application of the anti-CA-125 antibody OC125. They can easily be adapted to other therapeutic antibodies if they are available in labeled form (*see* **Note 5**). Fc-specific anti-human antibodies immobilized on agarose gel are used as capture antibodies (*see* **Note 10**). To exclude interferences by serum components such as the original antigen that may inhibit binding of the detector antibody, a two-step assay design was chosen with a separate detection step after removal of unbound serum components by washing (*see* **Note 11**).

Internal image antibodies can be quantified indirectly as a subgroup of antiidiotypic antibodies. To this end, binding of detector antibodies is measured in the presence of a high concentration of the original antigen, which inhibits binding of the detector antibodies to "internal image" antibodies (*see* **Note 12**).

3.1. Absorption of Interfering Antiiso/Allotypic Human Anti-Mouse Antibodies

1. For absorption of HAMA from serum samples, 200 μL of mouse IgG-agarose suspension (equivalent to 100 μL gel) is pipetted into a conical 4.5-mL polystyrene test tube (*see* **Note 13**).
2. Add 2 mL of PBS-T, mix each tube and centrifuge at 3500*g* for 15 min (*see* **Note 14**).
3. Carefully aspirate the buffer supernatant. Pay attention that the sedimented pellet is not destroyed (*see* **Note 15**).
4. Add 400 μL PBS-T to the washed agarose pellet followed by 100 μL of the respective serum sample.
5. Mix each tube and incubate for 2 h at room temperature on an orbital shaker with intensive agitation (*see* **Note 16**).
6. Stop incubation by centrifugation at 3500*g* for 15 min. The serum supernatant can be stored at 4°C until further processed for measurement of specific antiidiotypic antibodies (*see* **Note 17**).

3.2. Determination of Human Antiidiotypic Anti-OC125 Antibodies

1. For binding of human serum IgG, 100 μL of anti-human IgG-agarose suspension (equivalent to 50 μL gel; *see* **Note 18**) is pipetted into a conical 4.5-mL polystyrene test tube (*see* **Note 13**).
2. Add 2 mL of PBS-T, mix each tube and centrifuge at 3500*g* for 15 min (*see* **Note 14**).
3. Carefully aspirate the buffer supernatant. Pay attention that the sedimented pellet is not destroyed (*see* **Note 15**).
4. Add 200 μL of PBS-T to the washed agarose pellet followed by 10 μL of the serum supernatant obtained after absorption of HAMA (as described in **Subheading 3.1.**).
5. Mix each tube and incubate for 1 h at room temperature on an orbital shaker with intensive agitation (*see* **Note 16**).
6. Stop incubation by addition of 1 mL PBS-T followed by centrifugation at 3500*g* for 15 min.
7. Carefully aspirate the buffer supernatant and wash the agarose pellet by resuspension in 2 mL PBS-T. After centrifugation at 3500*g* for 15 min aspirate the buffer supernatant.

8. Add 300 μL of detector antibody solution, mix each tube and incubate over night at room temperature on an orbital shaker with intensive agitation (*see* **Note 16**).

9. Stop incubation by addition of 1 mL PBS-T followed by centrifugation at 3500*g* for 15 min.

10. Carefully aspirate the buffer supernatant and wash the agarose pellet two times by resuspension with 2 mL PBS-T, centrifugation at 3500*g* for 15 min and aspiration of the buffer supernatant (*see* **Note 19**).

11. The radioactivity bound to the washed pellet is measured in a γ-counter (*see* **Note 20**).

12. The respective antiidiotypic antibody concentration of a sample is calculated by interpolation from a standard curve measured in the same assay as the sample. The standard curve is generated processing the working standard solutions such as the samples. The radioactive counts measured for each working standard solution is plotted against the standard concentration (*see* **Note 21**). If samples have concentrations greater than the highest standard, they must be reanalysed after adequate dilution with the diluent.

3.3. Inhibition Assay

1. For indirect determination of internal image antibodies, the human IgG of the serum supernatant obtained after absorption of HAMA (as described in **Subheading 3.1.**) is bound to anti-human IgG agarose according to the procedure described in **Subheading 3.2.**, **steps 1–7**. Three replicates are performed for each serum sample.

2. Add 300 μL of one of the detector solutions A, B, and C to one of the three replicates, mix all tubes and incubate over night at room temperature on an orbital shaker with intensive agitation (*see* **Note 16**).

3. Stop incubation by addition of 1 mL PBS-T followed by centrifugation at 3500*g* for 15 min (*see* **Note 14**).

4. Furthermore the buffer supernatant is carefully aspirated, the agarose pellet is washed and the bound radioactivity is measured as described in **Subheading 3.2.**, **steps 10–11**.

5. The apparent antiidiotypic antibody concentrations of the three replicates are calculated by interpolation from a standard curve generated using the detector solution A (without antigen). The concentration of "internal image" antibodies is calculated as the difference between the apparent concentrations measured with (detector solution C) and without (detector solution A) addition of antigen (*see* **Note 22**).

4. Notes

1. For complete binding of HAMAs directed against the different iso/allotypic epitopes a polyclonal mouse IgG preparation is optimal *(21)*. We found this agarose gel suitable for HAMA absorption but numerous competitive reagents are available from other commercial sources.

2. Clear conical test tubes are used to have better control when the buffer supernatant is aspirated from sedimented agarose pellet.

3. We found this agarose gel suitable for binding human serum IgG but numerous competitive reagents are available from other commercial sources.

4. Humanized antibodies cannot be used as detector antibodies because they directly bind to the anti-human IgG antibodies employed as capture antibodies. To determine antiidiotypic antibodies developed in response to therapy with a humanized antibody, the original murine MAb, the humanized MAb is derived from, should be used as detector antibody.

5. This protocol can easily be adapted for other therapeutic antibodies. Instead of radio-labeling antibodies also can be conjugated to biotin using commercial available biotinylation kits (e.g., Biotin Tag™, Micro Biotinylation Kit, Sigma-Aldrich).

6. HAMAs may interfere with the determination of specific antiidiotypic antibodies by cross-linking capture and detector antibodies. Thus, a high amount of polyclonal mouse IgG is added to the detector antibody solution as a target for HAMA binding to prevent binding to the test antibodies. A polyclonal mouse IgG preparation is the best agent for blocking HAMA interferences because all allotypic epitopes are presented *(21)*. The supplementation with mouse IgG can be omitted when the antiiso/allotypic antibodies are completely removed by previous absorption with mouse IgG-agarose (*see* **Subheading 3.1.**).

7. Absorption of antiiso/allotypic antibodies can be performed as described (*see* **Subheading 3.1.**). To get a sufficient volume of master standard, a greater serum volume can be absorbed with an accordant amount of gel (e.g., 1 mL serum diluted with 4 mL PBS-T is absorbed with 1 mL gel).

8. For inhibition of the binding of detector antibodies to the "internal image" antibodies the relevant antigen, the therapeutic antibody is developed against, should be used. The antigen concentration of the detector solutions B and C should be high enough to achieve a complete inhibition of "internal image" antibody binding.

9. For determination of human antibodies developed against murine iso/allotypic epitopes (HAMA) various test kits are commercially available (e.g., ImmuSTRIP HAMA Test Kit, Immunomedics, Morris Plains, NJ or HAMA-ELISA medac, MEDAC, Wedel, Germany). In our experience the HAMA-ELISA medac, which use polyclonal mouse IgG as both capture and detector antibodies is a reliable test for simple quantification of those HAMAs.

10. We use capture antibodies immobilized on agarose gel instead by coating on 96-well plates to get a high binding capacity for human serum IgG, which is a limitation of assay sensitivity. Insufficient binding capacity of the solid phase can be compensated in part by increasing the amount of gel used in the first incubation step.

11. There are alternative assay formats, in which the antiidiotypic antibodies are captured by the immobilized therapeutic antibody. Subsequently the bound antiidiotypic antibodies are detected by incubation with labeled anti-human immunoglobulin G antibodies *(17,22)*. In a homologous "sandwich"-assay format the therapeutic antibody can be used as both capture and detector antibodies *(23)*. However, because in these assay formats the immobilized therapeutic antibodies are incubated with whole serum, possible interferences are to be expected for serum samples containing the original antigen. In contrast, the assay procedure

described here allows the correct quantification of antiidiotypic antibodies in the presence of the original antigen because in a first step the human serum IgG is selectively extracted and interfering serum components including circulating antigen, which may react with the detector antibodies are removed before specific detection of the anti-idiotypic antibodies by labeled therapeutic antibodies.

12. It is a well-accepted principle that "internal image" antibodies are identified by inhibition of their binding to the original antibody by the corresponding antigen. However, also binding of antiidiotypic antibodies recognizing paratope associated idiotopes, which do not present an internal image of the antigen can be inhibited by the antigen, probably owing to alteration of the three-dimensional structure of the paratope *(24)*.

13. Distribution of agarose gel in test tubes may be done with a multidispensing device (e.g., Eppendorf Multipipette), but pipetting time should not exceed 10–15 s to avoid sizable sedimentation of gel.

14. Conditions of centrifugation can be modified to assure the formation of a pellet compact enough for removal of buffer supernatant.

15. Alternatively, tubes can be decanted to remove the buffer supernatant, but in our hand, supernatant can be aspirated more exhaustively.

16. To prevent sedimentation of agarose gel, the incubation is performed with agitation at 1600 rounds per min. We use the orbital shaker IKA Vibrax VXR with the suitable attachment VX2 for 16-mm test tubes.

17. The absorbed supernatants may be stored at 4°C for 2 d. For prolonged storage (up to 1 wk) they should be kept at –20°C.

18. To ensure complete binding of human IgG from 2 μL serum we use 50 μL anti-human IgG agarose gel with a binding capacity of 3 mg human IgG per mL. We found this agarose gel suitable for IgG binding but numerous competitive reagents are available from other commercial sources.

19. This washing step is very important. Insufficient removal of the detector solution grossly affects accuracy and precision of test results.

20. If a biotin labeled detector antibody is used, determination of the bound biotin can be done using commercial available detection kits (e.g., Avidin-Peroxidase and Sigma*F*ast™ OPD, Sigma-Aldrich).

21. For data reduction we use the computer assisted data reduction program of the γ-counter LB 2111 (Berthold, Bad Wildbad, Germany), but other programs appropriate to reduction of immunoassay data also can be used.

22. The replicate with the detector solution B is not used for calculation. It only serves as control to indicate how far the antigen concentration of the detector solution C is sufficient to inhibit the binding of "internal image" antibodies completely.

Acknowledgments

The author would like to thank Dietlind Ackermann for excellent technical assistance.

References

1. Trail, P. A. and Bianchi A. B. (1999) Monoclonal antibody drug conjugates in the treatment of cancer. *Curr. Opinion Immunol.* **11,** 584–588.

2. Milenic, D. E. and Brechbiel, M. W. (2004) Targeting of radio-isotopes for cancer therapy. *Cancer Biol. Ther.* **3,** 361–370.
3. DiJoseph, J. F., Armellino, D. C., Boghaert, E. R., et al. (2004) Antibody-targeted chemotherapy with CMC-544: a CD22-targeted immunoconjugate of calicheamicin for the treatment of B-lymphoid malignancies. *Blood* **103,** 1807–1814.
4. Wiedmann, M. W. and Caca, K. (2005) Molecularly targeted therapy for gastrointestinal cancer. *Curr. Cancer Drug Targets* **5,** 171–193.
5. Caponigro, F., Formato, R., Caraglia, M., Normanno, N., and Iaffaioli, R. V. (2005) Monoclonal antibodies targeting epidermal growth factor receptor and vascular endothelial growth factor with a focus on head and neck tumors. *Curr. Opinion Oncol.* **17,** 212–217.
6. Rueckert, S., Ruehl, I., Kahlert, S., Konecny, G., and Untch, M. (2005) A monoclonal antibody as an effective therapeutic agent in breast cancer: trastuzumab. *Expert Opinion Biol. Ther.* **5,** 853–866.
7. Nicodemus, C. F. and Berek, J. S. (2005) Monoclonal antibody therapy of ovarian cancer. *Expert Rev. Anticancer Ther.* **5,** 87–96.
8. Pimm, M. V., Perkins, A. C., Armitage, N.C., and Baldwin, R. W. (1985) The characteristics of blood-borne radiolabels and the effect of anti-mouse IgG antibodies on localization of radiolabeled monoclonal antibody in cancer patients. *J. Nucl. Med.* **26,** 1011–1023.
9. Reynolds, J. C., Carrasquillo, J. A., Keenan, A. M., et al. (1986) Human antimurine antibodies following immunoscintigraphy or therapy with radiolabeled monoclonal antibodies. *J. Nucl. Med.* **27,** 1022–1023.
10. Pastan, I. and Kreitman, R. J. (2002) Immunotoxins in cancer therapy. *Curr. Opinion Investig. Drugs* **3,** 1089–1091.
11. Chatterjee, M. B., Foon, K. A., and Kohler, H. (1994) Idiotypic antibody immunotherapy of cancer. *Cancer Immunol. Immunother.* **38,** 75–82.
12. Foon, K. A., John, W. J., Chakraborty, M., et al. (1999) Clinical and immune responses in resected colon cancer patients treated with anti-idiotype monoclonal antibody vaccine that mimics the carcinoembryonic antigen. *J. Clin. Oncol.* **17,** 2889–2895.
13. Pride, M. W., Shuey, S., Grillo-Lopez, A., et al. (1998) Enhancement of cell-mediated immunity in melanoma patients immunized with murine anti-idiotypic monoclonal antibodies (MELIMMUNE) that mimic the high molecular weight proteoglycan antigen. *Clin. Cancer Res.* **4,** 2363–2370.
14. Wagner, U., Schlebusch, H., Schmolling, J., Reinsberg, J., and Krebs, D. (1997) Anti-idiotypes in ovarian cancer. In: *Idiotypes in Medicine: Autoimmunity, Infection and Cancer,* (Shoenfeld, Y., Kennedy, R. C., and Ferrone, S., eds.), Elsevier, New York, pp. 475–485.
15. Jefferis, R. (1993) What is an idiotype? *Immunol. Today* **14,** 119–121.
16. Cerny, J. and Hiernaux, J. (1990) Concept of idiotypic network: description and functions. In: *Idiotypic network and Diseases,* (Cerny, J. and Hiernaux, J., eds.), American Society for Microbiology, Washington, DC, pp. 13–29.
17. Pavlinkova, G., Colcher, D., Booth, B. J., Goel, A., Wittel, U. A., and Batra, S. K. (2001) Effects of humanization and gene shuffling on immunogenicity and antigen binding of anti-TAG-72 single-chain Fvs. *Int. J. Cancer* **94,** 717–726.

18. Utset, T. O., Auger, J. A., Peace, D., et al. (2002) Modified anti-CD3 therapy in psoriatic arthritis: a phase I/II clinical trial. *J. Rheumatol.* **29,** 1907–1913.

19. Boscato, L. M. and Stuart, M. C. (1988) Heterophilic antibodies: a problem for all immunoassays. *Clin. Chem.* **34,** 27–33.

20. Krika, L. J. (1999) Human anti-animal antibody interferences in immunological assays. *Clin. Chem.* **45,** 942–956.

21. Reinsberg, J. (1998) Interferences with two-site immunoassays by human anti-mouse antibodies formed by patients treated with monoclonal antibodies: comparison of different blocking reagents. *Clin. Chem.* **44,** 1742–1744.

22. Ferroni, P., Milenic, D. E., Schlom, J., and Colcher D. (1990) Assay for detection of anti-idiotypic antibodies to monoclonal antibody B72.3. *J. Clin. Lab. Anal.* **4,** 465–473.

23. Reinsberg, J., Schmolling, J., and Ackermann, D. (1996) A simple and sensitive assay for determination of human anti-idiotypic anti-B72.3 antibodies not affected by TAG-72. *Eur. J. Clin. Chem. Clin. Biochem.* **34,** 237–244.

24. Bona, C. A. (1996) Internal image concept revisited. *Proc. Soc. Exp. Biol. Med.* **213,** 32–42.

15

Measuring Allergen-Specific IgE

Where Have We Been and Where Are We Going?

M. Michael Glovsky

Summary

About 40 yr ago, two groups of investigators identified a new class of immunoglobulins, IgE. By exchanging their results and reagents, they proved that the immunoglobulin responsible for immediate hypersensitivity was IgE. From that day forward the science of allergy was greatly advanced. Within a few years of the IgE discovery, an assay for IgE was developed. This test was named the radio allergosorbent test. The specific IgE testing methodology has matured in the last four decades. Different means of detecting IgE bound to allergen is the subject of this review. We have included methods for measuring specific IgE using the ImmunoCAP 1000 instrument. The methodology for measuring basophile histamine release is also detailed in this chapter.

Key Words: Allergy; RAST; immunoassay; allergen-specific IgE; ImmunoCAP.

1. Introduction

IgE, the immunoglobulin isotype related to immediate hypersensitivity (allergy), was identified by two groups of investigators in 1966 and 1967. The Ishizakas, in Denver, extracted a new class of immunoglobulins (not IgG, IgA, IgM, or IgD) from reaginic sera of individuals highly allergic to ragweed pollen *(1)*. When the isolated immunoglobulin was passively injected into human skin and the skin was challenged with ragweed extract, a wheal and flare reaction occurred. Within the same years Bennisch and Johanson in Sweden had identified a patient, N. D., with an unusual myeloma protein not identified by antisera to the known immunoglobulin isotypes *(2)*. They called this myeloma protein Ig N. D. The two groups compared the myeloma protein with the isolated immunoglobulin and proved that the reagenic antibody and IgE N.D. were similar in structure, antibody reactivity, and function, and named the allergy antibody "IgE" *(2)*.

From: *Methods in Molecular Biology, vol. 378: Monoclonal Antibodies: Methods and Protocols*
Edited by: M. Albitar © Humana Press Inc., Totowa, NJ

Diagnostic testing for allergy has progressed since the discovery of IgE. In 1967, Wide and colleagues introduced an in vitro test for specific allergens *(3)*. They produced antibody to human IgE in rabbits and coupled specific allergen protein (such as ragweed or ryegrass extract) to cellulose discs. Next, they added sera of individuals allergic to ragweed, ryegrass, or other allergens to the specific allergen-coated cellulose discs. After washing the discs to remove unbound antibody, they added I^{125} labeled anti-IgE to the paper discs. The I^{125} that bound to the discs was analyzed to determine the quantity of specific IgE. This test was named the Radio Allergo Sorbent Test, or RAST (**Fig. 1**). Since its initial development, the RAST has been modified and automated. Other versions of the specific IgE test have been formulated, such as the MAST, AlaSTAT®, and Hycor-EIA tests. All are based on similar methodologies. This review will focus on the ImmunoCAP–FEIA methodology, thought by some investigators to be the most accurate and best-validated in vitro specific IgE test available.

ImmunoCAP is a third-generation quantitative test developed by Pharmacia Diagnostics from the original RAST technology *(4)*. Also included in this chapter is an overview of newer methods, including flow cytometry, upregulation of basophile receptors CD_{63} and CD_{203}, and silica chip evaluation of specific IgE using recombinant allergens.

2. Specific IgE Testing With ImmunoCAP

The third-generation Pharmacia ImmunoCAP-specific IgE technology uses an activated sponge-like matrix to absorb specific allergens. The tests are sandwich immunoassays using a flexible, hydrophilic carrier polymer encloses in a capsule as the solid phase (the ImmunoCAP). Serum is added to the ImmunoCAP and incubated, and the cap tube is then washed. Enzyme-labeled anti-IgE is added to the cap, and after further washing the bound IgE is quantified using a fluorescent substrate. Results are reported quantitatively using a kU/L scale. The calibrator is IgE bound to anti-IgE caps using a six-point quantitative curve. Calibration ranges from <0.35 kU/L to >100 kU/L. Results can be reported by a second system using six classes (0, 1, 2, 3, 4, 5, and 6) (**Table 1**).

CAP testing has been highly automated on several instruments such as the AutoCAP 100, ImmunoCAP 250, and ImmunoCAP 1000; the numeric suffixes indicate the numbers of tubes that can be analyzed.

2.1. Method for Measurement of Specific IgE Using the Unicap 1000 Instrument

2.1.1. Analytical Principle—UniCAP Specific IgE

The UniCAP-specific IgE FEIA is an in vitro quantitative assay that measures the concentration of circulating allergen-specific IgE in human blood samples.

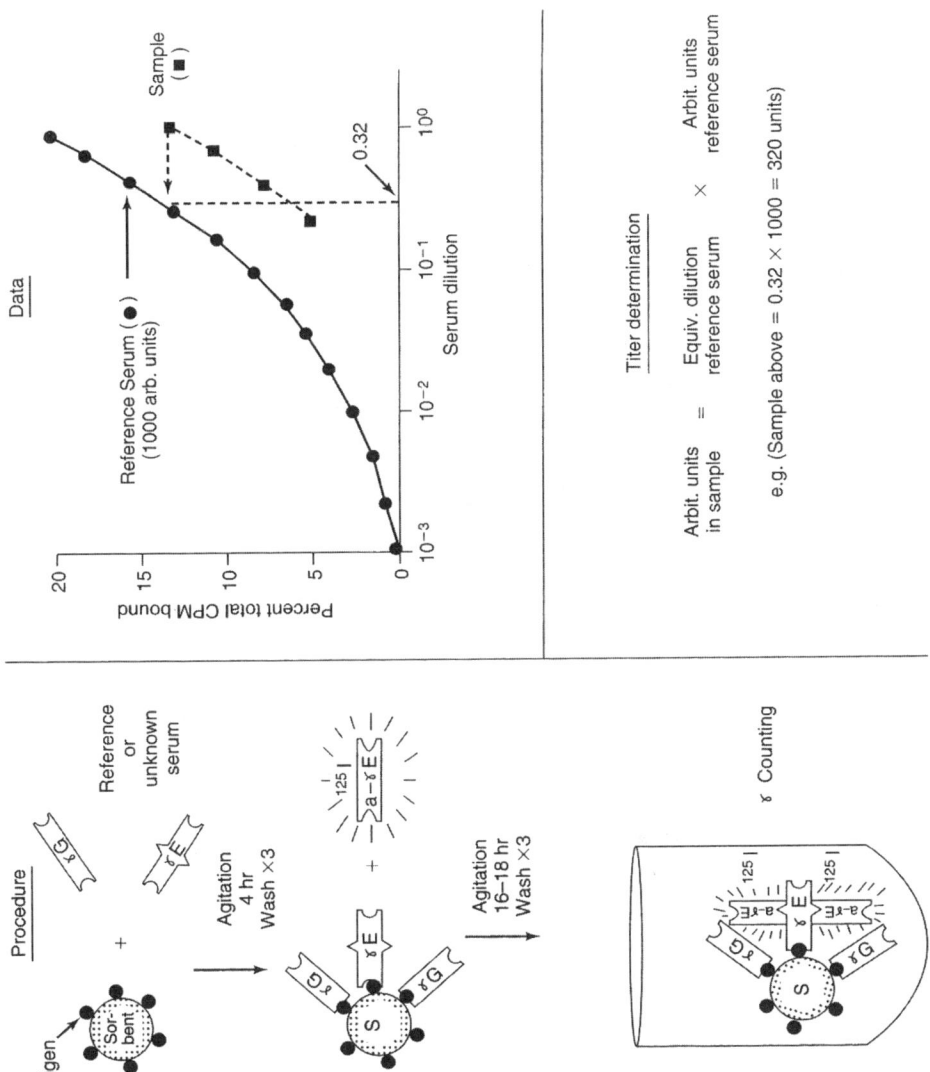

Fig. 1. Schematic of original radioallergosorbent test reported in 1967. In the first assay incubation, human antibodies of different isotypes (e.g., IgG, IgE) in reference and unknown sera bind to antigens coupled to the sorbent (allergosorbent). After isotonic buffer washes to remove unbound serum proteins, bound IgE antibody is detected with ^{125}I-labeled rabbit anti-human IgE detection antibody. The percentage of total radioactivity in counts per minute (CPM) bound to the allergosorbent is then measured in a gamma counter and plotted against the serum dilution analyzed. The amount of specific IgE in reference and original sera is proportional to the amount of radioactivity bound. Interpolated units of antibody are corrected for sample dilution and reported as the number of arbitrary units of allergen-specific IgE in the original serum. (Reproduced with permission from **ref. *18*.**)

Table 1
Relative Concentration of Specific IgE

Class	Relative activity	kU_A/L
Class 0	Undetectable	<0.35
Class 1	Low	0.35–0.70
Class 2	Moderate	0.71–3.50
Class 3	High	3.5–17.5
Class 4	Very high	17.6–50
Class 5	Very high	51–100
Class 6	Very high	>100

The calibration reflects total IgE bound and not specific IgE. Specific IgE to ryegrass, short ragweed, and cat extract would be ideal for use as a standard for each assay. However, such specific standards for over 400 assays would be technically impractical. For that reason, bound IgE is used as a relative calibrator for both specific and total IgE.

In principle, the allergen of interest, covalently coupled to ImmunoCAP, captures the specific IgE in the patient specimen. Nonspecific IgE is washed away and enzyme-labeled antibodies against IgE are then added to form a complex. After incubation, unbound enzyme-anti-IgE is washed away and the bound complex is incubated with a developing agent. The reaction is then stopped and the fluorescence of the eluate is measured. To evaluate the test results, the response units for patient samples are compared directly to the response of the calibrators.

The IgE calibrators are traceable to the Second International Reference Preparation 75/502 of Human Serum Immunoglobulin E from the World Health Organization (WHO). The UniCAP 1000 Instrument calculates the concentration in kU/L and the instrument software automatically calculates the concentration.

2.1.2. Equipment and Supplies

1. UniCAP 1000 instrument (cat. no. 12-3800-01).
2. UniCAP 1000 pipet tips in racks (cat. no. 12-3805-04).
3. Solid waste container bags (cat. no. 12-3807-36).

2.1.3. Reagent Summary, Preparation, and Storage (see **Note 1**)

All reagents are manufactured by Pharmacia and Upjohn Diagnostics, Uppsala, Sweden. **Note:** date and initial all reagents upon opening. Each container should be labeled with substance name, lot number, date of preparation, expiration date, and any special storage instructions.

1. Anti-IgE ImmunoCAP (cat. no. 14-4417-01). Anti-IgE Mouse monoclonal antibodies. 16 ImmunoCAP/carrier. Store at 2–8°C.

2. Allergen-specific ImmunoCAP (refer to catalog for specific allergen product number). Each ImmunoCAP is specific for detecting IgE antibodies against one or multiple types of allergen. Store at 2–8°C.

3. UniCAP-specific IgE conjugate 400 (cat. no. 10-9310-02). β-galactosidase-anti-IgE (mouse monoclonal antibodies) approx 1μg/mL. Color-coded blue. Six vials, 20.5 mL/vial. Store at 2–8°C.

4. UniCAP-specific IgE calibrator strip (cat. no. 10-9386-01). Human IgE in buffer, concentrations 0.35, 0.70, 17.5, 50, and 100 kU/L (0.2 mL/vial), five strips, one curve per strip. Store at 2–8°C.

5. UniCAP-specific IgE positive control (cat. no. 10-9446-01). Prepared from selected pooled human serum and contains IgE antibodies to a number of different allergens. Each kit contains six bottles with four determinations per bottle (0.3 mL each). Store at 2–8°C.

6. UniCAP-specific IgE negative control (cat. no. 10-9445-01). Prepared from human serum. Each kit contains six bottles with four determinations per bottle (0.3 mL each). Store at 2–8°C.

7. UniCAP development solutions (cat. no. 10-9439-01): 4-methylumbelliferyl-β-D-galactosidase 0.01%. Six bottles with 1200 determinations per bottle (64 mL per bottle). Store at 2–8°C.

8. UniCAP stop solutions (cat. no. 34-2271-51): sodium carbonate 4%, one bottle with 1200 determinations per bottle (850 mL per bottle). Store at 2–8°C.

9. UniCAP/Pharmacia CAP System washing solution set (cat. no. 10-9202-01). Set contains two bottles each of washing solution additive (86 mL) and washing solution concentrate (400 mL). Store at 2–8°C. To prepare for use, reconstitute using 10 L of distilled water per kit. Shake gently to mix. Prepared washing solution may be kept on the instrument. The washing solution bottle must be emptied and rinsed with distilled or ionized water. Water during weekly maintenance. Store at room temperature.

2.1.4. Testing of New Lots of Reagents

New lots of reagents and kits must be tested for performance, and the results of such testing recorded, before being placed in service. Include patient samples in parallel. To be acceptable, the new lot must perform the same as the old lot. New vendor shipments of in-use lots are also tested prior to use.

2.1.5. Calibrators and Standards

UniCAP-specific IgE calibrator strip (cat. no. 10-938601): human IgE in buffer, concentrations 0.35, 0.70, 3.50, 17.5, 50, and 100 kU/L. The IgE calibrators are traceable to the Second International Reference Preparation 75/505 of human serum IgE from WHO. Date and initial all calibrators upon opening. Each *aliquot tube* should be labeled with (1) substance name, (2) lot number, (3) date of preparation, (4) expiration date, and (5) any special storage instructions. Store at 2–8°C.

3. Procedure

3.1. Calibration Procedure

A six-point reference curve is set up along with the patient samples each time, and results are calculated by comparing the fluorescence of the unknown to that of the reference. The UniCAP 1000 Instrument measures specific IgE concentrations in kU/L and the instrument software automatically calculates the concentration.

3.2. Procedure

Follow the manufacturer's instructions.

4. Calculations

All calculations are preformed by the UniCAP operator software. For complete details, refer to the UniCAP 1000 system manual.

4.1. Other Commercial IgE Tests

4.1.1. AlaSTAT

The AlaSTAT IgE assay (Diagnostic Products Corp., Los Angeles, CA) employs biotin-labeled allergen extracts that bind in the fluid phase to specific IgE (5). The biotin–IgE complexes are added to microtiter wells or plastic tubes where biotin-albumin is coated to the surface. Avidin is added to the solution and the IgE–biotin complexes are linked to the biotin solid phase. An enzyme-linked anti IgE is used to calibrate the specific IgE.

Quantitative IgE calibrators are used to assess specific IgE in the complexes and the results are calculated and classified as kU/L bound or with specific classes. The results of the AlaSTAT-specific IgE are similar, though not necessarily identical, to those of the ImmunoCAP IgE. Like the ImmunoCAP system, the AlaSTAT system has been automated.

The specific IgE bound in the AlaSTAT system depends on the individual extracts (such as cat dander, perennial ryegrass, and so on) that are coupled with biotin. The specific extract and or the coupling procedure may, by altering the binding of the allergen or the extract content of major allergens, give different values than the ImmunoCAP procedure.

4.2. Hycor Test

The Hycor EIA and the Hycor Turbo-MP RIA (Hycor Stratogene, Garden Grove, CA) methods for specific IgE detection are both FDA cleared (6). In these tests, allergens are linked to cellulose discs and serum IgE is tested after incubation with the allergen-coated discs. The Hycor-EIA uses a modified RAST scheme in which low-level specific IgE is recorded as positive. These low-level tests may be clinically unimportant. The Hycor test is similar to the original RAST technology, but may be less well standardized owing to the purity of the extracts and the comparative validity of the specific IgE.

4.3. MAST Test

In a chemiluminescent system from Hitachi Chemical Diagnostics (formerly called MAST), the allergens are linked to a thread *(7)*. After incubation with sera containing IgE antibodies, the threads are washed, incubated with anti IgE, washed again, and then developed with a chemiluminescent indicator. The test results are reported as specific classes, 0–6, and the assay is considered a qualitative rather than a quantitative test.

5. Cell- and Microarray-Based Technologies to Detect Allergen-Specific IgE

5.1. Basophile Histamine Release

Histamine release using leukocytes from atopic individuals has been studied for the last half century *(8,9)*. Leukocytes are separated from heparinized blood to remove red blood cells, and the volume of the leukocyte preparation is restored to the initial blood volume. The specific allergen under study is added to the leukocyte preparation (containing 0.5–1.0% basophiles) as well as controls. After an appropriate incubation, the cells are separated from the supernatant. Released histamine is then determined by comparing lysed basophiles (100% histamine) to buffer and other controls. A good correlation (~90%) between histamine release and skin testing as well as specific IgE is usually found with pollen allergens. With venoms and B-lactam drugs, the sensitivity vs skin testing is approx 50% *(10)*. This discordance may be related to false-positive skin test reactivity or secondary to relative nonsensitivity of separated basophiles. In any event, basophile histamine release is more time-consuming and difficult to perform than specific IgE immunoassays, but is a relevant confirmatory test for unclear allergen biologic activity.

5.1.1. Method for Basophil Histamine Release: Evaluation of Allergic Status

Basophil histamine release in response to allergens (e.g., antigen E or Amb a1, Fel d1) correlates well with the severity of clinical symptoms suffered by individuals who are allergic to these proteins. In fact, allergen sensitivity is related to the serum of specific IgE, with very low concentrations of allergen often causing basophil histamine release in vitro when allergen-specific IgE antibody levels are high. As a result, release of histamine from basophils in vitro can serve as a dependable and precise indicator of an individual's allergic status, with few false-positive results when compared with skin testing techniques. Also, because many dilutions of antigens can be readily tested for reactivity, the assay can be more quantitative than skin testing, which often relies on a somewhat less precise endpoint.

5.1.2. Histamine Release From Washed Human Leukocytes

5.1.2.1. Materials

1. 50-mL Polypropylene centrifuge tubes (Corning Inc. Corning, NY; cat. no. 25330).
2. 12×75-mm Polystyrene test tubes.
3. 2-mL Auto analyzer cups.
4. 1,4-piperazinebis (ethane sulfonic)-buffered saline containing 0.003% human serum albumin, 0.1% D-glucose (PAG) buffer.
5. 1,4-piperazinebis (ethane sulfonic)-buffered saline containing 0.003% human serum albumin, 0.1% D-glucose 10–M $CaCl_2$ and 0.1 mM $NaCl_2$ (PAGCM) buffer.

5.1.2.2. Methods

The techniques described herein are, for the most part, used when histamine is analyzed by automated fluorimetry.

1. Blood is drawn into a plastic syringe, preferably using a butterfly infusion set with a needle size reflecting the desired volume required for the assay. Usually 1 mL of blood per reaction tube will provide total histamine levels of approx 20 ng with some variation occurring among donors.
2. Whole blood is immediately transferred to disposable 50-mL polypropylene centrifuge tubes, each containing 12.5 mL dextran, 5.0 mL 0.1 M EDTA, and 375 mg dextrose, which allows proper mixing for up to 20 mL of blood.
3. After sitting for 60–90 min at room temperature (23–25°C), or until a sharp interface develops between the plasma and erythrocyte pellet, the leukocyte-rich plasma layer is carefully removed using a disposable plastic pipet and transferred to a clean tube. The plasma is then centrifuged for 8 min at 110g in a refrigerated centrifuge at 4°C.
4. The upper plasma is carefully decanted (or aspirated) and discarded. The leukocyte pellet is gently resuspended and approx 40 mL (or twice the amount of blood used) of cold PAG buffer and centrifuged as previously listed.
5. The centrifugation and washing done in this manner are sufficient to remove most of the platelet contamination. It is sometimes useful to do one or more washes in PAG containing EDTA (~4 mM) because this reagent chelates calcium and prevents platelet clumping. However, it is important that the final wash be done in the absence of EDTA because histamine release requires calcium, and residual EDTA may prevent the reaction cascade. After the final wash, the cell pellet is resuspended in PAGCM buffer.
6. Histamine release is performed in polystyrene test tubes (12×75 mm). Total reaction volumes usually range from 0.1 to 1.0 mL. In practice, most experiments are run in a total volume of 0.1 mL. Because the sample volume necessary for automated fluorimetry is 0.5–1.0 mL, reactions performed in smaller volumes are brought up to 1.0 mL with PAG buffer at the end of the reaction, prior to harvesting the supernatants for histamine analysis.
7. For simple histamine release experiments, 0.02 mL each of 5X concentrations of antigen, buffer, perchloric acid, or other reagents are added to test tubes and kept at 4°C.

8. The washed leukocytes in PAGCM buffer and the reaction tubes are then warmed separately by incubating them for 5 min in a 37°C water bath before adding 0.08 mL of the cell suspension to each tube.

9. The total histamine content (called "completes") is obtained by lysing the cells in a duplicate set of reaction tubes using perchloric acid at a final concentration of 1.6%. It is also important that tubes containing only cells and buffer (blanks) be included in each experiment as a measure of the spontaneous release of histamine (usually less than 5% of the total).

10. All conditions are tested in duplicate. During the reaction, the tubes are mixed by vigorously shaking the test tube racks every 15 min. At the end of 45 min at 37°C, reaction tubes are removed from the water bath and 0.9 mL of PAG buffer is added to each tube.

11. The tubes are then immediately centrifuged for 2 min at 1000g. Alternatively, the tubes can be centrifuged at 150g for 10 min.

12. The cell-free supernatants are decanted into 2 mL auto analyzer cups and stored at 4°C in plastic racks (Elkay Products Inc., Shrewsbury, MA). To prevent evaporation, samples should be frozen at –20°C if histamine cannot be analyzed within 2 wk. Alternatively, histamine can be measured using a histamine immunoassay.

5.2. Histamine Autoanalyzer Method (11)

The fluorometric technique remains the most popular method of assessing histamine release and is capable of consistently producing accurate and sensitive measurements of this histamine. Automation of this technique by Siraganian allowed analysis of up to 30 samples per hour *(11)*; with more modern machines, as many as 45–60 samples can be analyzed per hour. The procedure is based on the extraction of histamine and its coupling with *o*-phthalaldehyde at a highly alkaline pH to form a fluorescent product. Samples tested must be relatively free of protein and other interfering compounds such as histidine. This is achieved by first extracting histamine into *n*-butanol from a salt-saturated, alkalinized solution before the condensation step with OPT, histamine is back-extracted into an aqueous solution of dilute HCl by adding heptane. The histamine–ophthaldehyde complex is stable at an acid pH, which increases the fluorescent intensity of the compound. The automated technique requires a sample volume of 0.6–1.0 mL and is capable of detecting histamine levels in the range of 0.5 to >100 ng/mL. Although the automated methodology for histamine measurement is preferable, similar results can be obtained manually with minor loss of sensitivity and precision. The assay is linear from 0.5 to 1000 ng/mL. The advantage of automated fluorimetry over other systems is its ability to rapidly process a large number of samples. However, this is the method of choice only when samples are obtained from studies using low-protein buffer systems such as the in vitro release of histamine from basophile or mast cell cultures.

5.2.1. Special Reagents and Equipment for Flow Analyzer of Histamine

1. RFA 300 Rapid Flow Analyzer for histamine measurement by fluorimetry (Astoria-Pacific International, Clackamas, OR).
2. Filtered reagents for fluorimetry.
   a. 0.73 *M* Phosphoric acid.
   b. 30% NaCl.
   c. 5 *N* NaOH.
   d. 1 *N* NaOH containing 1 m*M* EDTA.
   e. 0.1 *N* HCl.
   f. Brij-saline-EDTA: 0.17 *M* NaCl, 1.5 m*M* EDTA, 0.015% Brij-35 (Perstorp Analytical, Silver Spring, MD).
   g. Heptane.
   h. Butanol.
   i. OPT solution: 50 mg of OPT (Sigma, St. Louis, MO) recrystallized in Ligoine solvent (Eastman Kodak Co., Rochester, NY), 1 mL of spectranalyzed methanol (Fisher Scientific, Pittsburgh, PA), and 0.5 *M* 99 mL of borate buffer.
3. Histamine standards (for fluorimetry).
   a. Histamine dihydrochloride (molecular weight = 184.1).
   b. Histamine (molecular weight = 111.0).
   c. 1 mg/mL Histamine solution. (**Note:** 1 mg of histamine equals 1.66 mg of histamine dihydrochloride.)
   d. Dilute the 1 mg/mL solution 1:1000 in 2% $HClO_4$ to give 1 µg/ mL stock and store at –20°C in 6-mL aliquots.
   e. 6 mL of 1 µg/mL histamine added to 294 mL of 2% perchloric acid = 20 ng/mg.
   f. 50 mL of ~20 ng/mL standard added to 50 mL of 2% perchloric acid = 10 ng/mL.

5.2.2. Buffer for Basophil Histamine Release

1. 10X PIPES buffer, pH 7.4: 250 m*M* PIPES (Sigma), 1.10 *M* NaCl, and 50 m*M* KCl.
2. PAG buffer: 10% 10X PIPES, 0.003% human serum albumin (Calbiochem~Bering Corp., La Jolla, CA), and 0.1% D-glucose.
3. PAG-EDTA buffer: PAG containing 4 m*M* EDTA.
4. PAGCM buffer: PAG containing 1 m*M* $CaCl_2$ and 1 m*M* $MgCl_2$.
5. Isotonic Percoll: nine parts Percoll (Pharmacia, Piscataway, NJ) plus one part 10X PIPES.

5.3. Going With the Flow

In the last decade, basophiles have been found to upregulate cell surface markers (CD_{45}, CD_{63}, CD_{69}, and CD_{203}). CD_{63} is a transmembrane marker of basophiles, mast cells, macrophages, and platelets. The flow cytometry assay measures upregulation of CD_{63} concentration on basophiles after incubation of specific allergens (drug, food, or pollen) with heparinized blood supplemented with the cytokine IL-3. The relative upregulation of CD_{63} on basophiles is then determined by flow histograms after stimulation with allergen, compared to

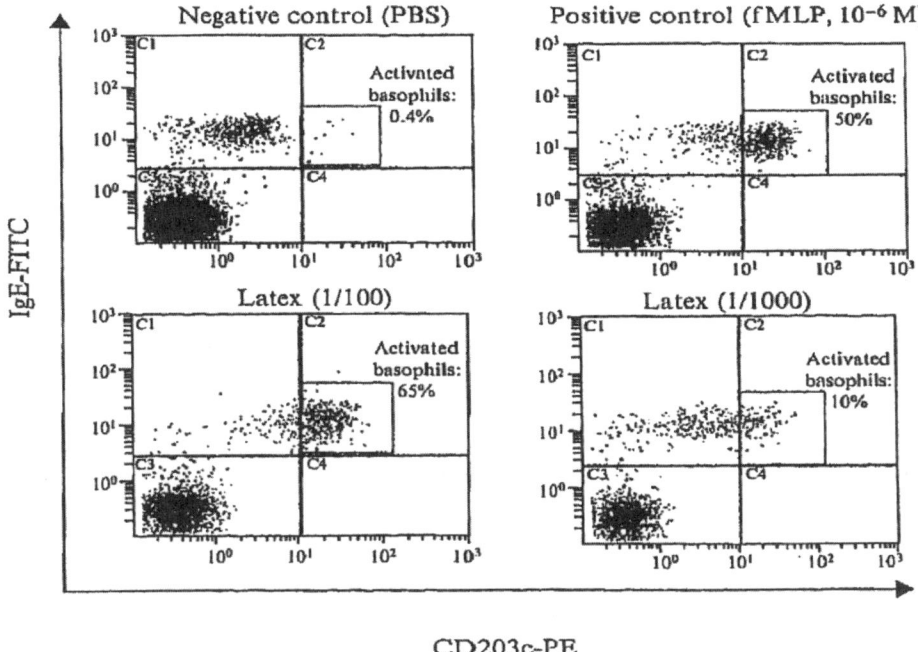

Fig. 2. Representative increased expression of CD203c after fMLP or allergen challenge. Gated cells are presented on the basis of CD203c-IgE staining: before stimulation (upper left dot-plot), after fMLP challenge (upper right), and after latex challenge at two different concentrations (lower dot-plots). (Reproduced with permission from **ref. 12.**)

appropriate controls. In one study of penicillin allergy, about 50% of the patients had a positive CD_{63} increase compared to controls.

CD_{203} is a neural cell surface biomarker found on IgE-bearing basophiles and mast cells. The advantage is that it is found primarily on basophiles. In a study of allergy to *Hymenoptera* (honeybee) venom, CD_{203} was found to be upregulated from 4.2- to 13.5-fold in patients relative to normal controls. The CD_{203} flow assay was found to confirm the presence of venom-specific IgE in 91% (20/22) of skin test positive patients who had clinical symptoms of honeybee sensitivity *(12)*. In another study, latex-specific sensitivity was 63% and CD_{203} upregulation was better than CD^{63} *(13)* (**Fig. 2**).

A limitation of CD_{203} studies with specific allergens is the viability of basophiles in human blood. Some investigators estimate that basophile function may last 24–36 h in heparinized blood. For transport of blood to a distant reference laboratory, the ability to receive the sample within a short time is a limiting factor. Partial separation of basophiles from other blood products could prolong the basophile viability. With certain classes of specific allergen reactivity

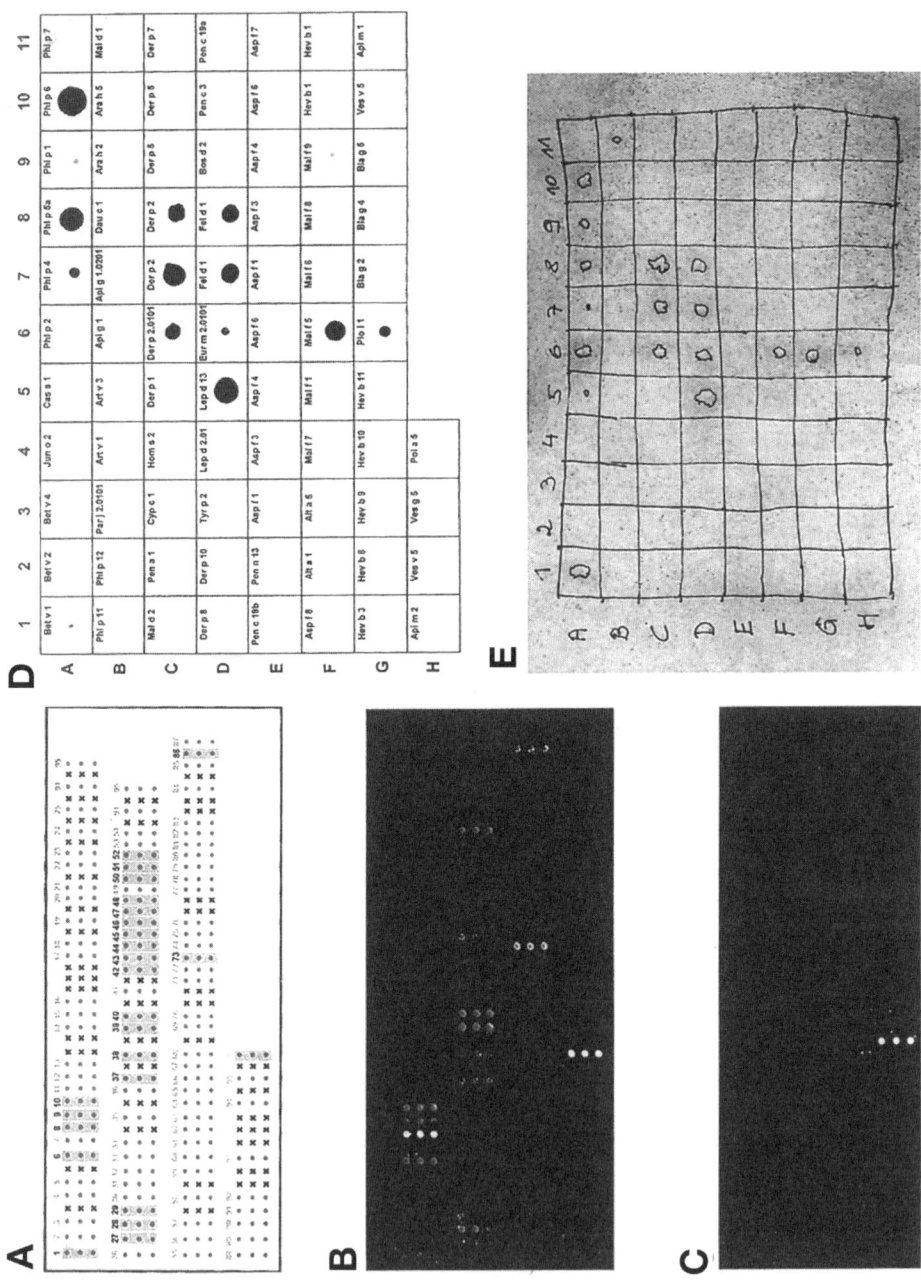

such as drug and food allergy, where skin testing may be inadequate, flow cytometry may provide valuable clues for patients sensitive to these allergens.

5.4. Microarray-Bound Allergens

The availability of recombinant allergens and recent advances in chip technologies have led to the development of new systems for the identification of specific IgE antibody. The ordered array with micrometer spacing could accommodate more than 1000 allergens and controls bound to the microchip surface *(14)*.

Jahn-Schmid and colleagues in Vienna studied IgE binding to recombinant ryegrass and birch allergens linked to silica chips. In a study of 51 sera from atopic patients, the results obtained with microarray technology correlated well with those of the ImmunoCAP assay *(15)*. An advantage of microarray methodology is the relatively small serum specimen required (<40 µL). **Fig. 3** shows the relative activity of microarray vs skin testing and immunoblot techniques. Because the current validated ImmunoCAP tests have over 400 specific allergen extracts available and each extract may contain five or more major allergens, validating and comparing hundreds of recombinant allergens will await future comparative studies.

6. Conclusion

In the last 40 yr we have witnessed amazing advances in the science of identifying allergy antibodies and in the understanding of the immunology of allergic diseases. Since the discovery of IgE and the development of recombinant technologies, the in vivo and in vitro diagnosis of allergic reactivity has rapidly progressed. In vitro techniques are currently approaching in vivo (skin test) accuracy and time frames. Skin tests take 15–20 min from application of the allergen extract to final reading of the wheal and flare endpoint. Because skin tests are usually performed with nonstandardized extracts, the results may vary from lot to lot of the tests performed. Also, many of the tests, especially for environmental allergens such as house dust, molds, and animal dander, may show positive wheal swelling and negative IgE-specific results with ImmunoCAP. This discordance could be due to greater sensitivity of the skin tests or false-positive results secondary to an irritant response. In any event, the ImmunoCAP and other IgE tests are highly specific for the allergen tested. The specific IgE

Fig. 3. Allergen microarray. (**A**) Scheme of environmental allergens spotted in triplicate in vertical columns. (**B,C**) Scanned images from a microarray chip-based IgE assay obtained with serum from an allergic (**Fig. 2**) (**B**) and nonallergic (**Fig. 2**) (**C**) individual. (**D**) Dot-blot IgE reactivity to the same allergens bound to nitrocellulose. (**E**) Skin reactivity to allergens and histamine (H6; wheal circled for visualization). (Reproduced with permission from **ref. 14.**)

tests may, however, be too sensitive: patients with class 3 or higher specific IgE (3.5–17.5 kU/L) may have food-related anaphylaxis *(16)* to important food allergens, whereas class 1 or 2 specific IgE (0.35–3.50 kU/L) to food allergens may not correlate with skin test positivity and or a history of food allergy *(16)*. Thus, the relative clinical importance of skin testing, relevant clinical history and provocative tests, and specific IgE testing needs to be sorted out.

Current in vitro testing takes 2–4 h from the time serum is added to the analytical system until readout of the quantitative results. Patient time and discomfort can be minimized by a single venipuncture, and the time required to obtain results from in vitro tests may be similar to that for in vivo (skin) tests. It is not unreasonable to assume that allergy laboratory testing will take less time in the future. Laboratory testing is likely to be more accurate and nearly as quick, if not quicker than current skin test procedures. Currently, skin tests for drug allergy are not reliable because of the relative absence of purified drug metabolites that may be relevant in causing drug allergies. The lack of positive control subjects also limits the validity of drug testing. Flow cytometry may provide a highly specific and sensitive methodology to test relative drug sensitivity. In the future, a combination of biological testing (skin tests and or provocative tests) and specific IgE testing should provide important information for therapeutic intervention. However, the new technologies require careful validation to develop paradigms that encompass relevant clinical scenarios.

7. Notes

1. Date and initial all reagents upon opening. Each container should be labeled with substance name, lot number, date of preparation, expiration date, and any special storage instructions.

References

1. Ishazaka, K. and Ishizaka, T. (1967) Physiochemical properties of reaginic antibody. I. Association of reaginic activity with an immunoglobulin other than gamma A or gamma G globulin. *J. Allergy.* **37,** 169.
2. Bennich, H., Ishizaka, K., Ishizaka, T., and Johansson, S. G. O. (1969) A comparative antigenic study of gamma E globulin and myeloma IgND. *J. Immunol.* **102,** 826–831.
3. Wide, L., Bennich, H., and Johansson, S. G. O. (1967) Diagnosis of allergy by an in vitro tests for allergen-specific IgE antibodies. *Lancet* **2,** 1105–1107.
4. Paganelli, R., Ansoteugi, I. J., Sastre, J., et al. (1998) Specific IgE antibodies in the diagnosis of atopic disease. Clinical evaluation of a new in vitro test system, UniCAP, in six European allergy clinics. *Allergy* **53,** 763–768.
5. Ownby, D. R. and McCullough, J. (1994) Testing for latex allergy. *J. Clin. Immunoassay* **16,** 109–113.
6. Biagini, R. E., Krieg, E. F., Pinkerton, L. E., and Hamilton, R. G. (2001) Receiver operating characteristics analyses of Food and Drug Administration-cleared

serological assays for natural rubber latex-specific immunoglobulin E antibody. *Clin. Diagn. Lab. Immunol.* **8,** 1145–1149.

7. Hamilton, R. G. and Franklin Adkinson, N., Jr. (2004) In vitro assays for the diagnosis of IgE-mediated disorders. *J. Allergy Clin. Immunol.* **114,** 213–225.

8. Crockard, A. D. and Ennis, M. (2001) Basophil histamine release tests in the diagnosis of allergy and asthma. *Clin. Exp. Allergy* **31,** 345–350.

9. Nolte, H. (1993) The clinical utility of basophil histamine release. *Allergy Proc.* **14,** 251–254.

10. Maly, F. E., Marti-Wyss, S., Blumber, S., Cuhat-Stark, I., and Wuthrich, B. (1997) Mononuclear blood cell sulpholeukotriene generation in the presence of interleukin 3 and whole blood histamine release in honeybee and yellow jacket venom allergy. *J. Invest. Allergy Clin. Immunol.* **7,** 217–224.

11. Siraganian, R. P. (1974) An automated continuous-flow system for the extraction and fluorometric analysis of histamine. *Anal. Biochem.* **57,** 383–394.

12. Boumiza, R., Monneret, G., Forissier, M. F., et al. (2003) Marked improvement of the basophil activation test by detecting CD203c instead of CD63. *Clin. Exp. Allergy* **33,** 259–265.

13. Ebo, D. G., Hagendorens, M. M., Bridts, C. H., Schuerwegh, A. J., De Clerk, L. S., and Stevens, W. J. (2004) In vitro allergy diagnosis: should we follow the flow? *Clin. Exp. Allergy.* **34,** 332–339.

14. Hiller, R., Laffer, S., Harwanegg, C., et al. (2002) Microarrayed allergen molecules: diagnostic gatekeepers for allergy treatment. *FASEB J.* **16,** 414–416.

15. Jahn-Schmid, B., Harwanegg, C., Hiller, R., et al. (2003) Allergen microarray: comparison of microarray using recombinant allergens with conventional diagnostic methods to detect allergen-specific serum immunoglobulin E. *Clin. Exp. Allergy* **33,** 1443–1449.

16. Sampson, H. A. and Ho, D. G. (1997) Relationship between food-specific IgE concentrations and the risk of positive food challenges in children and adolescents. *J. Allergy Clin. Immunol.* **100,** 444–451.

17. Lichtenstein, L., Norman, P., and Winkenwereder, W. (1968) Clinical and in vitro studies on the role of immunotherapy in ragweed hay fever. *Am. J. Med.* **44,** 514–524.

18. Adkinson, N. F., Jr. (1976) Measurement of Total Serum Immunoglobulin E and Allergen-Specific Immunoglobulin E Antibody. In: *Manual of clinical laboratory Immunology*, (Rose, N. R. and Friedman, H., eds.), American Society for Microbiology, Washington, DC, p. 590.

Index

A

AlaSTAT, immunoglobulin E
measurement, 210
Alemtuzumab,
flow cytometry quantification in
plasma with bead-based assay,
bead conjugation and preparation,
161, 162, 164
data acquisition and analysis, 164
free antibody detection, 162, 164
instrument setup, 161
materials, 160, 161
overview, 159, 160
sample preparation, 162, 164
total antibody detection, 162
indications, 159, 160
mechanism of action, 159, 160
Allergy, see Immunoglobulin E
Aminopeptidase N, see CD13
Anti-CA-125 antibody, see
Antiidiotypic antibodies
Antiidiotypic antibodies,
antiiso/allotypic immune response,
196
immunoassay,
anti-OC125, 198—202
antiiso/allotypic anti-murine
antibodies, 198, 199, 201
inhibition assay, 200—202
materials, 197, 198, 200, 201
internal image antibodies, 196
therapeutic monoclonal antibody
response, 195, 196
Anti-OC125, see Antiidiotypic
antibodies

B

Basophil,
flow cytometry markers, 214, 215,
217
histamine release assay
automation in flow analyzer, 213,
214
fluorometry, 212, 213
materials, 212
overview, 211
B-cell, immunohistochemistry, 101,
103
Bcl-2,
CD10/Bcl-2/Bcl-6/MUM-1
immunohistochemistry in
diffuse large B-cell lymphoma,
112
immunohistochemistry, 110, 111
Bcl-6,
CD10/Bcl-6 immunohistochemistry
in follicular lymphoma, 111,
112
CD10/Bcl-2/Bcl-6/MUM-1
immunohistochemistry in
diffuse large B-cell lymphoma,
112
BCR-ABL, see Leukemia
Bone marrow,
cell subsets,
erythroid cells, 93
granulocytes, 93
lymphocytes, 95
megakaryocytes, 93
monocytes, 93
precursor cells, 95